Recent Advances in Wound Healing

Edited by Shahin Aghaei

Published in London, United Kingdom

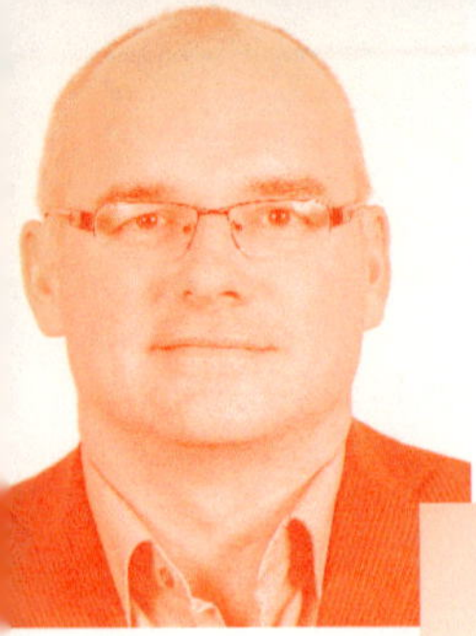
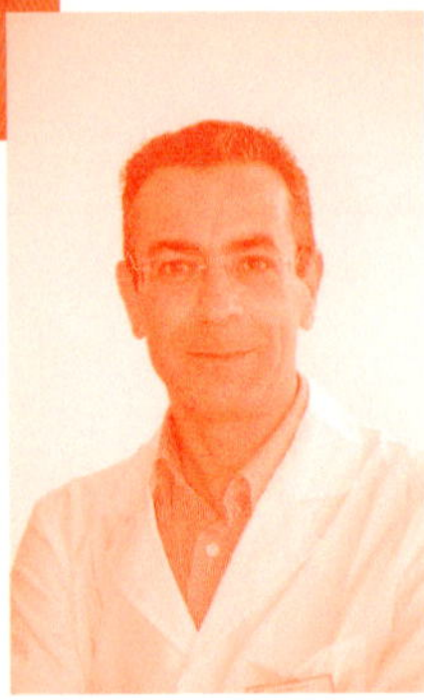
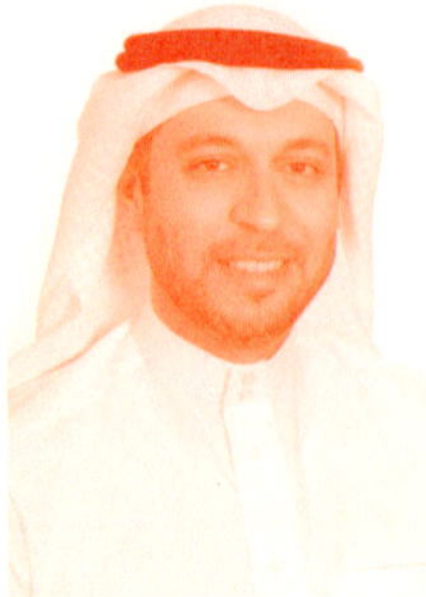
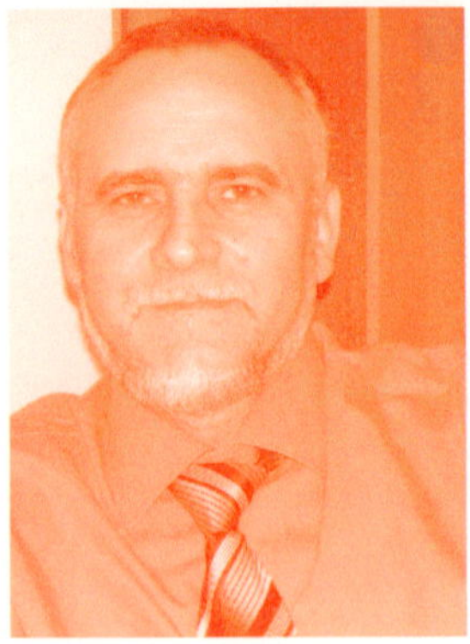
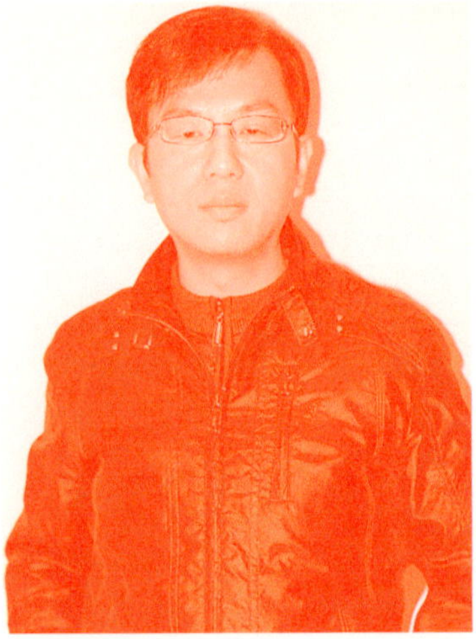
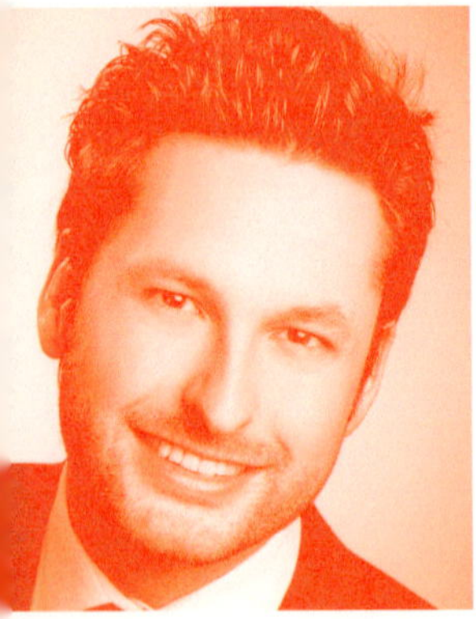
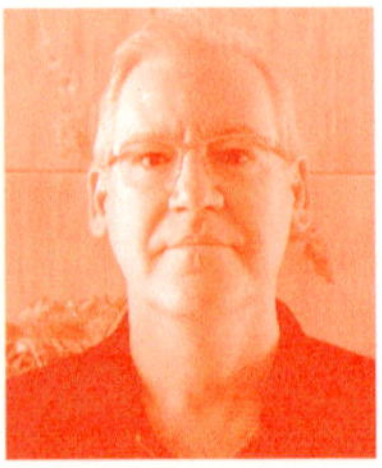

IntechOpen

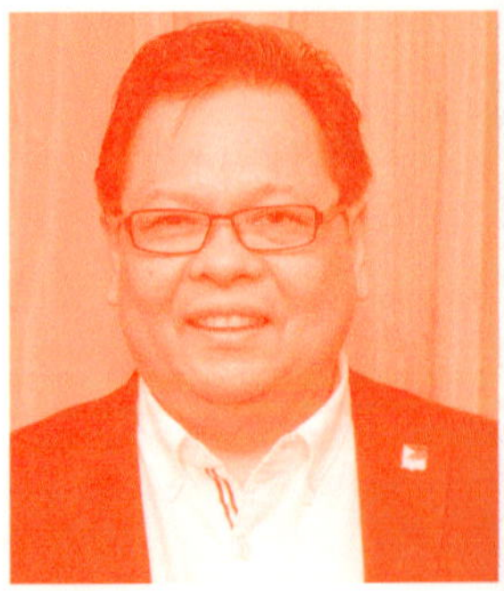
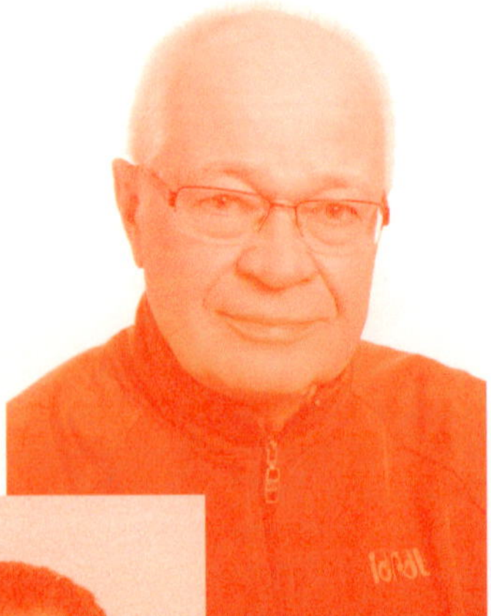
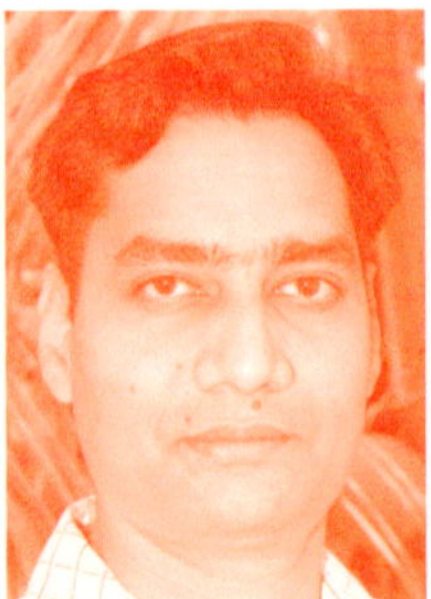
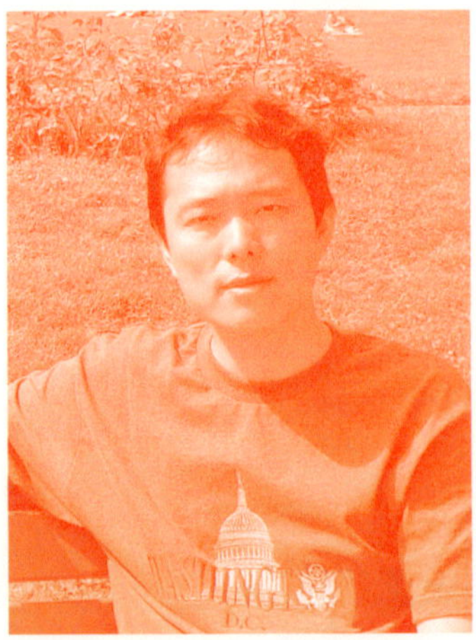
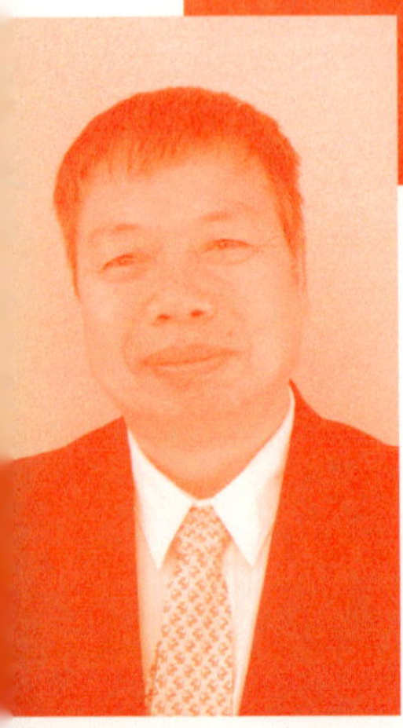
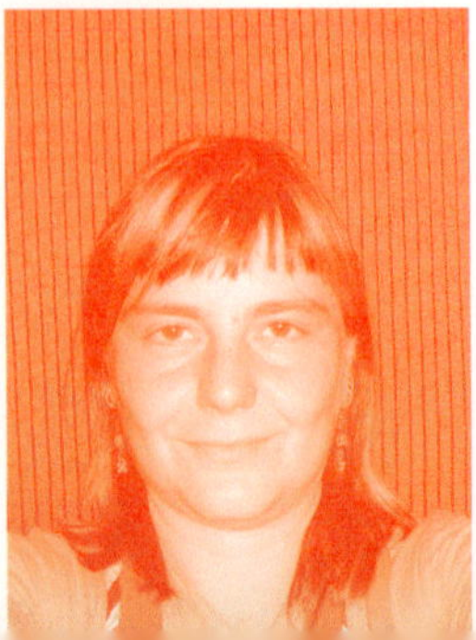

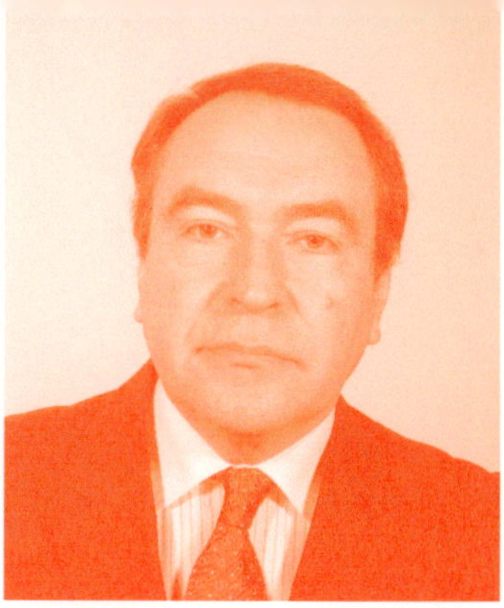
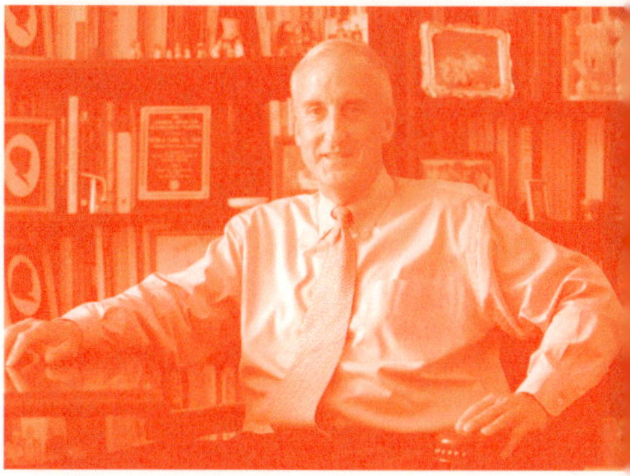
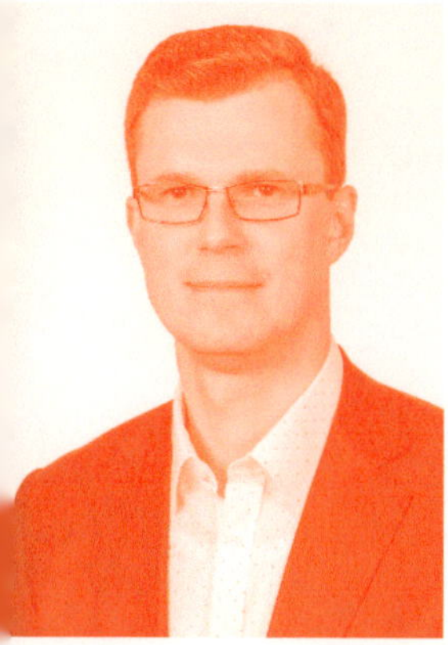
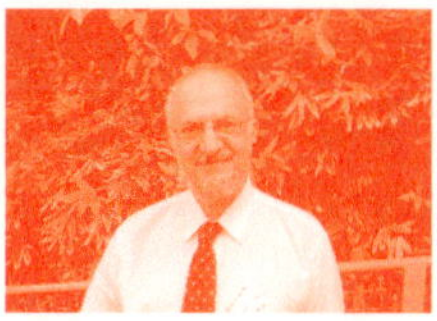
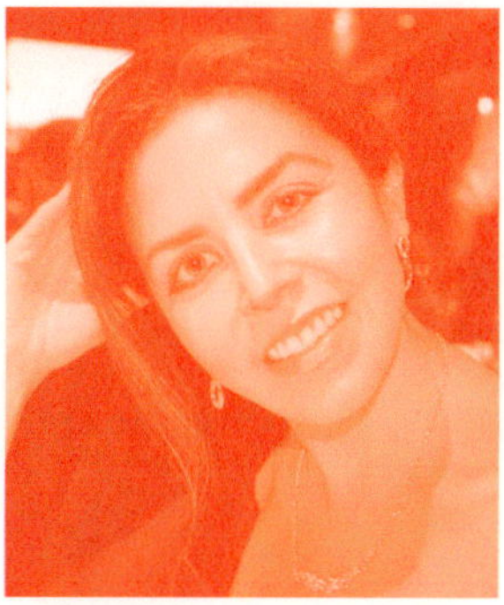

Supporting open minds since 2005

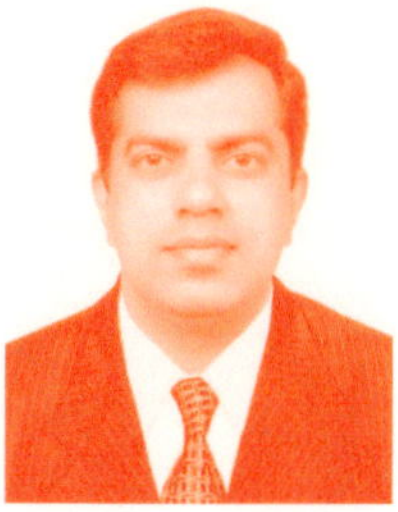
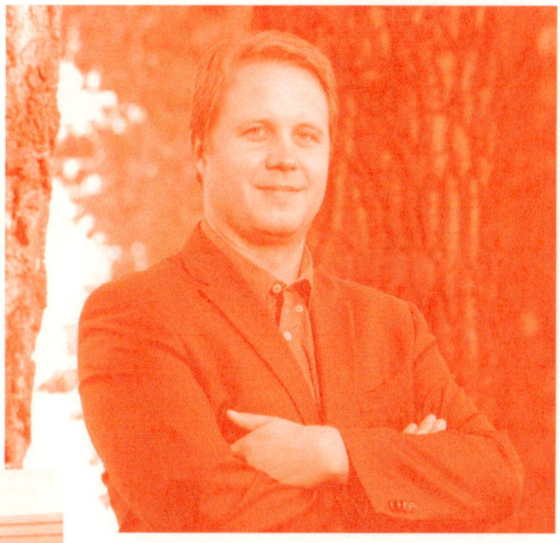
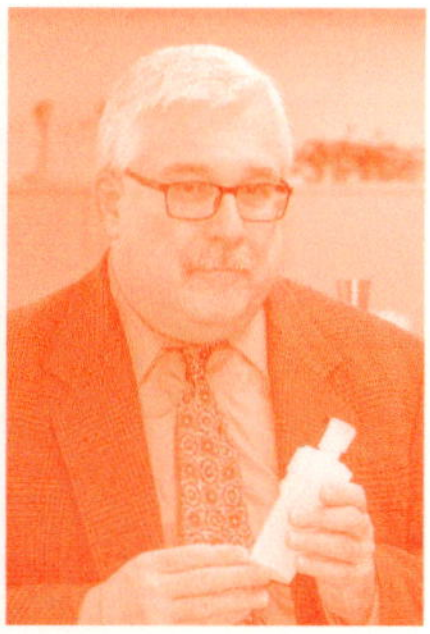
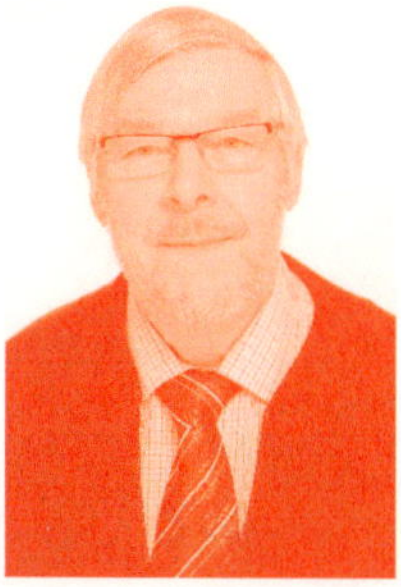
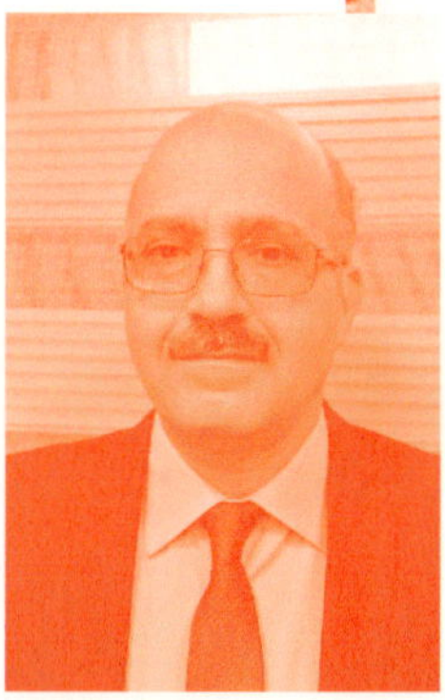
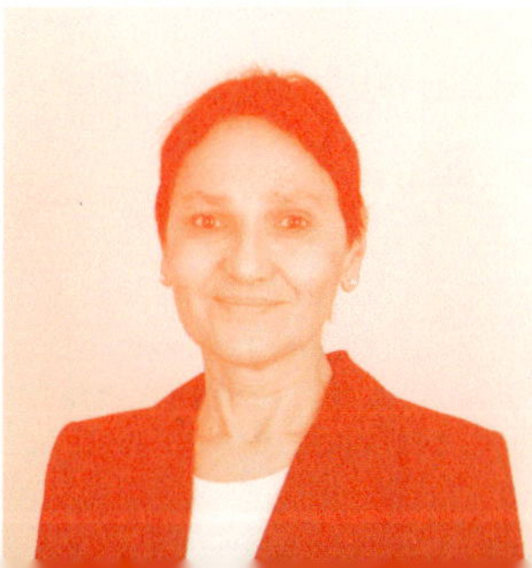
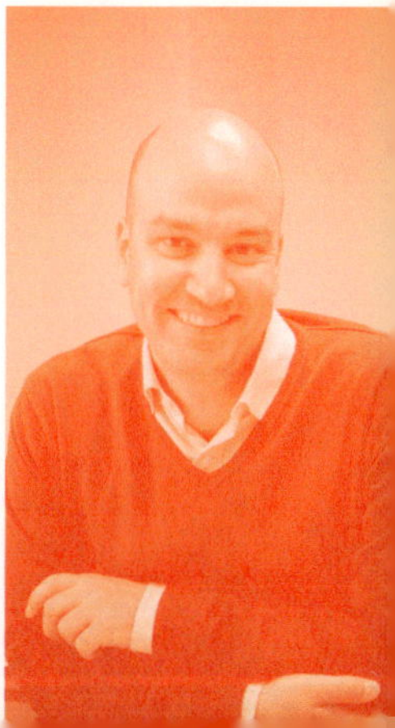

Recent Advances in Wound Healing
http://dx.doi.org/10.5772/intechopen.83072
Edited by Shahin Aghaei

Contributors
Bonnie C. Carney, Taryn E. Elise Travis, Jeffrey W. Shupp, Santhini Elango, Amalorpava Mary Loordhuswamy, Priyanka Chhabra, Kajol Bhati, Margaret O. Ilomuanya, Uloma N. Ubani-Ukoma, Adannaya C. Adebona, Ibilola M. Cardoso-Daodu, Mohammad Bayat, Sufan Chien, Gadi Borkow, Şerban V.G. Vifor Gabriel Berteşteanu, Raluca Grigore, Mihnea Cojocarita-Condeescu, Alexandru Nicolaescu, Catrinel Simion-Antonie, Popescu Bogdan, Paula Bejenaru, Gloria Munteanu, Shravan Kumar Paswan, Sunil Kumar, Pritt Verma, Akanksha, Sajal Srivastava, Chandana Venketeswara Rao, Walid A.M. Ganod, Danijela Semenič, Tadej Voljč, RamKishor Sah, Eyal Melamed

First published in London, United Kingdom, 2022 by IntechOpen
IntechOpen is the global imprint of INTECHOPEN LIMITED, registered in England and Wales, registration number: 11086078, 5 Princes Gate Court, London, SW7 2QJ, United Kingdom
Printed in Croatia

British Library Cataloguing-in-Publication Data
A catalogue record for this book is available from the British Library

Additional hard and PDF copies can be obtained from orders@intechopen.com

Recent Advances in Wound Healing
Edited by Shahin Aghaei
p. cm.
Print ISBN 978-1-83968-572-9
Online ISBN 978-1-83968-573-6
eBook (PDF) ISBN 978-1-83968-574-3

For EU product safety concerns:
IN TECH d.o.o., Prolaz Marije Krucifikse Kozulić 3, 51000 Rijeka, Croatia, info@intechopen.com or visit our website at intechopen.com.

Meet the editor

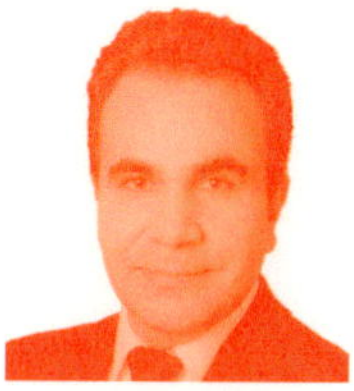

Shahin Aghaei, MD, graduated from Shiraz University of Medical Sciences, Shiraz, Iran, in 2004. He was awarded a fellowship of International Society of Dermatopathology (ISD) from Charles University in Prague, Czech Republic, in 2008 and a fellowship of Dermatologic Surgery from the Medical University of Graz, Austria, in 2010. He is currently editor in chief of the *Journal of Surgical Dermatology* in Singapore and associate professor of Dermatology and Dermatologic Surgery at Iran University of Medical Sciences School of Medicine, Tehran, Iran. He is also a member of the following medical societies: American Academy of Dermatology, European Academy of Dermatology and Venereology, American Society for Laser Medicine and Surgery, International Society of Dermatology, International Hyperhidrosis Society, and Iranian Society of Dermatology.

Contents

Preface

Wound healing is a multifaceted and dynamic procedure of revitalizing lost cellular organizations and flesh layers in the human body [1]. The human wound-healing process could be divided into three or four discrete phases. Formerly, contributors denoted three phases, that is, inflammatory, fibroblastic, and maturation, but the human wound-healing process has also been indicated as inflammatory, proliferation, and remodeling [2]. In the four-phase model, there are the hemostasis, the inflammatory, the proliferation, and the remodeling phase. In the three-phase approach, the hemostasis phase is enclosed within the inflammatory phase [3].

For a wound to be healed efficaciously, all four phases must sequentially happen at an expected time setting. Numerous aspects can hinder one or more stages of this procedure and thus can cause inappropriate or diminished wound healing. This book reviews the recent literature on the most significant factors that affect wound healing and the potential cellular and/or molecular mechanisms involved. The factors discussed include physiology of wound healing, interferon, stem cells and photobiomodulation, a chronic venous ulcer, chronic fistula, bionanomaterials, topical antiseptic agents, including silver and sodium hypochlorite solution, diabetic ulcers, and nutritional supplements such as copper. A better understanding of the effects of these elements on wound mending may lead to therapeutics that progress wound healing and resolve compromised wounds [4]. This book includes 4 sections and 10 chapters as follows:

Section 1: Hypertrophic Scars and Keloids

Chapter 1 "Interferon Therapy for Hypertrophic Scars and Keloids"

Interferons (IFNs) from the family of cytokines are widely used to treat keloids because of their ability to increase collagenase activity, thereby reducing the production of collagen and other extracellular matrices (ECM). In this chapter, the benefits and limitations of IFN-mediated therapy for the treatment of scars and keloids and the advantages of combinatorial therapy with the appropriate literature support are discussed.

Chapter 2 "The Need for Basic, Translational, and Clinical Research in the Field of Hypertrophic Scars"

Hypertrophic scar (HTS) is a fibrotic skin disorder marked by excessive inflammation and extracellular matrix deposition in response to cutaneous traumatic injuries such as burns, lacerations, incisions, and abrasions. Additional fibrotic skin disorders such as keloid scars are often thought of as being the same pathophysiology existing along the continuum of severity of HTS and hence are often studied as one scar type, despite their varied etiology. This chapter will review current in vitro and in vivo modeling and highlight research needs to address gaps in the study of HTS.

Section 2: Chronic Ulcers

Chapter 3 "Pharyngocutaneous Fistulas Following Total Laryngectomy"

Total laryngectomy is still the final therapeutic solution for locally advanced laryngeal cancer cases. Following excision of the larynx, the remaining pharynx is reconstructed to obtain continuity of the upper digestive tract. One of the most common complications seen in patients, despite constant refinement of the procedure, is the development of a pharyngocutaneous fistula. The development of the fistula prolongs hospital stay and often requires a second surgical procedure, increasing hospitalization cost and morbidity and impairing the quality of life of patients. Only some among the risk factors identified before surgery may be corrected. Managing the fistula once present depends on multiple factors, essential being the size of the fistula as well as the position and concomitant factors. Understanding the healing mechanisms of these structures is important in the proper management of this complication.

Chapter 4 "Combined Administration of Stem Cells and Photobiomodulation on Wound Healing in Diabetes"

Wound healing is an active and compound biological course divided into four steps: hemostasis, inflammation, proliferation, and remodeling. Diabetes mellitus induces weakened wound healing by disturbing one or more of the biological functions of these steps. And based on the current study that analyzes results from studies that used separate and combined administrations of stem cells and photobiomodulation for diabetic wound healing in patients and animal models, we hypothesize that the combined application of photobiomodulation and stem cells will accelerate the repair process and assist the healing of foot ulcers in diabetes mellitus patients.

Chapter 5 "Chronic Venous Ulcer"

This research review is endeavoring to shed light on the cause and effect of chronic venous ulcer (CVU) in line with its therapeutic procedures. In the last two decades, a lot has changed in the strategy of wound management due to the development of adjunctive therapy that supported wound healing. Eventually, the latest development was in platelet concentration technology that produced platelet-rich fibrin (PRF). The first therapeutic procedure used in the treatment of venous leg ulceration (VLU) was compression therapy where the application of effective graduated compression decreased the overload in the venous system and venous reflux. Furthermore, it accelerated blood flow and decreased fluid leakage in the capillary, which in return alleviated limb edema.

Section 3: Biomaterials for Wound Healing

Chapter 6 "Polymeric Biomaterials for Wound Healing Incorporating Plant Extracts and Extracellular Matrix Components"

Biomaterials are constructed to promote or stimulate the processes of wound healing. Polymeric biomaterials can be used to hydrate the wound and serve as a barrier to pathogens, with plant extracts, antimicrobial agents, and extracellular components incorporated to stimulate the healing process. The biological and physical augmentation provided by extracellular matrix–derived implants continues to facilitate innovation in biomaterials utilized in the management of nonhealing wounds. Extracellular matrix components and plant extracts have been shown to possess pharmacological properties with potential for use in the treatment of skin diseases and wound healing. Antioxidant, anti-inflammatory assays, and wound-healing assays have been shown to support the dermatological and wound-healing usage of these medicinal plant extracts.

Chapter 7 "Bionanomaterials: Advancements in Wound Healing and Tissue Regeneration"

Abnormal wound healing is an indication of a major healthcare issue owing to an upsurge in a number of traumas and morbid physiology that ultimately posed a health-care burden on patients, society, and health-care organizations. As wound healing is a complex process, effective management of chronic wounds is often hard. Recently, in addition to many conventional wound treatments, advances in bionanomaterials are attaining much attention in wound care and skin tissue engineering. In this chapter, we highlight the sources, biological role, and bioengineering approaches adapted for biopolymers for the facilitation of the wound-healing process.

Chapter 8 "Current Understanding to Accelerate Wound Healing: Mechanism and Clinical Importance"

Wound mending is a complex organic cycle that brings about the reclamation of tissue honesty. Physiologically, it may be very well separated into four particular periods: hemostasis, inflammation, proliferation, and tissue remodeling (redesigning). This chapter portrays the cellular premise of wound mending and extracellular flagging cycles that are responsible for controlling the periods. The capacity of fibroblasts, neutrophils, platelets, and macrophages is contemplated exhaustively.

Section 4: Wound Healing and Treatments

Chapter 9 "Copper, an Abandoned Player Returning to the Wound Healing Battle"

Copper has two key properties that endow it as an excellent active ingredient to be used in the wound-healing battle. First, copper plays a key role in angiogenesis, dermal fibroblasts proliferation, upregulation of collagen, and elastin fiber production by dermal fibroblasts, and it serves as a cofactor of lysyl oxidase needed for efficient dermal extracellular matrix (ECM) protein cross-linking. Second, copper has potent wide-spectrum biocidal properties. Both Gram-positive and Gram-negative bacteria, including antibiotic-resistant bacteria and hard-to-kill bacterial spores, fungi, and viruses, when exposed to high copper concentrations are killed. Copper has been used as a biocide for centuries by many different civilizations. The positive outcome at all wound-healing stages of using copper-impregnated wound dressings is shown, indicating the neglected critical role copper plays in wound healing.

Chapter 10 "Contribution of Topical Agents to Wound Healing"

The process of wound healing is often accompanied by a bacterial infection or critical colonization, which leads to an extension of the inflammatory response phase and delayed epithelization. In the review of scientific articles, we found the description and mode of action of topical antiseptic agents, including silver and sodium hypochlorite solution, in controlling the spread of microorganisms. The value of hyaluronic acid for wound healing is described. Furthermore, a novel treatment option with microspheres is mentioned.

Shahin Aghaei, MD
Associate Professor of Dermatology and Dermatologic Surgery,
Department of Dermatology,
Iran University of Medical Sciences,
Tehran, Iran

References

[1] Sorg H, Tilkorn DJ, Hager S, Hauser J, Mirastschijski U. *Skin Wound Healing: An Update on the Current Knowledge and Concepts*. Eur Surg Res. 2017. 58 (1-2):81-94.

[2] Gilmore MA. *Phases of Wound Healing*. Dimens Oncol Nurs. 1991. 5(3):32-4.

[3] Romo T, Al Moutran H, Pearson JM, Yalamanchili H, Pafford W, Zoumalan RA. *Skin Wound Healing*. Medscape Reference. June 20, 2012.

[4] Guo S. and DiPietro LA. *Factors Affecting Wound Healing*. J Dent Res. 2010 Mar; 89(3): 219-229.

Section 1

Hypertrophic Scars and Keloids

Chapter 1

Interferon Therapy for Hypertrophic Scars and Keloids

Amalorpava Mary Loordhuswamy and Santhini Elango

Abstract

Interferons (IFNs) belong to the family of cytokines are widely used to treat keloids owing to their ability to increase collagenase activity thereby reducing the production of collagen and other extracellular matrix (ECM). Intralesional injection of IFN-α – 2b increases the collagenase level by inhibiting the secretion of metalloproteinases, an inhibitor of collagenase. Moreover, the anti-fibrotic activity of IFNs, interfere with fibroblast mediated collagen synthesis. On the other hand, combinatorial therapy has been preferred recently along with IFN due to its side effects observed in various clinical trials conducted only with IFN. Triamcinolone acetonide (TAC) and CO_2 lasers along with IFNs are found to be the potential therapy for the treatment of scars and keloids. In this chapter, IFN mediated therapy for the treatment of scars and keloids, its benefits and limitations and the advantages of combinatorial therapy with the appropriate literature support are discussed.

Keywords: *hypertrophic* scars, keloids, interferon, collagen synthesis, combinatorial therapy

1. Introduction

Hypertrophic scars and keloids are the most common skin disease associated with aesthetically disfiguring morphology, pain, itching, discomfort as well as psychological stress and affect individual life style [1]. This disease is characterized by over production of extracellular matrix collagen and proteoglycans [2]. The development of keloids involves unpredictable irregular arrangement of collagen and other extra cellular proteins in the milieu of wound healing. Wound healing is a well orchestrated sequential process happening through the four distinct steps such as hemostasis, inflammation, proliferation and tissue remodeling [3]. In hemostasis, immediately after an injury, platelet degranulation and activation of compliments initiates blood clotting and forms fibrin network at the site of injury which act as a scaffold for wound repair [4]. Platelet degranulation is crucial step for the release and activation of cytokines including epidermal growth factor (EGF), insulin like growth factor (IGF-I), platelet-derived growth factor (PDGF) and transforming growth factor β (TGF-β). These cytokines acts as chemotactic agents for the recruitment of neutrophils, macrophages, epithelial cells, mast cells, endothelial cells and fibroblasts [5–7]. The recruited fibroblast, synthesis granulation tissue made up of procollagen, elastin, proteoglycans, hyaluronic acid and forms a structural repair framework to bridge the wound and allow vascular in growth. At that time, myofibroblast which contain actin filament initiates wound contraction. Once the wound is closed, the abundant Extra Cellular Matrix (ECM) is then degraded and the immature type III collagen of the early wound is modified into mature type I collagen. Proper balance between ECM protein deposition and degradation is required for wound healing with minimal scarring. Once this balance is disrupted, abnormalities in scarring appear, resulting in the formation of either hypertrophic scar or keloids [8, 9]. The mechanism of *Hypertrophic* scar and keloid formation is given in the **Figure 1**. Both lesions are formed by the occurrence of imbalance between anabolic and catabolic process of wound healing, however keloids seems to be more aggressive fibrotic disorder compared to *hypertrophic* scars [10]. Keloids are more prevalent in Dark skinned individuals of Africa, Asia and Hispanic descents compared to Caucasians [11]. The occurrence of keloids in these population is found to be in the range of 5–16%. The risks of developing keloids are equal in both male and females. Due to the cosmetic procedures such as ear and nose piercing and physiological conditions like puberty and pregnancy, females have more risk for developing keloids compared to male. Persons with the age around 10 to 30 are more prone to develop keloids compared to other age groups [12, 13]. Apart from sex and age, additional risk factor include having blood group A, hyper-IgE and hormonal peaks during pregnancy and puberty also play a role in developing keloids [14]. In recent days, numbers of gene and gene loci associated with keloid development have been identified. Single nucleotide polymorphism has identified in certain loci of NEDD4 genes by genome wide association studies and admixture mapping studies which is genetically linked to keloid development. In addition to that, several human leucocyte antigen (HLA) alleles, p53, bcl-2 and fas genes have also involved in keloid development [15–17]. Studies have also reported that people with rare genetic disorders including Dubowitz syndrome, Bethlem myopathy, Rubinstein-Taybi syndrome, Noonan syndrome and Geominne syndrome have the risk of developing keloids [15].

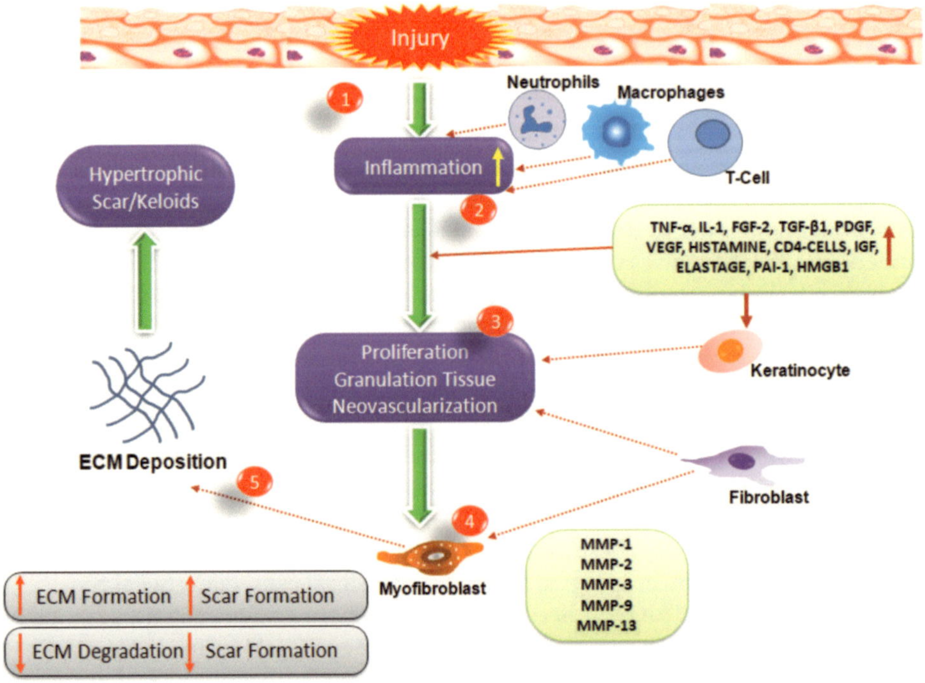

Figure 1.
Mechanism of Hypertrophic *scars and keloid formation.*

2. Currently available treatments

At present, various forms of treatment for keloids are available but no single therapeutic modality is best for all keloids. The size, location, depth of lesion, age,

S. No	Current and emerging therapies available for *hypertrophic* scars and keloid treatments	Types	Mode of action	Limitations
1.	Corticosteroids [19–22]	Triamcinolone acetonide (TAC), hydrocortisone acetate, dexamethasone and methyl prednisolone	Inhibit the growth of fibroblast, attenuate the synthesis of procollagen and glycosaminoglycan, reduce endothelial budding and enhance the degeneration of collagen and fibroblast, inhibit TGF - β1 expression in fibroblast, inhibit VEGF and alphaglobulins.	Telangiectasis, atrophy, steroid acne, pigmentary changes, necrosis, ulcerations
2.	Surgical exsition [23–25]	Linear closure and flap coverage, excision with grafting, W-plasty and Z-plasty	Surgical removal of excessive fibrous tissue growth	Higher recurrence rate, needs additional treatments like intralesional injection of TAIL, Interferon, pressure therapy etc.
3.	Silicone based products [19, 26–28]	Creams, sprays, gel cushion and liquid	Enhance hydration and provide an occlusive environment which regulates proliferation of fibroblast there by decreases collagen synthesis.	Local irritation and lack of clinical trials.
4.	Pressure therapy [29–31]	Variety of materials are used to apply pressure such as adhesive plaster moulds, pressure earrings and custom-fitted splints	Applying pressure to the scar surface reduces perfusion and oxygen supply which in turn reduces collagen synthesis and angiogenesis.	Depends on patients compliance, site specific and discomfort to the patients
5.	Radiotheraphy [32–34]	X ray radiation	Reduce fibroblast proliferation, induce cell senescence and apoptosis there by reducing collagen production and suppress keloid formation	Oedema, necrosis, ulceration, desquamation, erythema, pigmentary changes, atrophy, telangiectasis and alopecia

S. No	Current and emerging therapies available for *hypertrophic* scars and keloid treatments	Types	Mode of action	Limitations
6.	Cryotherapy [35–37]	Low temperature treatment including spray and contact probes, or Intralesional-needle cryoprobe method	Destroying the core of the keloid by sparing the surface epithelial cells including melanocytes there by reducing the volume of keloids.	Hypopigmentation, blistering, pain, delayed healing and infection
7.	Laser therapy [38–40]	Ablative laser: 2940-nm erbium doped yttrium aluminium garnet (Er:YAG) laser and the 10,600-nm carbon dioxide (CO2) laser Non ablative laser: 585-nm or 595-nm PDLs, 1064-nm neodymium-doped:yttrium-aluminium-garnet (Nd:YAG) laser, 532-nm neodymiumdoped-vanadate (Nd:Van) laser and 1064 nm Q-switched Nd:YAG laser with low fluence	Laser beam is absorbed by water present in the skin leading to local tissue destruction and reduction of lesion volume	Itching, pigmentary changes, blister formation and postoperative purpura
8.	Anti cancer drugs [41–43]	5-Flurouracil	Pyrimidine analogue that inhibits thymidylate synthase enzyme leading to suppression of nucleic acid synthesis and inhibits fibroblast proliferation	Skin erythema, pain and ulceration
9	Stem cell therapy [44–46]	Exposure of adipose derived stem cells (ASCs) by fat grafting method	Modulating fibrogenesis through increased collagen production and inhibiting fibroblast proliferation	Mechanism is not clear
10.	Anti cancer drugs [47–49]	Mitomycin C (MMC)	MMC inhibits nucleic acid and protein synthesis thereby decrease the proliferation of fibroblast	Larger randomized clinical trials are needed to elucidate the efficacy of MMC towards keloid treatment.

S. No	Current and emerging therapies available for *hypertrophic* scars and keloid treatments	Types	Mode of action	Limitations
11.	Anticancer drugs [50–52]	Bleomycin	Diminish TGF-β1-induced collagen expression, decrease the levels of lysyl-oxidase, a cross-linking enzyme involved in collagen maturation and increase apoptosis	Pain at injection site, hyperpigmentation, ulceration and dermal atrophy
12	Drugs that lowers blood pressure and angina [53–55]	Verapamil	Inducing pro collaginase secretion. Alters fibroblast shape, induces TGF-β1 apoptosis, reduces ECM production and depolymerises actin filaments	Combinational therapy such as pressure therapy, PDL, TAIL and nifedipine is needed to effectively treat keloids.
13	Botulinum toxin type A [56–58]	Intralesional Injection	Decreasing tension at the wound edge while contraction, accumulating fibroblasts in GO and G1 of the cell cycle, reducing TGF-β1 expression	Extensive studies need to prove the efficacy towards keloid treatment.
14	ACE inhibitors [59–61]	Intraleisional injection.	Reduce the expression of Ang II, TGF-β1, PDGF-BB, heat shock protein and inhibit fibroblast proliferation and collagen synthesis.	Extensive Clinical investigation is needed.

Table 1.
Current and emerging therapies available, mode of action and their limitations.

response to the previous treatment determines the type of therapy need to cure keloids. Treatments including corticosteroids, surgical exsition, pressure therapy, radiotherapy, cryotherapy, laser therapy, 5- flurouracil, stem cell therapy, mitomycin C application, Verapamil, Bleomycin, Botulinum toxin type A and ACE inhibitors are available [18]. The current and emerging therapy for *hypertrophic* scars and keloids are briefly discussed in **Table 1**.

3. Interferons

In 1957, Isaacs and Lindeman identified a new substance which has the capacity to interfere with viral replication and coined the term "Interferon". Interferons are the group of naturally occurring cytokines produced by the cells upon exposure to various stimuli such as viruses, double – standard RNA and Polypeptides. Owing to its immunomodulatory, antiviral, antiangiogenic, anti-proliferative and antitumor activities, interferons are used to treat various diseases including Hairy Cell Leukemia, Follicular Lymphoma, Renal cell carcinoma, melanoma, chronic hepatitis, AIDS-related Kaposi Sarcoma etc. In addition to their therapeutic properties, it is used to study the mechanism of mammalian signal transduction and transcriptional regulation.

4. Types of interferons

Currently, interferons are categorized in to four types namely alpha (α), beta (ß), gamma (ɣ) and Lambda (λ) interferon [62]. More recently, IFNs were divided into three major subgroups by virtue of their ability to bind to common receptor types namely type I, type II and type III. Type I IFNs bind to a type I IFN receptor and IFN-α, IFN-β belongs to type I IFN family. IFN-γ is the sole type II IFN, and binds to a distinct type II receptor. IFN-λ belongs to Type III IFN and binds to – IFNλR receptor [63–65]. Various types of IFN and their receptors and biological properties are given in the **Table 2**.

Alpha interferons are also called as 'leukocyte interferon' is a cytokine produced by innate immune system in response to external stimuli including viral infections [65–68]. Alpha interferons are categorized under type I interferons which processes antiviral, immunomodulatory as well as anti-proliferative properties. It was reported that at least 20 copies of genes which encodes alpha interferons in human genome and standard recombinant interferons alfa-2a, alfa-2b and alfa-con1 ("consensus" interferon) have been produced [69].

Beta interferons (IFN β) are type I interferon produced by fibroblasts and possesses anti viral, anti proliferative and immunomodulatory effects. There are two forms of IFN β, IFN β- 1a and, IFN β- 1b both are used therapeutically. INF β -1b SC is produced by bacterial expression system and this was the first developed recombinant interferon for clinical use [63, 70].

Gamma interferon (IFN γ) is the only interferon categeroized under type II IFNs. IFN γ is produced by CD4T helper cell type 1 (Th1) lymphocytes, CD8 cytotoxic lymphocytes, NK cells, B cells and professional antigen-presenting cells (APCs). INF γ is acid liable where as other interferons are acid stable. IFN γ involved in various biological activity such as promotes natural killer (NK) cell activity, increase

Interferon Type	Interferon categories	Receptor Type	Cell of origin	properties
Type I	Alpha (α) Beta (β)	Type I	Leukocyte Fibroblast	Direct anti proliferative effects on cells, Stimulation of MHC Class I expression and activation of Natural Killer (NK) Cells
Type II	Gamma (γ)	Type II	T cells and NK cells	Direct anti proliferative effects on cells, Stimulation of MHC Class I & II expression, delayed activation of NK cells.
Type III	Lamda (λ)	Type III	Intestinal epithelial cells	Anti tumor activity and amplify the induction of anti viral activity of type I IFN, Up regulation of MHC Class I expression

Table 2.
Interferon Classification and properties.

APS and lysosome activity of macrophages, activates inducible nitric oxide synthase (iNOS), induces the production of IgG2a and IgG3 from activated plasma B cells, Promotes adhesion and binding required for leukocyte migration [71–73].

Interferon lamda (IFN λ) was discovered in early 2003 and were categorized under type III interferon. There are three different interferon genes encodes and produce three different interferon λ proteins namely IFN λ1, INF λ2 and INF λ3. These proteins are also called as interleukin – 29 (IL-29), IL- 28 A and IL-28 B respectively [74]. IFN λ differ from other type I and type II interferon by signaling mechanism. IFN λ, signals through heterodimeric acceptor complex. IFN λ is responsible for the development of anti tumor immune response and amplify the induction of antiviral activity of type I interferon. IFN λ processes anti viral activity and up regulate major histocompatibility complex (MHC) class I antigen expression on many cell types [75].

5. Interferon therapy for *hypertrophic* scars and keloids

Keloid is benign fibrous growth that extends outside the original wound and invades adjacent dermal tissue due to the excessive production of extra cellular matrix, especially collagen. Histologically, keloids are characterized by disorganized deposition of thick collagen fibers along with abundant lymphocytes, eosinophils and macrophages [76]. Although numerous attempts made to understand the pathophysiology and molecular abnormalities behind keloid formation, the exact pathogenesis of keloid formation is yet to be understood. Literature reports revealed that keloid shows an elevated expression of collagen mRNA, upregulation of TGF-β genes which results in excessive production of collagen and other ECM components especially fibronectin. TGF-β, especially the TGF-β1 isoform, is a key mediator of variety of processes including cell growth, proliferation, differentiation, apoptosis and responsible in many fibrotic diseases including keloids through its role in promoting extracellular matrix (ECM) production and tissue fibrosis [77]. TGF-β belongs to the member of cytokine family which binds and activates dimerization of TGF-β type II receptors and the subsequent phosphorylation of TGF-β type I receptors, which phosphorylate and activate Smad2/3 leading to the translocation of Smad4 to the nucleus and activate the expression of target genes [78]. TGF-β receptors and Smad proteins are over expressed in keloids and *hypertrophic* scars compared to normal skin.

Matrix metalloproteinases (MMPs) or matrix metallopeptidases are calcium dependent zinc containing endopeptidases that plays a critical role in ECM formation. The major function of MMPs is to catabolize ECM and cleave regulate the activity of many other extracellular bioactive substrates [79]. MMPs are classified into 4 subsets namely collagenases, gelatinases, stromelysins, and membrane type. The collagenases including MMP-1, MMP-8, and MMP-13, cleave types I and III collagens present in scar tissue. The activity of MMPs is regulated by tissue inhibitors of metalloproteinases (TIMPs) including TIMP-1, TIMP-2, TIMP-3, and TIMP-4, which inhibit MMPs. MMPs participate in inflammation, proliferation and remodeling phase of wound healing and MMPs involved in scars and keloid formation are also secreted by fibroblasts itself. An imbalance between MMP and TIMP leads to cause disturbance in collagen synthesis and degradation resulting in keloid and hypertrophic scar development [80–82].

Fibroblasts derived MT1-MMP and active MMP-2 play crucial roles in keloid formation and tumor invasion. Excessive synthesis and deposition of collagen contribute to the development of keloids with prolonged and excessive presence of TGFβ-1. Downregulation of TIMP-2 leads to the progression of keloids because of relative increase of MT 1-MMP activity. MT 1-MMP increases the activity of TGFβ-1 lead to collagen synthesis and collagen deposition in keloid development [83]. Schematic of keloid formation with respect to TGFβ-1 and MMP and role of interferon therapy in preventing TGFβ-1 and MMP mediated keloid development is given in the **Figure 2**.

Although many treatments and therapies are available for treating *hypertrophic* scars and keloids, the most efficient and successful treatment is yet to be achieved. Interferon therapy is one of the emerging therapies which have potential therapeutic effect against keloids by decreasing the synthesis of collagen types I and III and increasing collagenase activity [84]. It has been reported that Interferon alpha and gamma decrease procollagen messenger RNA levels of fibroblasts both in normal and scleroderma patients and enhance collagenase activity. Interferon not only influences collagen synthesis in skin but also reduces the inflammatory reaction. Generally, Transforming Growth Factor (TGF) which is released by platelets at the site of injury is highly chemotactic to macrophages and monocytes during the inflammatory reaction. TGF also induces collagen and fibronectin production. Interferon antagonizing the effects of TGF-β and histamine there by reducing inflammatory reaction. Among the three isoforms of interferons, IFN-α and IFN-γ have been found to be very effective for keloid treatment since it decreases collagen and other ECM expression and increasing collagenase activity [85, 86].

Specifically, IFN - α2b is widely used in the treatment of keloids owing to its anti-proliferative property and reduce dermal fibrosis directly or antagonizing the effects of TGF-β and histamine. In addition, it was reported that IFN - α2b, increase collagenase levels and to inhibit the secretion of collagenase inhibitors such as metalloproteinases. Anti proliferative properties of IFN-α2b was demonstrated by Berman and Duncan. They have intralesionally injected 1.5 million IU IFN α-2b, twice over 4 days and found that size of the keloid was reduced to 50%. Post operative injection of IFN α-2b reduce the rate of recurrence to 19% as compared with that of intralesional steroid, where the rate of recurrence was 51% [87].

Injection of IFN into the suture line of keloid excision may be prophylactic for reducing recurrences. Post operative IFN- α2b injection treatment (5 million U, 1 million U injected per cm of scar) into keloid excision sites in 124 patients, fewer keloid recurrence rate (18%) was observed compared to excision site alone (51.1%) [88].

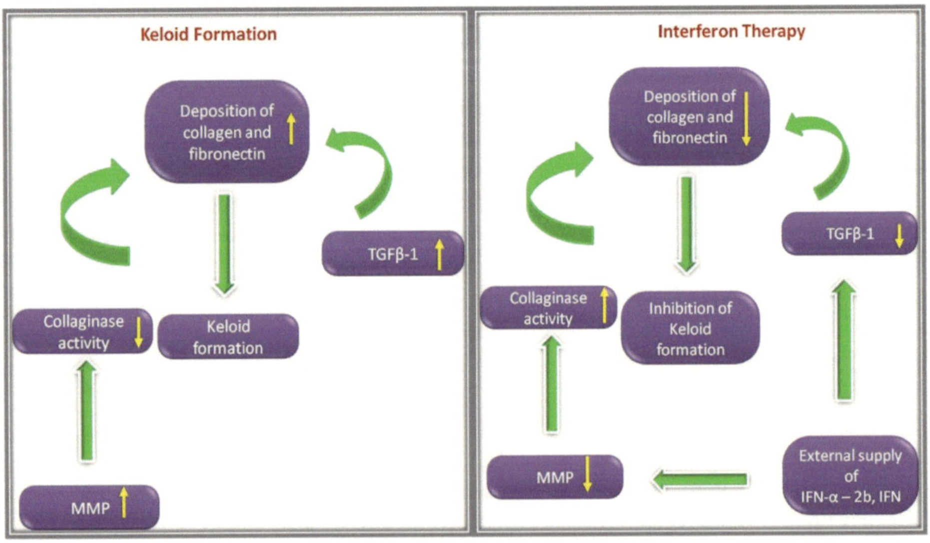

Figure 2.
Mechanism of IFN therapy.

Subcutaneous injection of human recombinant IFN- α2b (1x10^6 units) for 7 days on a daily basis to patients with hypertrophic scars and then 2x10^6 units for 24 weeks in 3 times per week basis showed significant increase in the rate of scar improvement with control. Scar assessment and scar volume also improved after 3 months of treatment and no recurrences were observed after stopping IFN therapy.

Pittet et al. reported that intralesional injections of human recombinant IFN-γ 200 mcg (6 X 10^6 U) per injection for 4 weeks to 7 patients with *hypertrophic* scar and observed that 7 of 7 patients showed decrease in redness, swelling, firmness, and lesion area. In addition to that, the reappearance of symptoms was minimal in only 2 of 7 patients and a small increase in the lesion area occurred in 4 of 7 patients, although these lesions remained smaller than the original area was observed in 16th week [89].

IFN-γ play an important role in reducing fibrosis by inhibiting TGF-β via initial activation of Jak1, which in turn stimulates the negative regulator of collagen YB-1 (Y-box protein-1), which activates Smad7, eventually leading to TGF-β1 suppression. Intralesional injection of IFN-γ has been shown to be effective in improving the appearance of keloids and hypertrophic scars, and also reducing keloid recurrence after excision along with variable treatment regimens [85].

6. Source and production of interferons

Commercially available interferons are human interferons manufactured by using recombinant DNA technology. There are many forms of interferons commercialized including interferon alfa-2a (Roferon-A), interferon alfa-2b (Intron-A), interferon alfa-n3 (Alferon-N), peginterferon alfa-2b (PegIntron, Sylatron), interferon beta-1a (Avonex), interferon beta-1b (Betaseron), interferon beta-1b (Extavia), interferon gamma-1b (Actimmune), peginterferon alfa-2a (Pegasys ProClick), peginterferon alfa-2a and ribavirin (Peginterferon), peginterferon alfa-2b and ribavirin, (PegIntron/Rebetol Combo Pack), peginterferon beta-1a (Plegridy). Among these interferons, interferon alfa-2b (Intron-A)

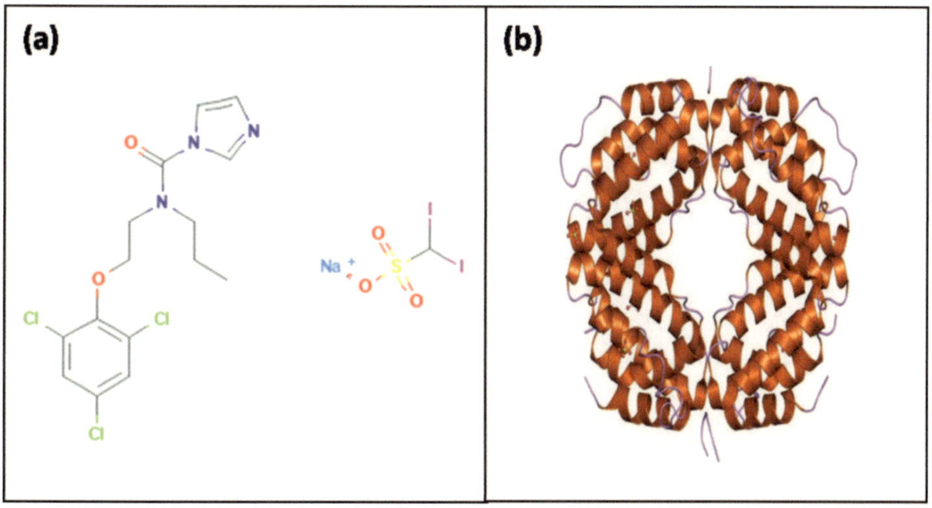

Figure 3.
Structure of human recombinant interferon (a) INTRON® A (b) ACTIMMUNE®. (Reproduced from pubchem and EMBL-EBI respectively).

and interferon gamma-1b (Actimmune) is used in the treatment of *hypertrophic* scars and keloids [90].

Interferon alfa-2b is commercialized under the trade name INTRON® A. It is a recombinant IFN available in the form of injection and molecular formula is $C_{16}H_{17}Cl_3I_2N_3NaO_5S$. The structure of this recombinant IFN is given in **Figure 3**. This IFN is water soluble proteins produced by recombinant DNA technology and possess molecular weight around 19000 Daltons. It is obtained from bacterial fermentation of *E.coli* bearing genetically engineered plasmid containing an interferon alfa2b gene from human leukocytes. The specific activity of this recombinant IFN (INTRON® A) is approximately 2.6×10^8 IU/mg [91].

Interferon Gamma is commercialized under the trade name ACTIMMUNE®. It is a recombinant interferon produced by cloning of hIFNγ cDNA and expressed the recombinant in *E.coli*. Production and purification of recombinant IFNγ is cost effective. Molecular weight of the recombinant IFNγ in monomeric form is around 17 kDa and dimeric form is around 35 kDa. The specific activity of this recombinant IFNγ is 3×10^6 IU/mg [92].

7. Combinatorial therapy

The most commonly employed treatment for keloid is Triamcinolone acetonide intralesional injection (TAIL). Major disadvantage of this therapy is limited success and adverse effects such as atrophy, telangiectasia, depigmentation, ulceration, and systemic effects, including cushingoid changes. In order to increase the success rate, TAIL is injected along with IFN – α 2 b. Twenty lesions (combined TAIL + IFN – α 2 b group) and 20 control lesions (TAIL-only group) were studied in 19 patients. Both groups were treated with TAIL once in 2 weeks. The combined TAIL + IFN-alpha2b group was treated with intralesional injection of IFN – α 2 b, twice a week. Lesion measurements were noted. Statistically significant decreases in depth (81.6%, $P = 0.005$) and volume (86.6%, $P = 0.002$) were observed in lesions of the combined TAIL IFN – α 2 b group. In the TAIL-only group, the decreases in depth (66.0%, $P = 0.281$) and volume (73.4%, $P = 0.245$) were less statistically significant. Hence, injection of IFN – α 2 b enhances the healing potential of TAIL [93].

Combinatorial therapy of laser ablation in conjugation with IFN – α 2 b injection, showed better healing and reduction in recurrence rate towards keloid treatment. 30 patients with keloids were chosen for the study. Among them, 16 patients have keloids on the ear and 14 patients on trunk. The duration of the study was 12 to 24 months and the size of the keloids was ranged from 1 to 3 cm in diameter. Keloids were ablated using ultra pulse carbon dioxide laser followed by sublesional and perilesional injections of 3 million IU of IFN-α 2b three times per week. By this combinatorial therapy, the recurrence rate was reduced and observed that 66% of lesions did not recur after three years. In particular, no recurrence was observed in the auricular area [94].

Though IFN therapy is successful, treatment associated adverse effects including fever, headache, arthralgias, fatigue, chills, and confusion were observed and the treatment is expensive.

8. Summary and conclusion

Keloids are problematic disfiguring scars arises due to abnormal wound healing and excessive fibrosis. Un controlled proliferation of fibroblast results in over production and deposition of collagen and other ECM components responsible for keloid development. There are many treatments available for *hypertrophic* scars and keloids including corticosteroid injections, surgical excision, pressure therapy, radiotherapy, laser therapy etc. Efficient and successful treatment for keloids is yet to be developed. Interferon therapy is one of the emerging therapies which have potential therapeutic effect against keloids by decreasing the synthesis of collagen types I and III and increasing collagenase activity. Recombinant IFN-α2b (INTRON® A) and IFN-γ (ACTIMMUNE®) is commercially available and used for the treatment of keloids. Significant improvement in rate of scar reduction and recurrence % was also decreased. In order to further improve the efficacy of IFN treatment, combinatorial therapy was attempted. IFN-α2b along with TAIL injection and CO2 laser ablation showed higher success rate. Hence, IFN and/or the combinatorial therapy would be a better treatment options to the patients with *hypertrophic* scars and keloids.

Acknowledgements

The authors are thankful to Dr. Prakash Vasudevan, Director, SITRA and Shri. S. Sivakumar, Head, Centre of Excellence for Medical Textiles, SITRA for providing permission to write the book chapter.

Author details

Amalorpava Mary Loordhuswamy and Santhini Elango*
Centre of Excellence for Medical Textiles, The South India Textile Research Association (SITRA), Coimbatore, India

*Address all correspondence to: se@sitra.org.in

References

[1] Bayat A, McGrouther D. A,Ferguson M.W.J. Skin scarring. Bmj. 2003; *326*:88-92. Doi:10.1136/ bmj.326.7380.88

[2] Gauglitz G.G, Korting H.C, Pavicic T, Ruzicka T,Jeschke M.G. Hypertrophic scarring and keloids: pathomechanisms and current and emerging treatment strategies. Molecular medicine. 2011; *17*:113-125. Doi: 10.2119/ molmed.2009.00153

[3] Berman B, Maderal A, Raphael B. Keloids and hypertrophic scars: pathophysiology, classification, and treatment. Dermatologic Surgery. 2017; *43*:3-18. Doi: 10.1097/ DSS.0000000000000819

[4] Tredget E.E, Nedelec B, Scott P.G, Ghahary A. Hypertrophic scars, keloids, and contractures: the cellular and molecular basis for therapy. Surgical Clinics of North America. 1997; *77*: 701-730. Doi.org/10.1016/ S0039-6109(05)70576-4.

[5] Slemp A.E, Kirschner R.E. Keloids and scars: a review of keloids and scars, their pathogenesis, risk factors, and management. Current opinion in paediatrics. 2006; 18:396-402. Doi: 10.1097/01.mop.0000236389.41462.ef

[6] Niessen F.B, Spauwen P.H, Schalkwijk J, Kon M. On the nature of hypertrophic scars and keloids: a review. Plastic and reconstructive surgery. 1999;*104*:1435-1458.

[7] Gong Z.H, Ji J.F, Yang J, Xiang T, Zhou C.K, Pan X.L, Yao J. Association of plasminogen activator inhibitor-1 and vitamin D receptor expression with the risk of keloid disease in a Chinese population. The Kaohsiung Journal of Medical Sciences. 2017; *33*:24-29. Doi. org/10.1016/j.kjms.2016.10.013.

[8] Tanriverdi-Akhisaroglu S, Menderes A, Oktay G. Matrix metalloproteinase-2 and-9 activities in human keloids, hypertrophic and atrophic scars: a pilot study. Cell Biochemistry and Function: Cellular biochemistry and its modulation by active agents or disease. 2009;*27*: 81-87. Doi.org/10.1002/cbf.1537.

[9] Zhu Z, Ding J Tredget E.E. The molecular basis of hypertrophic scars. Burns & trauma. 2016; *4*: 1-12.Doi. org/10.1186/s41038-015-0026-4

[10] Brown J.J, Bayat A. Genetic susceptibility to raised dermal scarring. British Journal of Dermatology, 2009;*161*:8-18. Doi. org/10.1111/j.1365-2133.09258.x

[11] Coppola M.M, Salzillo R, Segreto F, Persichetti P.Triamcinolone acetonide intralesional injection for the treatment of keloid scars: patient selection and perspectives. Clinical, cosmetic and investigational dermatology. 2018;*11*:387. Doi: 10.2147/CCID. S133672.

[12] Shih B, Bayat A. Genetics of keloid scarring. Archives of dermatological research, 2010; *302*:319-339. DOI: 10.1007/s00403-009-1014-y

[13] Bayat A, Arscott G, Ollier W.E.R, Mc Grouther D.A, Ferguson M.W.J. Keloid disease: clinical relevance of single versus multiple site scars. British journal of plastic surgery. 2005; 58:28-37. Doi.org/10.1016/j.bjps.2004.04.024

[14] Arno A. I, Gauglitz G.G, Barret J.P, Jeschke M.G. Up-to-date approach to manage keloids and hypertrophic scars: a useful guide. Burns. 2014:*40*;1255-1266. https://doi.org/10.1016/j. burns.2014.02.011

[15] Glass II D.A.2017, October. Current understanding of the genetic causes of keloid formation. In Journal of Investigative Dermatology Symposium

Proceedings (Vol. 18, No. 2, pp. S50-S53). Elsevier.

[16] Fujita M, Yamamoto Y, Jiang J.J, Atsumi T, Tanaka Y, Ohki T, Murao N, Funayama E, Hayashi T, Osawa M T. NEDD4 is involved in inflammation development during keloid formation. Journal of Investigative Dermatology. 2019: *139*: 333-341. Doi.org/10.1016/j.jid.2018.07.044.

[17] Lu M.Z, Ang Q.Q, Zhang X, Zhang L.F, Ya X.H, Lv H, Zheng X.D, Lu W.S. Genomic risk variants at 3q22. 3 are associated with keloids in a Chinese Han population. American journal of translational research, 2018:*10*;554.

[18] Ojeh N, Bharatha A, Gaur U, Forde A.L. Keloids: Current and emerging therapies. Scars, Burns & Healing. 2020;*6*:2059513120940499. Doi.org/10.1177/2059513120940499

[19] Ud-Din S, Bayat A. New insights on keloids, hypertrophic scars, and striae. Dermatologic clinics. 2014; *32*;193-209. Doi.org/10.1016/j.det.2013.11.002

[20] Arno A.I, Gauglitz G.G, Barret J.P, Jeschke M.G. Up-to-date approach to manage keloids and hypertrophic scars: a useful guide. Burns. 2014: *40*;1255-1266. Doi: 10.1016/j.burns.2014.02.011.

[21] Hochman B, Locali R.F, Matsuoka P.K, Ferreira L.M. Intralesional triamcinolone acetonide for keloid treatment: a systematic review. Aesthetic plastic surgery. 2008;*32*: 705-709. DOI 10.1007/s00266-008-9152-8

[22] Roques C, Téot L. The use of corticosteroids to treat keloids: a review. The international journal of lower extremity wounds, 2008; *7*:137-145. Doi.org/10.1177/1534734608320786

[23] McGoldrick R.B, Theodora kopoulou E, Azzopardi E.A, Murison M. Lasers and ancillary treatments for scar management Part 2: Keloid, hypertrophic, pigmented and acne scars. Scars, burns & healing. 2017; *3*:2059513116689805.

[24] Park T.H, Rah D.K. Successful eradication of helical rim keloids with surgical excision followed by pressure therapy using a combination of magnets and silicone gel sheeting. International wound journal. 2017:*14*;302-306. Doi.org/10.1177/2059513116689805

[25] Reish R.G, Eriksson E. Scar treatments: preclinical and clinical studies. Journal of the American College of Surgeons. 2008: *206*; 719-730. Doi.org/10.1016/j.jamcollsurg.2007.11.022.

[26] Mustoe T.A, Cooter R.D,Gold M.H, Hobbs F.R, Ramelet A.A, Shakespeare P.G, Stella M, Téot L, Wood F.M, Ziegler U.E. International clinical recommendations on scar management. Plastic and reconstructive surgery. 2002; *110*: 560-571.Doi: 10.1097/00006534-200208000-00031

[27] Puri N, Talwar A, The efficacy of silicone gel for the treatment of hypertrophic scars and keloids. Journal of cutaneous and aesthetic surgery. 2009; *2*: 104. Doi: 10.4103/0974-2077.58527

[28] Katz B.E. Silicone gel sheeting in scar therapy. Cutis. 1995;*56*:65-67.

[29] Trace A.P, Enos C.W, Mantel A, Harvey V.M. Keloids and hypertrophic scars: a spectrum of clinical challenges. American journal of clinical dermatology. 2016; *17*:201-223.Doi: 10.1007/s40257-016-0175-7

[30] Goldenberg G, Luber A.J. Use of intralesional cryosurgery as an innovative therapy for keloid scars and a review of current treatments. The Journal of clinical and aesthetic dermatology, 2013; *6*;23.

[31] Macintyre L, Baird M. Pressure garments for use in the treatment of

hypertrophic scars—a review of the problems associated with their use. Burns. 2006; *32*; pp.10-15.Doi: 10.1016/j.burns.2004.06.018

[32] Klumpar D.I, Murray J.C, Anscher M, Keloids treated with excision followed by radiation therapy. Journal of the American Academy of Dermatology. 1994;*31*: 225-231.Doi: 10.1016/s0190-9622(94)70152-0.

[33] Ji J, Tian Y, Zhu Y.Q, Zhang L.Y, Ji S.J, Huan J, Zhou X.Z, Cao J.P. Ionizing irradiation inhibits keloid fibroblast cell proliferation and induces premature cellular senescence. The Journal of dermatology. 2015; *42*:56-63. Doi.org/10.1111/1346-8138.12702

[34] Lee K.S, Jung J.B, Ro Y.J, Ryoo Y.W, Kim O.B, Song J.Y. Effects of x-irradiation on survival and extracellular matrix gene expression of cultured keloid fibroblasts. Journal of Dermatological Science. 1994; *8*:33-37. Doi.org/10.1016/0923-1811(94)90318-2

[35] Har-Shai Y, Amar M, Sabo E. Intralesional cryotherapy for enhancing the involution of hypertrophic scars and keloids. Plastic and reconstructive surgery, 2003;*111*:1841-1852. Doi: 10.1097/01.PRS.0000056868.42679.05

[36] Har-Shai Y, Zouboulis C.C. Intralesional cryotherapy for the treatment of keloid scars: a prospective study. Plastic and reconstructive surgery. 2015;*136*: 397e-398e. Doi: 10.1097/PRS.0000000000001511

[37] Rusciani L, Rossi G, Bono R. Use of cryotherapy in the treatment of keloids. The Journal of dermatologic surgery and oncology. 1993; *19*: 529-534.Doi.org/10.1111/j.1524-4725.1993.tb00386.x

[38] Mamalis AD, Lev-Tov H, Nguyen DH, Jagdeo JR. Laser and light-based treatment of Keloids–a review. Journal of the European Academy of Dermatology and Venereology. 2014:*28*;689-699. Doi.org/10.1111/jdv.12253

[39] Forbat E, Ali F.R, Al-Niaimi F. Treatment of keloid scars using light-, laser-and energy-based devices: a contemporary review of the literature. Lasers in Medical Science, 2017; *32*:2145-2154. Doi.org/10.1007/s10103-017-2332-5

[40] Anderson R.R,Parrish J.A. Selective photothermolysis: precise microsurgery by selective absorption of pulsed radiation. Science. 1983; *220*: 524-527. DOI: 10.1126/science.6836297

[41] Bijlard E, Steltenpool S, Niessen F.B. Intralesional 5-fluorouracil in keloid treatment: a systematic review. Acta dermato-venereologica, 2015; *95*: 778-782. Doi.org/10.2340/00015555-2106

[42] Hietanen K.E, Järvinen T.A, Huhtala H, Tolonen T.T,Kuokkanen,H.O, Kaartinen I.S. Treatment of keloid scars with intralesional triamcinolone and 5-fluorouracil injections–a randomized controlled trial. Journal of Plastic, Reconstructive & Aesthetic Surgery, 2019: *72*; 4-11. Doi.org/10.1016/j.bjps.2018.05.052

[43] Mari W, Alsabri S.G, Tabal N, Younes S, Sherif A, Simman R. Novel insights on understanding of keloid scar: article review. Journal of the American College of Clinical Wound Specialists. 2015; *7*:1-7. Doi.org/10.1016/j.jccw.2016.10.001.

[44] SILVA V.Z.D, Albacete Neto A, Horacio G.D.S, ANDRADE G.A, Procopio L.D, Coltro P.S,Farina Junior J.A. Evidences of autologous fat grafting for the treatment of keloids and hypertrophic scars. Revista da Associação Médica Brasileira. 2016;*62*:862-866. Doi.org/10.1590/1806-9282.62.09.862

[45] Lee G, Hunter-Smith D.J, Rozen W.M. Autologous fat grafting

in keloids and hypertrophic scars: a review. Scars, burns & healing. 2017: *3*; p.2059513117700157. Doi.org/10.1177/2059513117700157

[46] Williams E.A, Thaller S.R, The role of fat grafting in the treatment of keloid scars and venous ulcers. Journal of Craniofacial Surgery. 2019; *30*:696-697. Doi: 10.1097/SCS.0000000000005208

[47] Shin J.Y, Yun S.K, Roh S.G, Lee N.H, Yang K.M. Efficacy of 2 representative topical agents to prevent keloid recurrence after surgical excision. Journal of Oral and Maxillofacial Surgery, 2017; *75*:401. Doi.org/10.1016/j.joms.2016.10.009

[48] Sewall G.K, Robertson K.M, Connor N.P, Heisey D.M, Hartig G.K. Effect of topical mitomycin on skin wound contraction. Archives of facial plastic surgery. 2003; *5*: 59-62.

[49] Stewart IV C.E, Kim J.Y. Application of mitomycin-C for head and neck keloids. Otolaryngology—Head and Neck Surgery, 2006;*135*: 946-950. Doi.org/10.1016/j.otohns.2005.07.026

[50] Hendriks T, Martens M.F.M.W, Huyben C.M.L.C, Wobbes T. Inhibition of basal and TGF β-induced fibroblast collagen synthesis by antineoplastic agents. Implications for wound healing. British journal of cancer. 1993;*67*: 545-550.

[51] Templeton S.F, Solomon A.R, Swerlick R.A. Intradermal bleomycin injections into normal human skin: a histopathologic and immunopathologic study. Archives of dermatology.1994; *130*:577-583. doi:10.1001/archderm.1994.01690050045006

[52] Camacho-Martínez F.M, Rey E.R, Serrano F.C, Wagner A. Results of a combination of bleomycin and triamcinolone acetonide in the treatment of keloids and hypertrophic scars. Anais brasileiros de dermatologia. 2013;*88*:387-394. Doi.org/10.1590/abd1806-4841.20131802

[53] Alexandrescu D, Fabi S, Yeh L.C, Fitzpatrick R.E, Goldman M.P. Comparative Results in Treatment of Keloids With Intralesional 5-FU/Kenalog, 5-FU/Verapamil, Enalapril Alone, Verapamil Alone, and Laser: A Case Report and Review of the Literature. Journal of drugs in dermatology. 2016;*15*:1442-1447.

[54] Boggio R.F, Boggio L.F, Galvão B.L, Machado-Santelli G.M. Topical verapamil as a scar modulator. Aesthetic plastic surgery. 2014; *38*:968-975.

[55] Kant S.B, Van den Kerckhove E, Colla C, Tuinder S, Van der Hulst R.R.W.J. de Grzymala, A.P. A new treatment of hypertrophic and keloid scars with combined triamcinolone and verapamil: a retrospective study. European journal of plastic surgery, 2018;*41*:69-80. DOI 10.1007/s00266-014-0400-9

[56] Gassner H.G, Sherris D.A, Otley C.C. Treatment of facial wounds with botulinum toxin A improves cosmetic outcome in primates. Plastic and reconstructive surgery. 2000;*105*: 1948-1953. Doi:10.1097/00006534-200005000-00005

[57] Xiao Z, Zhang F, Lin W, Zhang M, Liu Y. Effect of botulinum toxin type a on transforming growth factor β1 in fibroblasts derived from hypertrophic scar: a preliminary report. Aesthetic plastic surgery. 2010: *34*;424-427. DOI 10.1007/s00266-009-9423-z

[58] Freshwater M.F. Botulinum toxin for scars: Can it work, does it work, is it worth it? . Journal of Plastic, Reconstructive & Aesthetic Surgery. 2013:*66*; 92-93. DOi.org/10.1016/j.bjps.2012.11.034.

[59] Colafella K.M.M, Bovée D.M, Danser A.J. The renin-angiotensin-aldosterone system and its therapeutic

targets. Experimental eye research. 2019: *186*; 107680. Doi.org/10.1016/j.exer.2019.05.020

[60] Iannello S, Milazzo P, Bordonaro F, Belfiore F. Low-dose enalapril in the treatment of surgical cutaneous hypertrophic scar and keloid-two case reports and literature review. Medscape General Medicine. 2006; *8*:60.

[61] Buscemi C.P, Romeo C. Wound healing, angiotensin-converting enzyme inhibition, and collagen-containing products: a case study. Journal of Wound Ostomy & Continence Nursing. 2014; *41*:611-614. Doi: 10.1097/WON.0000000000000074

[62] Jonasch E, Haluska F.G, Interferon in oncological practice: review of interferon biology, clinical applications, and toxicities. The oncologist. 2001; *6*:34-55. Doi: 10.1634/theoncologist.6-1-34

[63] Isaacs A, Lindenmann J, Virus interference I. The interferon. Proceedings of the Royal Society of London. Series B-Biological Sciences, 1957: *147*; 258-267. Doi.org/10.1098/rspb.1957.0048

[64] Pestka S. 1997, June. The human interferon-alpha species and hybrid proteins. In *Seminars in oncology* (Vol. 24, No. 3 Suppl 9, p. S9).

[65] Haque S.J, Williams B.R. 1998, February. Signal transduction in the interferon system. In *Seminars in oncology* (Vol. 25, No. 1 Suppl 1, pp. 14-22).

[66] Aguet M, Gröbke M, Dreiding P. Various human interferon a subclasses cross-react with common receptors: their binding affinities correlate with their specific biological activities. Virology, 1984:*132*; 211-216. Doi.org/10.1016/0042-6822(84)90105-3

[67] Merlin G, Falcoff E, Aguet M. 125I-labelled human interferons alpha, beta and gamma: comparative receptor-binding data. Journal of general virology. 1985:*66*;1149-1152. Doi.org/10.1099/0022-1317-66-5-1149

[68] Pfeffer L.M, Dinarello C.A, Herberman R.B, Williams B.R, Borden E.C, Bordens R., Walter M.R, Nagabhushan T.L, Trotta P.P, Pestka, S. Biological properties of recombinant α-interferons: 40th anniversary of the discovery of interferons. Cancer research. 1998; *58*:2489-2499.

[69] Sang Y, Bergkamp J, Blecha F. Molecular evolution of the porcine type I interferon family: subtype-specific expression and antiviral activity. PLoS One. 2014; *9*:112378. Doi.org/10.1371/journal.pone.0112378

[70] Lopušná K, Režuchová I, Betakova T, Skovranova L, Tomašková J, Lukáčiková L, Kabat P. Interferons lambda, new cytokines with antiviral activity. Acta Virol. 2013; *57*: 171-179. Doi:10.4149/av_2013_02_171

[71] Zaidi M.R, Merlino, G. The two faces of interferon-γ in cancer. Clinical cancer research. 2011; *17*:6118-6124. DOI: 10.1158/1078-0432.CCR-11-0482

[72] Tau G, Rothman P. Biologic functions of the IFN-γ receptors. Allergy. 1999; *54*: 1233.

[73] Kim K, Cho S.K, Sestak A, Namjou B, Kang C, Bae S.C. Interferon-gamma gene polymorphisms associated with susceptibility to systemic lupus erythematosus. Annals of the rheumatic diseases, 2010; *69*:1247-1250. Doi.org/10.1136/ard.2009.117572

[74] Ank N, West H, Bartholdy C, Eriksson K, Thomsen A.R, Paludan S.R. Lambda interferon (IFN-λ), a type III IFN, is induced by viruses and IFNs and displays potent antiviral activity against select virus infections in vivo. Journal

of virology, 2006; *80*: 4501-4509. DOI: 10.1128/JVI.80.9.4501-4509.2006

[75] Vilcek J. Novel interferons. Nature immunology. 2003; *4*:8-9.

[76] Bayat A, Arscott G, Ollier W.E.R, Ferguson M.W.J. Mc Grouther D.A. Description of site-specific morphology of keloid phenotypes in an Afrocaribbean population. British journal of plastic surgery. 2004;57:122-133. Doi.org/10.1016/j.bjps.2003.11.009

[77] Jagadeesan J, Bayat A. Transforming growth factor beta (TGFβ) and keloid disease. International journal of surgery, 2007; *5:278*-285. Doi.org/10.1016/j.ijsu.2006.04.007

[78] Zhang T, Wang X.F, Wang Z.C, Lou D, Fang Q.Q, Hu Y.Y, Zhao W.Y, Zhang L.Y, Wu L.H, Tan W.Q. Current potential therapeutic strategies targeting the TGF-β/Smad signaling pathway to attenuate keloid and hypertrophic scar formation. Biomedicine & Pharmacotherapy, 2020;129: 110287. Doi.org/10.1016/j.biopha.2020.110287

[79] Gill S.E,Parks W.C. Metallo proteinases and their inhibitors: regulators of wound healing. The international journal of biochemistry & cell biology, 2008: *40*; 1334-1347. Doi.org/10.1016/j.biocel.2007.10.024

[80] Armstrong D.G, Jude E.B.The role of matrix metalloproteinases in wound healing. Journal of the American Podiatric Medical Association, 2002; *92*: 12-18. Doi.org/10.7547/87507315-92-1-12

[81] Wolfram D, Tzankov A, Pülzl P, PIZA-KATZER H.I.L.D.E.G.U.N.D.E. Hypertrophic scars and keloids—a review of their pathophysiology, risk factors, and therapeutic management. Dermatologic surgery, 2009: *35*;171-181. Doi:10.1111/j.1524-4725.2008.34406.x

[82] Eto H, Suga H, Aoi N, Kato H, Doi K, Kuno S, Tabata Y, Yoshimura K. Therapeutic potential of fibroblast growth factor-2 for hypertrophic scars: upregulation of MMP-1 and HGF expression. Laboratory investigation. 2012: *92*;214-223.

[83] Dohi T, Miyake K, Aoki M, Ogawa R, Akaishi S, Shimada T, Okada T, Hyakusoku H. Tissue inhibitor of metalloproteinase-2 suppresses collagen synthesis in cultured keloid fibroblasts. Plastic and reconstructive surgery Global open. 2015; 3:9. Doi: 10.1097/GOX.0000000000000503

[84] Granstein R.D, Flotte T.J, Amento E.P. Interferons and Collagen Production. Journal of investigative dermatology. 1990: *95*; 75-80.

[85] Dooley S, Said H.M, Gressner A.M, Floege J, En-Nia A. Mertens P.R. Y-box protein-1 is the crucial mediator of antifibrotic interferon-γ effects. Journal of Biological Chemistry, 2006;281:1784-1795. Doi: 10.1074/jbc.M510215200

[86] Berman B. Biological agents for controlling excessive scarring. American journal of clinical dermatology, 2010;11:31-34. Berman, B. (2010). Doi:10.2165/1153419-s0-000000000-00000

[87] Berman B. Duncan M.R. Short-term keloid treatment in vivo with human interferon alfa-2b results in a selective and persistent normalization of keloidal fibroblast collagen, glycosaminoglycan, and collagenase production in vitro. Journal of the American Academy of Dermatology, 1989: *21*;694-702. Doi.org/10.1016/S0190-9622(89)70239-5

[88] Berman B.Flores F. Recurrence rates of excised keloids treated with postoperative triamcinolone acetonide injections or interferon alfa-2b injections. Journal of the American Academy of Dermatology.

1997:37; 755-757. Doi.org/10.1016/S0190-9622(97)70113-0

[89] Pittet B, Rubbia-Brandt L, Desmoulière A, Sappino A.P, Roggero P, Guerret S, Grimaud J.A, Lacher R, Montandon D, Gabbiani G. Effect of gamma-interferon on the clinical and biologic evolution of hypertrophic scars and Dupuytren's disease: an open pilot study. Plastic and reconstructive surgery. 1994;*93*:1224-1235. DOI: 10.1097/00006534-199405000-00018

[90] Panahi Y, Davoudi S.M, Madanchi N, Abolhasani E. Recombinant human interferon gamma (Gamma Immunex) in treatment of atopic dermatitis. Clinical and experimental medicine. 2012;12 :241-245. DOI 10.1007/s10238-011-0164-3

[91] Volberding P.A, Mitsuyasu R.T, Golando J.P, Spiegel R.J. Treatment of Kaposi's sarcoma with interferon alfa-2b (Intron® A). Cancer. 1987:*59*;620-625. Doi.org/10.1002/1097-0142(19870201)

[92] Green D.S, Nunes A.T, Tosh K.W. David-Ocampo V, Fellowes V.S, Ren J, Jin J. Frodigh S.E, Pham C, Procter J,Tran C. Production of a cellular product consisting of monocytes stimulated with Sylatron®(Peginterferon alfa-2b) and Actimmune®(Interferon gamma-1b) for human use. Journal of translational medicine, 2019;*17*:82. Doi:10.1186/s12967-019-1822-6

[93] Lee J.H, Kim S.E, Lee A.Y. Effects of interferon-α2b on keloid treatment with triamcinolone acetonide intralesional injection. International journal of dermatology, 2008; *47*;183-186. Doi:10.1111/j.1365-4632.2008.03426.x

[94] Conejo-Mir J.S, Corbi R, Linares M. Carbon dioxide laser ablation associated with interferon alfa-2binjections reduces the recurrence of keloids. Journal of the American Academy of Dermatology, 1998:*39*;1039-1040. Doi:10.1016/s0190-9622(98)70295-6

Chapter 2

The Need for Basic, Translational, and Clinical Research in the Field of Hypertrophic Scars

Bonnie C. Carney, Jeffrey W. Shupp and Taryn E. Travis

Abstract

Hypertrophic scar (HTS) is a fibrotic skin disorder that is marked by excessive inflammation and extracellular matrix deposition in response to cutaneous traumatic injuries such as burns, lacerations, incisions, and abrasions. HTS has various risk factors, available treatments, and treatment effectiveness. Research at the basic, translational, and clinical levels are in their infancy compared to fibrotic diseases in other organ systems. This chapter will review current in vitro and in vivo modeling, and highlight research needs to address gaps in the study of HTS. The following topics will be discussed in the chapter: a. Basic Science Research i. Seminal findings ii. Limitations to these models iii. Suggestions for topics of future research b. Translational Science Research i. Seminal findings ii. Limitations to these models iii. Suggestions for topics of future research c. Clinical Research i. Seminal findings ii. Limitations to these models iii. Suggestions for topics of future research.

Keywords: hypertrophic scar, basic and translational research, clinical research

1. Introduction

Hypertrophic scar (HTS) is a fibrotic skin disorder that is marked by excessive inflammation and extracellular matrix deposition in response to cutaneous traumatic injuries such as burns, lacerations, incisions, and abrasions. Additional fibrotic skin disorders such as keloid scars are often thought of as being the same pathophysiology existing along a continuum of severity with HTS, and hence are often studied as one scar type, despite their varied etiology. HTS is one possible outcome of wound healing and has various risk factors, available treatments, and treatment effectiveness. Research at the basic, translational, and clinical levels are in their infancy compared to fibrotic diseases in other organ systems and compared to the study of keloids. This chapter will review current *in vitro* and *in vivo* modeling, and highlight research needs to address gaps in the study of HTS.

The following topics will be discussed in the chapter:

Modeling of HTS

a. Basic Science Research

i. Seminal findings

ii. Limitations to these models

iii. Suggestions for topics of future research

b. Translational Science Research

i. Seminal findings

ii. Limitations to these models

iii. Suggestions for topics of future research

c. Clinical Research

i. Seminal findings

ii. Limitations to these models

iii. Suggestions for topics of future research

2 Basic science research

2.1 Seminal findings

Hypertrophic scar (HTS) can be defined through its hallmark clinical, histologic, cellular, and molecular features. Each of these categories are intertwined and contribute to the complex nature of HTS (**Figure 1**). HTS has been examined in the laboratory in studies of basic science for decades, and these findings have led to a number of discoveries about the features of HTS as described below. Despite this plethora of findings, there are some limitations to current knowledge and plentiful area for future research. HTS and keloid scar are often grouped together into one scar phenotype, and research focused on keloid scar is often thought to be applicable to HTS as well. Despite the similarities in these two fibrotic skin phenotypes, HTSs exhibit distinct histologic, cellular, and molecular features from keloids. The focus of this chapter is on HTS and not keloids, as the comparison of these two scar types would warrant its own review.

2.1.1 Histologic features

At a structural histologic level, there are several features of HTS including increased epidermal thickness, greater number of epidermal cell layers, and profound dermal thickness where HTS can reach up to several centimeters thick [1, 2]. HTS resulting from full thickness injuries lack dermal appendages such as hair follicles, eccrine glands, and apocrine glands. They also lack rete ridges and associated dermal papillae [1], and have increased cellularity and vascularity [3, 4]. Disorganized collagen with decreased inter-fibrillar spacing is a hallmark feature of HTS. Collagen changes its organization from the basket weave structure of normal skin to the nodular and whorl-like structure of HTS (**Figure 2**) [5–9].

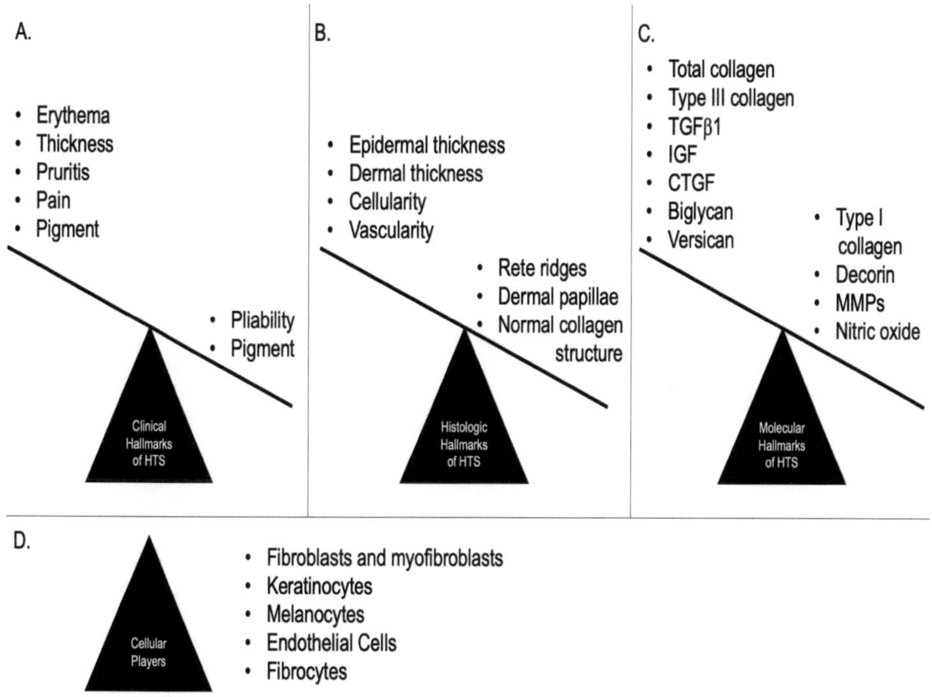

Figure 1.
There are four categories of hallmarks of HTS. These are clinical (A) histologic (B) molecular (C) and cellular (D).

2.1.2 Cellular features

2.1.2.1 Fibroblasts

Mesenchymal-derived fibroblasts are often thought of as the main contributors to the development of HTS due to the fact that they are the primary cell type which makes up the dermis. Since the dermis of HTS is thickened, and therefore comprises the large majority of the HTS volume, fibroblasts are the most populous cell type within HTSs. Fibroblast proliferation is upregulated in HTS and apoptotic processes are halted [10]. Fibroblasts are the cell type which deposit extracellular matrix (ECM). In normal skin, the processes of synthesis/deposition and remodeling of ECM exist in a delicate balance. In HTS, this balance is skewed towards synthesis with greatly reduced remodeling, resulting in scars with extreme elevation of ECM-related proteins (such as collagen types-1 and 2, tenascin, fibronectin, and tissue inhibitors of matrix metalloproteinase (TIMPS)) and downregulation of remodeling proteins (such as a multitude of matrix metalloproteinases (MMPs)) [11–13]. Fibroblasts participate in paracrine signaling with all of the other types of cells within HTS, and their production of proteins related to HTS is often regulated by these cells.

There is heterogeneity within fibroblasts with cells obtained from the papillary dermis having a different molecular signature compared to those derived from the reticular dermis [14]. Deep dermal fibroblasts are activated when a certain critical depth of injury is obtained [15]. Dunkin *et al.* used a graduated scratch model in 113 male and female healthy volunteers (ethnicity not reported) to determine this

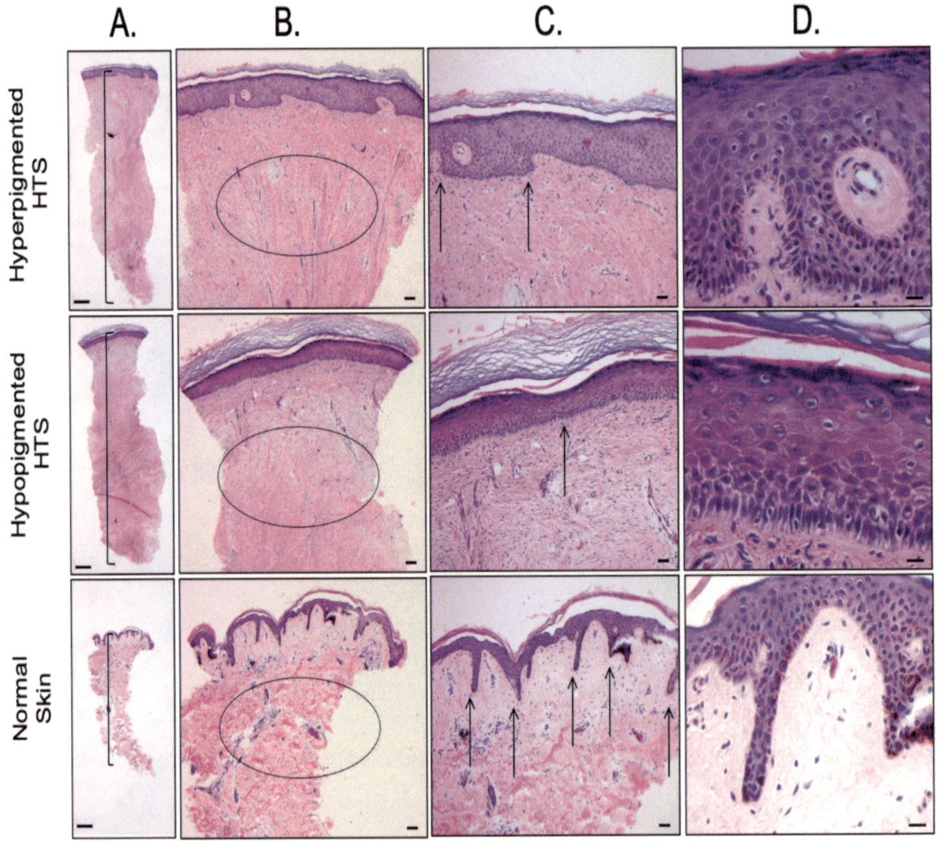

Figure 2.
Hematoxylin and &Eosin (H&E) showing histoarchitecture of HTS and skin. Regions of hyper- (top) and hypo (middle)-pigmentation share many of the hallmark characteristics of HTS compared to normal skin (bottom). Hyper- and hypo-pigmented scar and normal skin FFPE biopsies were stained with H&E. Scale bar= 500 μm at 1.25X (A) 100 μm at 5X (B) 50 μm at 10X (C) and 20 μm at 40X (D). Brackets indicate thickness (A) Circle indicates collagen organization (B) Arrows indicate rete ridges (C).

critical depth of 0.56 mm, or 33% of normal skin thickness at the hip where the wounds were created. HTS thickness was measured with high-frequency ultrasound scanning and showed that when wounds were made down into the deep dermis, HTS resulted, while injury to a superficial depth did not. The mechanistic reasoning behind this finding was elucidated when studying fibroblast cells derived from 5 different skin layers. Skin was collected from reductive plastic surgery cases (without demographic data reported), and a dermatome was used to section the skin into ~0.5 mm pieces. This study showed that fibroblasts of the deep dermis have a similar molecular signature to HTS fibroblasts [16]. This signature included increased alpha smooth muscle actin (α-SMA)-positive cells that produced more collagen and less collagenase, increased versican, and decreased decorin. Hence, injury depth within the dermis is a critical driving factor for the development of HTS.

Hypertrophic scars demonstrate increased numbers of myofibroblasts, with greater quantities in scars of earlier phases of remodeling as compared to late-stage remodeling scars [8, 9]. Myofibroblasts contribute to the increased contractility of fibroblasts, and their differentiation occurs through a transforming growth factor beta (TGFß)-mediated signaling pathway [17]. Myofibroblasts (which express α-SMA in a similar manner to vascular smooth muscle cells) have increased rates of ECM synthesis. Further compounding ECM synthesis is the contribution of mechanical tension and its ability to contribute to the mechano-sensitive regulation of differentiation processes of fibroblasts to myofibroblasts [18, 19]. This is why wounds that heal under tension, such as across joints, are at great risk for the development of scar-related contracture [20]. Many studies aimed at the development of potential treatments for HTS are intertwined with either the suppression of fibroblast to myofibroblast differentiation, or subsequent myofibroblast secretion of ECM [8, 21].

2.1.2.2 Keratinocytes

HTS keratinocytes are less well-studied in comparison to fibroblasts and in the past were thought to have a small role in HTS pathophysiology due to their small abundance compared to fibroblasts. However, they have been shown to be important drivers of HTS due to paracrine signaling with fibroblasts and melanocytes [22]. Their appearance in the healing wound often signals the transition from the proliferative phase to the remodeling phase, and HTS develops most often in wounds where there was delayed re-epithelialization, implying that these cells have a critical role to play.

Keratinocytes are found in the epidermis, which is the outermost layer of the skin and comprises only a small portion of its overall structure, less than 10% of normal skin volume [23]. Despite its limited volume, it is a complex structure that is composed of four layers of ectoderm-derived stratified epithelial cells that form a continuum of differentiated keratinocytes (basal, spinous, granular, and cornified layers). Epidermal cells are replenished from epidermal stem cells that reside in the basal layer and originate from the bulge of the hair follicle. Once an epidermal stem cell is a resident of the basal layer of the epidermis, it is unipotent and can only differentiate to produce daughter keratinocyte cells [24]. The main function of the epidermis is to act as a barrier from the external environment, and hence protect from damage. Epidermal integrity is maintained by cell-cell and cell-matrix connections made by desmosomes, adherens junctions, hemidesmosomes, and other structures comprised of a variety of integrins, glycoproteins, and proteoglycans [24]. Epidermal integrity is important for the maintenance of skin homeostasis, and yet damage can occur, especially during wounding or burn injury, due to bacteria, fungi, viruses, ultraviolet (UV) radiation, heat, or chemical exposure. The structure of the epidermis in normal skin is such that the basal layer of keratinocytes forms rete ridges in a predictable pattern which contribute to its attachment integrity.

It is known that keratinocyte-fibroblast (K-F) crosstalk is important during normal wound healing, and that keratinocytes can promote the development of fibroblast fibrotic processes. In an in-situ hybridization and immunohistochemical study of 22 Caucasian patients that had HTS resulting from partial thickness burns, expression of TGFß-1, TGFß-2, TGFß-3, basic fibroblast growth factor (bFGF), and vascular endothelial growth factor (VEGF) were evaluated at 1-, 4-, and 7-months post-burn [25]. Keratinocyte expression of all proteins was up-regulated at one month compared to normal site-matched skin from the same patients. At 4 months, some protein expression had returned to normal, and at 7 months, all growth factors were as expressed in normal skin. This data shows that keratinocyte cells are highly dynamic post-burn, and their signaling with growth factors is likely to significantly affect fibroblast cell processes. In a tissue-engineered model of 3D skin cultures, when keratinocytes derived from normal skin were seeded onto HTS fibroblasts, dermal thickness decreased. Similarly, when HTS keratinocytes were seeded onto normal fibroblasts, increased dermal thickness was likewise observed. This increase in thickness was regulated by collagen, MMPs, and apoptotic-related processes [26]. Another paper displayed the importance of K-F crosstalk when studying fetal keratinocytes of differing gestational ages and the effect of their co-culture with fibroblasts on pro-fibrotic proteins. The co-culture of HTS fibroblasts with fetal keratinocytes (fetuses are known to produce scarless healing phenotypes) decreased proliferation of fibroblasts and decreased expression of collagen-1, α-SMA, and fibronectin [27].

A number of different methods can be used when characterizing keratinocyte influence on fibroblast cells or vice versa. One simple method is growing each cell type in monoculture and collecting the conditioned media (CM) from these cultures and exposing the other cell type to the CM. Co-culturing of the two cell types can also be accomplished, however, differences in the optimum media properties for the two different cell types complicate this technique. Trans-well assays can be used to bypass this difficulty. 3D skin equivalents (either manufactured or lab-grown) can be used for a more complex system, and finally, organotypic cultures are also useful in the study of K-F crosstalk [22].

It has been suggested that HTS has altered expression of a number of keratin proteins and additional proteins related to proliferation and differentiation of keratinocytes. These alterations, which are contradictory in different reports, indicate a role for these processes in the pathophysiology of HTS development (**Table 1**) [2]. Keratin proteins make up a component of the cytoskeleton in the stratified epithelial cells of the skin epidermis [35]. They are an intermediate filament that are either classified as acidic (type I) or as neutral-basic (type II). Type I and type II keratins form heterodimers that interact with each other to contribute to mechanical resilience within keratinocytes. In addition, the basement membrane attachment proteins (such as collagen IV, laminin-5 and integrin ß4) of the epidermis to the dermis are known to be altered in HTS [2]. This alteration is evident in a lack of hemidesmosomes and focal adhesion proteins.

Lastly, keratinocytes are also critical as one component of the multicellular "epidermal melanin unit" [36]. They interact with melanocyte cells in the induction of constitutive pigmentation and acquired damage-associated pigmentation. Their response to thermal damage and secretion of protein signals to neighboring cells is altered in post-burn HTS as discussed below.

2.1.2.3 Melanocytes

Melanocytes are derived from the neural crest and ultimately reside in the skin, mucous membranes, and retinal pigmented epithelium [37]. Melanocytes distribute evenly along the dermal-epidermal junction and there is no difference in melanocyte cell number, size, or shape between light and dark skin [38]. There are, however, regional variations within individuals with the face and foreskin containing the largest number of melanocytes per area and the abdomen and lower extremities containing the fewest cells [36]. Melanocyte precursor cells, termed melanoblasts, reside in the hair bulb and can be mobilized upon injury to re-pigment healing skin. When dermal appendages are destroyed in full-thickness injuries, melanocytes repopulate healing wounds; however, the origin of these cells is not well studied and is currently unknown. Presumably, a pool of melanocytes migrates from the wound edges. It is also possible that blood-derived cells home to the wound bed, differentiate, and form a second pool of melanocytes. Melanocytes are characterized by the presence of two or more dendritic processes [36]. They are in contact with many keratinocytes and are able to interact with these cells through the extension of dendrites into a network of epidermal cells. One melanocyte can interacts with up to 30 keratinocytes.

The melanocyte and the keratinocytes with which it interacts form the multicellular "epidermal melanin unit" [36]. The two cell types work as a unit to determine the pigmentation phenotype of skin. Constitutive skin pigmentation is apparent

Protein	Type	Localization in epidermis of normal skin	Function	Role in HTS
Keratin-1	Neutral-basic (type II)	Spinous and granular layers	Interacts with K10 and desmoplakin.	Increased staining intensity towards the cornified layer compared to normal skin [28].
Keratin-2	Neutral-basic (type II)	Upper spinous layer	Associated with keratinocyte activation, proliferation, and keratinization.	Unknown
Keratin-5	Neutral-basic (type II)	Basal layer and suprabasal layer	Interacts with K14. Anchored to desmosomes via desmoplakin and plakophilin-1.	No different from normal skin [28]. Present In all layers of HTS with an increased number of epidermal cell layers [2]
Keratin-6	Neutral-basic (type II)	All layers	Interacts with K16 or K17. Activation of follicular keratinocytes during wound healing. Associated with hyper-proliferation. Induced by skin injury [29].	Up-regulated in HTS vs. normal skin throughout all suprabasal layers with strong staining [28]. Low or absent expression in normal skin [1].
Keratin-9	Acidic (type I)	Cornified layer	Expressed in palmo-plantar skin to relieve stress-bearing by increasing mechanical resilience.	Unknown
Keratin-10	Acidic (type I)	Suprabasal and cornified layers	Associated with differentiation.	Normal expression [1]. No different from normal skin [28]. More suprabasal staining compared to normal skin [2].
Keratin-14	Acidic (type I)	Basal layer and suprabasal, but not cornified layer	Interacts with K5	No different from normal skin [2, 28]. Present In all layers of HTS with an increased number of epidermal cell layers [2].
Keratin-15	Acidic (type I)	Basal layer	Interacts with K5	Present In all layers of HTS with an increased number of epidermal cell layers [2].
Keratin-16	Acidic (type I)	All layers	Interacts with K6. Associated with hyper-proliferation. Induced by skin injury [29].	Up-regulated in HTS vs. normal skin throughout all suprabasal layers [28, 30, 31]. Low or absent expression in normal skin [1].
Keratin-17	Acidic (type I)	All layers	Interacts with K6. Associated with hyper-proliferation and tumor growth [32].	Up-regulated in HTS vs. normal skin [28, 30]. Low or absent expression in normal skin [1].

Protein	Type	Localization in epidermis of normal skin	Function	Role in HTS
Keratin-19	Acidic (type I)	Basal layer	Does not interact with a type II keratin. Marker of epidermal progenitor cells [2].	Not detectable in HTS [2].
Involucrin	N/A	Spinous and granular layers	Transglutaminase substrate protein. Is a precursor to cornification in keratinocytes	In normal skin, common staining in the granular layer, HTS showed increased spinous layers and some basal layers [1].
Loricin	N/A	Cornified layers	Expressed in terminally differentiated keratinocytes [33].	Normal expression [1]
Filaggrin	N/A	Granular and cornified layers	Interacts with keratin proteins. Important for epidermal barrier function and homeostasis.	Normal expression [1]. Differential gradient density in HTS vs. NS [28].
Ki67	N/A	Basal layer	Proliferation marker	In HTS, percent of positive cells in basal layer was the same as normal skin [1]. Ki67 positive cells were increased in HTS from breast reduction surgery at 3 months compared to normotrophic scars [31]. Increased expression in suprabasal layers in HTS [34].

Table 1.
Keratinocyte proliferation and differentiation proteins. Localization in normal skin, function, and role in HTS.

and can be observed in people of different races where, at baseline, without response to damage, there are different levels of pigmentation in people with different genetic backgrounds [39]. The induction of pigmentation can also occur when keratinocytes regulate exposure to the outside environment by processing and secretion of damage-associated environmental signals. Melanocytes then receive these protein signals and respond by upregulating pigmentation machinery within the cell. When pigment is produced, melanocytes package it into melanosomes, transfer it back to keratinocytes along their dendritic processes, and keratinocytes house melanin where it is used in a variety of functions [39]. It is clear that pigmentation develops due to an increased rate of melanogenesis, and not proliferation of melanocytes [36].

Keratinocytes and melanocytes form the basis of investigation when attempting to develop treatments for dyschromia in burn-related HTS. Most pigmentation disorders such as Hermansky-Pudlak Syndrome, Waardenburg Syndrome, Type I Occulocutaneous albinism (OCA), Piebaldim, and Temperature-Sensitive OCA are genetic in origin and are a result of mutations to genes involved in melanogenesis [40]. Because burn dyschromia is a result of trauma, and not genetics, it is possible that it can be treated and potentially reversed. The first suggested treatments were reported in the 1980s [41, 42]. Onur *et al.* used a technique whereby they employed dermabrasion in the hypopigmented HTS area to ablate the epidermis and grafted this area with thin (0.2-0.3 mm) skin grafts. They were able to show "adequate repigmentation" in their case series of 18 patients. In 1991, investigators in the United States published a similar study where hypo-pigmented HTS area was also prepared using dermabrasion [43]. An "epidermal" sheet graft was then taken at a depth of 0.0006 inches (0.015 mm) using a dermatome. This method used a much thinner graft that contained only epidermis so as to limit donor site dyschromia. Eighty six percent of patients had a good result and 13% had an excellent result. The same group extended their findings in a 1996 publication of the same title where they added an additional 21 patients to their case series [44]. Their findings were similar and somewhat improved over their previous study. Similar studies continued to occur, one reported substituting dermabrasion with flash-scanned CO_2 laser to prepare the HTS area for thin split-thickness grafting (STSG) [45]. The papers described above report outcomes for patients treated exclusively for hypopigmented HTS. As time went on, this technique was also used to treat hyperpigmentation [46, 47]. In 1996 [48] and 1997 [49], concise reviews were published in *Burns* and the *Journal of Burn Care and Research*, respectively. They summarized the limited treatment options for postburn dyspigmentation. They described thin STSG after dermabrasion as the only surgical technique that was available at the time. The only other treatments that were mentioned were medical tattooing and temporary makeup [50–53]. Even as late as 2016, a paper was published showing the results of a retrospective chart review of patients who underwent dermabrasion and thin STSG from 1997-2007 [54]. Today, in many centers around the country, many patients are told that their only option for treatment of dyschromia is to use makeup or tattooing. Thin STSG treatment has benefits as discussed above; however, complications can occur. Some patients have experienced hyperpigmentation of the grafted site and donor site after sun exposure and cyst formation beneath grafts [42]. In addition, in patients with large TBSA injuries, who have extremely limited areas of normally pigmented skin, this sort of surgical correction is not an option. Lastly, there are only a few surgeons in the United States who perform this operation.

With this literature in mind, it is clear that none of these treatment methods are based on mechanistic reasoning. They rely on the transfer of cells or tissues from unaffected areas of the body to the HTS site. They can also lead to pigmentation abnormalities at the donor sites. As such, over the past many years, our lab has sought to investigate the mechanism of action of HTS dyschromia to develop treatments with a mechanistic basis that may be more efficacious, tissue sparing, and more widely applicable than prior methods.

Our group came upon the study of dyschromia while conducting a study on the effectiveness of pressure therapy in a Red Duroc pig model of HTS [55]. The scars for study also developed dyschromia with areas of hyper- and hypopigmentation. These scars closely resembled HTS that was observed in our patient population, and hence, samples were acquired for study. Grossly, the scars were hyperpigmented on the periphery with small islands of hyperpigmentation in the interior surrounded entirely by hypopigmentation. The inside of the scars were mostly hypopigmented. Unexpectedly and interestingly, due to the dogma that is currently reported in the literature, we discovered that melanocytes were present in equal amounts in regions of hyper- and hypo-pigmentation by immunofluorescent staining for a melanocyte marker, S100B [56]. This work also showed increases in staining for melanin by azure B and melanin activation proteins, alpha melanocyte stimulating hormone (α-MSH) and human melanoma black 45 (HMB45) in hyper- compared to hypopigmented scar. We next sought to further confirm the presence of melanocytes in regions of differential pigmentation, as well as look more in depth into the canonical pigmentation signaling cascade [57]. Melanocyte presence was confirmed by multiple assays including primary culture of these cells. In addition, a number of target molecules were shown to be up-regulated at the mRNA and protein levels in hyper- vs. hypopigmented scar, including pro-opiomelanocortin (POMC), adrenocorticotropin hormone (ACTH), stem cell factor (SCF), melanocortin 1 (MC1R), stem cell factor ligand (cKIT), tyrosinase (TYR), tyrosinase-related protein-1 (TYRP1), and tyrosinase-related protein-2 (TYRP2) or dopachrome tautomerase (DCT). While this work was useful in elucidating the molecules of interest that are up-regulated in hyperpigmented scar, and downregulated in hypopigmented scar, a mechanistic reasoning behind the dysregulation in the first step in the pigmentation signaling cascade was not revealed in this work. Canonical signaling by a DNA damage and p53-associated pathway were ruled out, as these moieties were not differentially regulated in different pigment phenotypes. In subsequent work, POMC was further investigated as a potential root cause of hyper- and hypopigmentation. Methylation of POMC's promoter was studied; however, there were no differences to suggest that methylation is the cause of dyschromia [58]. In addition, we used full transcriptome microarray analysis to identify a number of pathways that were differentially regulated between the two pigmentation phenotypes. These pathways provided us with additional and future avenues of study for preventing and treating dyschromia [58]. Some of this work is summarized in **Figure 3**. These studies are currently underway in our laboratory, and include treating areas of hypopigmentation with pigmentation stimulators as reviewed in our recent paper [59]. A recent paper by Dutta *et al.* is one of the few other mechanistic papers investigating

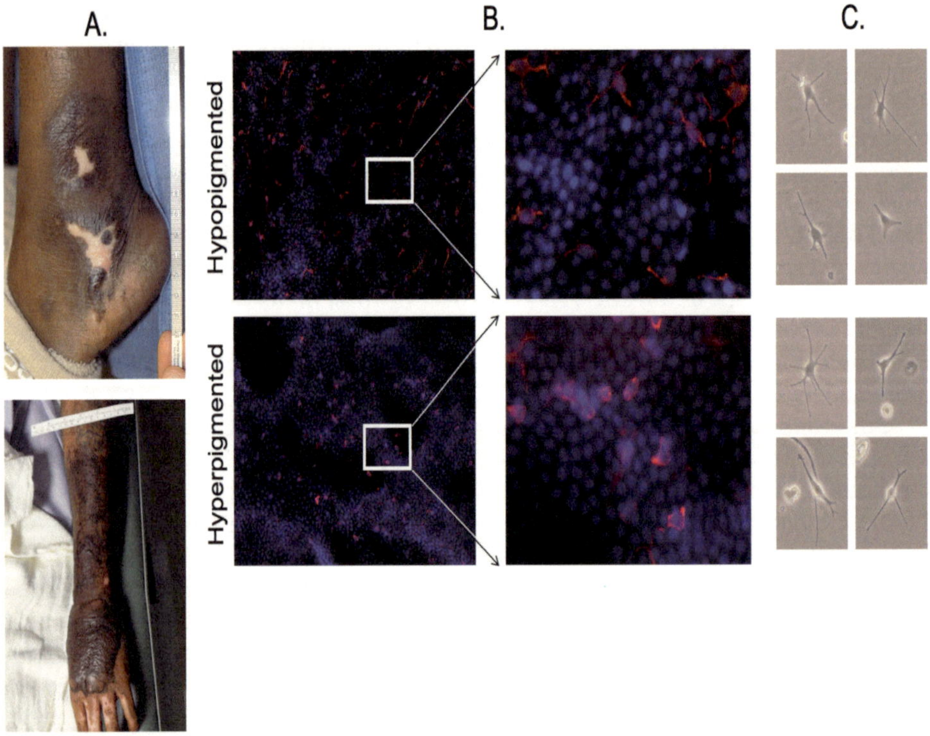

Figure 3.
Burn injury can result in dyspigmented scar that contains regions of hyper- and hypo-pigmentation with melanocytes in equal numbers. Examples of hyper- and hypo-pigmented burn HTS from two different patients (A) Epidermal sheets were stained for melanocyte marker S100β by en face staining. S100β (red), DAPI (blue). Scale Bar= 50μm at 10X (left) or 10μm at 40X (right) (B) Cells from regions of hyper- or hypo-pigmentation were isolated and imaged using phase contrast at 40X (B) Melanocytes and dendrite were counted in each region of pigmentation (C) Patient photographs were collected under an IRB-approved protocol and shared with patient consent.

hypopigmentation in burn patients [60]. This paper studied immunohistochemical staining for cytokeratin 5, MC1R, Ki67, loricrin, and TYRP1. They also showed that dendricity in melanocytes was altered in hypopigmented cells in cell culture. This is a valuable study of dyschromia in HTS, but also does not reveal a mechanistic cause of hypopigmentation as the work is mostly aimed at characterization. The study of HTS is still a relatively new area of research compared to some other organ systems where fibrosis has been studied extensively. Dyschromia in HTS is an even newer topic of study and should be a priority due to its psychosocial effects for patients with HTS.

2.1.2.4 Endothelial cells

Endothelial dysfunction is a newer topic of study in the setting of trauma [61], sepsis [62], and burn injury [63]. It is known to play a role in acute burns where circulating levels of a proteoglycan component of the glycocalyx which is shed upon injury, syndecan-1 (SDC-1), is up-regulated in a dose-dependent manner in relation to injury severity. The glycocalyx is a complex meshwork of proteoglycans that line the luminal surface of blood vessels [64]. Circulating SDC-1 levels measured by ELISA can predict mortality, and the amelioration of the shedding of the endothelial glycocalyx is a topic of current research in illuminating best practices for burn shock resuscitation [65, 66]. Due to the link between acute burn care and the long-term systemic effects of burn injury, it is hypothesized that endothelial dysfunction likewise plays a role in the development of HTS, and if it can be ameliorated, then HTS may be able to be prevented or treated.

One characteristic of HTS that provides evidence for this link is the erythematous nature that can result in purple, red, or pink scars that tend to improve over time. This erythema results from hyper-vascularity from an increased presence of blood vessels within these scars [67, 68]. Laser doppler imaging has shown an increased microcirculation and perfusion in HTS compared to surrounding unburned skin [69]. This data is somewhat contradictory to reports that; although there is increased blood vessel presence, these vessels are often totally or partially occluded through unknown mechanisms.

HTS are sometimes thought of as benign tumors that are "fed" by this vasculature [70]. In comparison to fibroblasts and keratinocytes, endothelial cells in HTS are less well-studied [71]. They gained recognition when a link between hypertension and increased hypertrophic and keloid scar severity was reported [72]. Hypertension can directly affect vascular function and as such, endothelial dysfunction is thought to play a role in scar development.

Pressure therapy is thought to work in part by "starving" the scar by inducing hypoxia [4]. Multiple non-pressure-related studies that target VEGF or angiogenesis have been studied to alleviate scar [73–75]. One such drug is endostatin which is a potent endothelial cell proliferation inhibitor. Endostatin inhibits angiogenesis and has also been shown to have an effect on tumor growth and metastasis. Its effects have been studied in a rabbit ear model of HTS where it was injected intralesionally [76]. Treatment with endostatin resulted in decreased scar elevation index, decreased thickness, decreased microvessel density, and changes to collagen organization. Interestingly, mechanistic studies have focused on the effect of endostatin treatment on fibroblasts, and not endothelial cells [77, 78]. In addition, it has been shown in keloid scar that not only epithelial to mesenchymal transition (EMT), but endothelial to mesenchymal transition (EndoMT) may play a role in scar development [79]. Endothelial pericytes may undergo EndoMT to become myofibroblasts which secrete ECM [80]. This concept should be further studied in the context of HTS as well.

2.1.2.5 Fibrocytes

Fibrocyctes are a peripheral blood mononuclear cell population (PBMC) making up 0.5% of total leukocytes. These cells home to tissues during wound repair and play a role in fibrosis [81]. They are termed as such due to their "fibroblast-like" properties and spindle shape in adherent cell culture. They are an interesting cell type because prior to their discovery in 1994, it was thought that all of the cells that contribute to wound healing migrated from surrounding areas of un-injured epidermis or dermis; however, blood-borne cells are now known to be critical for wound healing as well. When these cells differentiate, they lose hematopoietic markers and gain mesenchymal markers such as collagen, vimentin, cluster of differentiation 34 (CD34), and α-SMA. These cells target wound sites during the initial stages of injury and contribute to the inflammatory phase of healing by secreting a distinct profile of cytokines and chemokines, hence chemo-attracting other inflammatory cells. In addition, fibrocytes are known to be involved in numerous fibrotic diseases such as pulmonary fibrosis, asthma, atherosclerosis, and renal fibrosis [82–84]. They are present in post-burn HTS [85] where they are known to contribute to the proliferative phase by secreting ECM and the remodeling phase by secreting MMPs. They also regulate fibroblast activity through signaling with TGFß-1 and connective tissue growth factor (CTGF) by increasing cell proliferation, and migration, and increasing α-SMA expression, hence increasing the contractility of collagen [86]. Fibrocytes have been identified as circulating cells in burn patients with a dose-dependent response in the number of circulating cells with increasing injury severity [87] and in a model of HTS in Red Duroc pigs [88]. Fibrocytes are a potential cell type to focus on when developing targeted therapies for systemic or local treatments for HTS. Indeed, when patients with HTS were treated with interferon-alpha (IFN-α) 2b, which was shown to stop fibrocyte differentiation in a dose-dependent fashion, the number of fibrocytes in HTS tissues was reduced, and the activity of the remaining cells was likewise reduced [89]. There may also be additional blood-derived cells of importance in regulating HTS [90].

2.1.3 Molecular features

There are also several molecular hallmarks of HTS including upregulation of overall collagen [91] with shifts in the ratio of type I and type III collagens [11, 12] in superficial and deep dermis. This upregulation generally results in higher levels of type III collagen in HTS [12]. TGFβ1 [92], insulin-like growth factor 1 (IGF1) [93], CTGF [94], platelet-derived growth factor (PDGF) [95], biglycan, pleiotrophin [96], and versican [97] are all upregulated, while decorin [97], MMPs, IFN-α 2b [98], interferon-gamma, and nitric oxide are downregulated compared to normal, uninjured skin [96, 99–103].

The complexity of HTS development is not only in mRNA transcriptomes that code for proteins, but in non-coding RNAs such as micro-RNA (mi-RNA), circular RNAs, and other long-non-coding RNAs. mi-RNAs bind to mRNA and most often lead to their post-transcriptional degradation prior to protein coding. Hence, mi-RNA can have a drastic effect on protein expression. In the last 6 years, a flood of papers describing the effect of a multitude on mi-RNAs on HTS fibroblasts have been published. Dahai and colleagues have led the way with their work on mi-RNAs 21 [104], 130a [105], 155 [106], 192 [107], and 494 [108]. mi-RNA-21 is one of the most extensively studied with 3 papers claiming that aberrant mi-RNA expression has a role on the fibroproliferative effects of HTS fibroblasts [104, 109, 110]. Additional mi-RNAs 145 and 200b have also been studied by more than one group and have been connected to TGFß and Smad2/3 signaling pathways [111, 112]. Numerous others mi-RNAs have been studied such as mi-RNA 181b which regulates decorin production in fibroblasts [113], mi-RNA 22 which promotes fibroblast apoptosis [114], mi-143 which targets CTGF [115], mi-185 and mi-29 which both regulate TGFß and collagen-1 expression [116], and mi-137 which regulate pleiotrophin [117]. Circular RNA [118] and long-non-coding RNAs [119, 120] also seem to play a role in HTS.

2.2 Limitations to these models

2.2.1 Histologic

As shown above, a large number of studies use either freshly cut or formalin-fixed paraffin embedded tissue sections to study HTS at the histologic level. In patients, longitudinal biopsy studies are uncommon, though possible. As such, biopsies represent a snapshot in time and not the dynamic nature of HTS remodeling. Patients often have multiple hundreds of square centimeters worth of HTS. In addition, these areas of scar may look heterogeneous due to staged, variable acute burn interventions. Especially in large TBSA injuries, HTS phenotypes may differ regionally, and one small, often 3-mm tissue biopsy, is often not sufficient to display the heterogeneity (of color, thickness, elasticity) of scar within a particular patient.

2.2.2 Cellular

The co-culturing of keratinocyte and fibroblast cells is far more developed in the study of keloid scar compared to HTS where there are only a few papers which utilize these techniques [121, 122]. Due to the difficulty of obtaining HTS tissue from which to derive cells, and the lack of a universally agreed upon animal model to provide these cells, experiments attempting to understand HTS-related fibrotic processes often use skin cells from either immortalized lines (such as HaCat cells), or from normal skin donors from reductive plastic surgery cases [123]. These cells are inferior to using HTS-derived cells. Additionally, HTS resulting from cutaneous non-burn related trauma may have different mechanisms. Therefore, papers studying HTS from surgical incisions, such as in breast reduction surgery, may not apply to more severe HTS, such as that encountered post-burn injury [124]. Additionally, melanocytes are often not incorporated into *in vitro* models of HTS, under-emphasizing the importance of their role as photo-protectors of keratinocytes. Endothelial cells likewise are under-utilized in *in vitro* modeling of HTS, and should be added when attempting to model the full complexity of HTS. Fibrocytes and other blood-derived cells should also play a role in *in vitro* modeling for a more complete picture.

2.2.3 Molecular

After deriving primary cell cultures from HTS lesions and culturing cells *in vitro*, these cells often lose their molecular phenotype and don't secrete the same proteins as they do *in vivo*. With the addition of passaging of cells that further remove them from their *in* vivo environment, these cells become farther and farther from the pathology which researchers are attempting to study. Part of the loss of molecular signatures *in* vitro is most likely due to the paracrine signaling from a multitude of cell types that contribute to severe scar phenotypes. Non-coding RNA findings are very new, and should be validated and studied in the future and treatments related to these findings should be developed. Of note, all of these studies examine non-coding RNAs in fibroblast cells only.

2.3 Suggestions for topics of future research

2.3.1 Histologic

In studies utilizing patient tissue biopsies, time post-burn and post re-epithelialization, prior scar treatments, and demographic data including race and ethnicity should be judiciously reported. A large number of current studies report on Caucasian and Chinese populations, and future work should emphasize additional Asian, African, African American, Indigenous, and Hispanic patient populations. When one race or ethnicity makes up the large majority of samples, the title of the work should clearly indicate as such so as not to assert that all HTS contain these features. Blood collection should also be incorporated into prospectively-designed trials to evaluate the systemic responses to treatments or the natural systemic state that may contribute to HTS pathophysiology. Often, tissue biopsies are collected without companion blood samples. Details related to body location, and acute burn treatment of the particular biopsy site is likewise important for nuanced study of HTS at the histologic level. Longitudinal biopsies of scar can be performed in patients; however, large-scale studies should be reserved for animal modeling, and hint at the importance of both bench-to-bedside research, and bedside-(back)to-bench research.

2.3.2 Cellular

It is as yet unclear what is the best model for studying HTS *in vitro*, though it is clear from the described studies above that using cells in monoculture is the most commonly used method. In addition, these cultures are often carried out in 2D. While using these simplified techniques may be useful for some research questions, it is important not to over-simplify scar modeling. By utilizing co-culture models of multiple cell types, these *in vitro* systems become more sophisticated and more similar to the *in vivo* environment. An example of a co-culture system that should be developed is endothelial cells with fibroblasts. The contribution of endothelial cells to HTS development is an area ripe for study. A method for isolating and culturing dermal microvascular endothelial cells has been published, and reports a relatively simple antibody-based cell sorting method that could be easily incorporated into cell isolation protocols from HTS tissue samples derived from patients or animals [125]. In addition, 3D cell cultures can be used to more closely mimic the organization of skin as a tissue structure. Such "scar in a jar" models are likely to be useful moving forward [126]. It has also been suggested that media components may be altered to create a pseudo "crowded" environment in culture. Crowders such as ficolls and dextrans of differing molecular weights are meant to take up a fractional volume of the media to mimic fibrosis where ECM crowds cells *in vivo*. Such techniques, termed macromolecular crowding, should be incorporated into *in vitro* models in future work [127, 128].

2.3.3 Molecular

Future work should examine additional cell types when studying non-coding RNAs. The transcriptional profile of messenger RNA seems no longer adequate to explain the complexity of HTS. Non-coding RNAs should be incorporated into studies at the molecular level. As the scientific community progresses towards more sophisticated assaying capability in additional molecular components of the cells, these should all be likewise incorporated into our models. One such example is the discovery in 2020 of a novel tRNA-derived small RNA that plays a role in HTS fibrosis [129].

Non-coding RNAs are an example of a mechanism that could be studied in samples or cells of dyschromic HTS lesions. The molecular and cellular mechanisms behind the development of dyschromia have not yet been elucidated, and may be related to epigenetic pathways such as non-coding RNAs. The reasoning behind this hypothesis is due to the fact that dyschromia often persists over many years, and does not improve over time like many other scar symptoms. This phenomenon seems to hint that there are epigenetic modifications that contribute to its long-lasting nature. In addition, when moving from *in vivo* to *in vitro* systems, dyschromia persists in cells, further providing evidence that epigenetic mechanisms may be at play. There are a multitude of areas that could be studied in relation to dyschromia including global or gene-specific methylation of melanogenesis or keratinocyte-secreted proteins, acetylation patterns, or histone modifications. In addition, an interesting phenomenon is that HTS dyschromia does not improve over time even with treatment of scars that improve additional symptoms such as scar thickness or pruritis. The link between fibroblasts and melanocytes are an interesting area of future study due to the fact that treatments targeting the dermal cells do not seem to have an effect on melanocytes. HTS dyschromia is one area of research that should be prioritized due to its importance to patient populations for whom dyschromia is a factor in their psychosocial health.

3. Translational science research

3.1 Seminal findings

3.1.1 Patient samples and the need for animal models

Patient samples and patient-derived cells are often used to study HTS at the translational level. While these techniques can be useful, longitudinal and large-scale studies likely need to occur in animal models. There is no perfect animal model for the study of HTS [130, 131]. Murine species are not acceptable models because of the "loose-skinned" nature of these animals (**Figure 4**) [132]. They also have a panniculus carnosus which allows them to heal by contraction instead of by granulation tissue deposition and re-epithelialization. As such, murine species do not form HTS and are not an acceptable model. Non-animal models for wound healing and scar formation have also been suggested [133]. These models include in vitro models utilizing co-cultures of HTS-derived cells and organotypic culturing of biopsies of HTS. *Ex vivo* models utilizing excised human skin have also been proposed. While these models are useful for certain research questions, the drawback of not having the full *in vivo* system is clear.

A number of animal models for HTS have been proposed, including nude mouse models of xenografted human normal skin or HTS, the rabbit ear model, the Yorkshire pig model, and the red Duroc pig model. Each of the models has its own inherent pros and cons and each can be useful depending on the details of the specific research question. In addition, some papers claim that there is no universally accepted animal model for HTS, and hence, there is discord in the literature about methods for HTS creation even within the same species.

3.1.2 Nude mouse models

Nude mouse models of xenografted normal human skin have been used to create human-like HTS [134–136]. Although the skin was normal, and not HTS when it was xenografted, the skin forms scar that has many of the morphologic

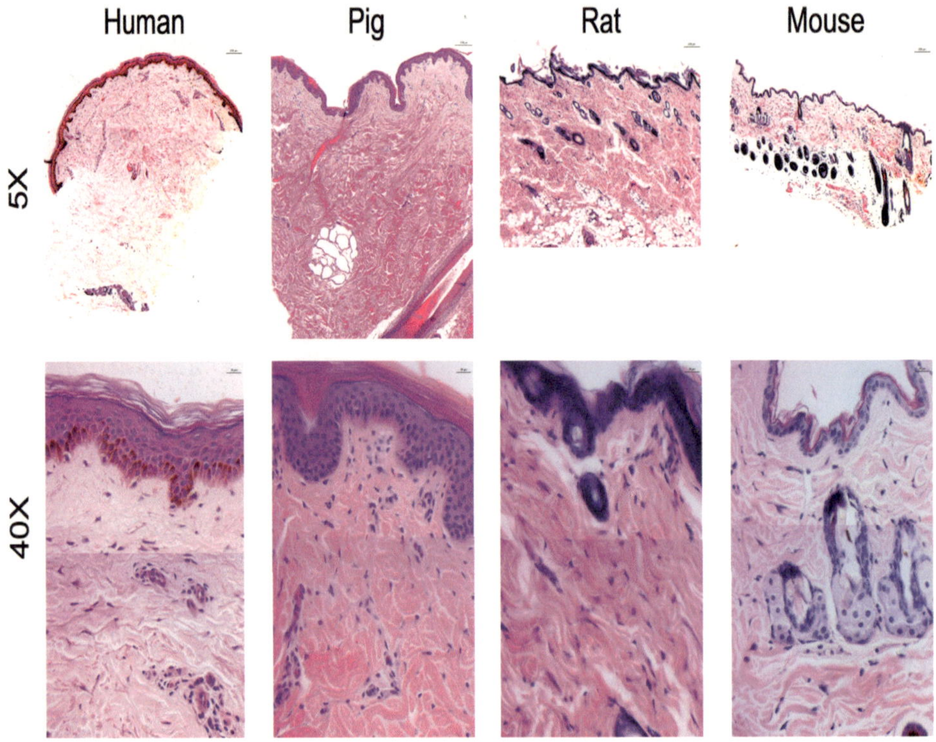

Figure 4.
Porcine skin most closely resembles human skin compared to rat and mouse skin. Epidermal and dermal thickness are similar and dermal appendages are present in similar densities. All animal work was conducted under IACUC-approved protocols.

and histologic criteria of HTS. Additional models have been developed over time where the normal skin is "scratched" to create a wound in the skin that then forms additional HTS [137].

3.1.3 Rabbit ear

The rabbit ear model likewise has its pros and cons [138]. It involves creating a small (6-8 mm) full thickness excisional wound in the ear of New Zealand white rabbits. Because the rabbit ear does not contain a panniculus carnosus, the small wounds heal with fibrosis and share some of the hallmarks of HTS including increased thickness, vascularity, and cellularity. In most papers, 6-8 scars are created on each ear and treatments are applied to each HTS as individual biologic replicates.

3.1.4 Yorkshire pig

The Yorkshire pig model is useful for modeling HTS similar in phenotype to scars from patients with baseline light skin pigmentation [139–144]. These scars are often described as "port-wine" scars due to their erythematous nature due to increased vascularity. They have increased thickness compared to normal skin (~2X), decreased tensile strength, different collagen architecture, increased vascularity, increased TGFβ expression, increased presence of myofibroblasts, and decreased presence of rete ridges [140]. This model is useful for certain research questions related to the prevention and treatment of scars that are present in patients with light skin pigmentation.

3.1.5 Duroc pig

In the 1970s, Silverstein *et al*. reported HTS development in red Duroc pigs after deep dermal wounding. They never published their model however, and it was not widely adapted. In 2003, Zhu *et al.* published an examination of a number of wound thicknesses and the resulting HTS that developed under different conditions in female red Duroc pigs [145]. They found that the creation of 8 cm by 8 cm (3.1 inches by 3.1 inches) deep partial thickness or full thickness wounds with a total dermatome setting of 0.06" to 0.09" led to the development of HTS that was thick, hypercontracted, and hyper-pigmented. In addition, there was disorganized collagen structure and many of the genes of interest known to be dysregulated in human HTS were appropriately dysregulated. The same group went on to publish a number of papers demonstrating the clinical, histologic, and molecular similarities of Duroc pig HTS to human HTS [68, 146–149]. Around the same time period, another group published similar findings in Duroc pigs [150, 151]. Gallant *et al.* used females or castrated males and created 2 cm by 2 cm (0.8 inches by 0.8 inches) full thickness wounds using a scalpel to remove the full thickness skin down to subcutaneous fat. Multiple small wounds were created in 2 rows of 10 wounds per flank. These HTSs ultimately progressed to become hyper-pigmented at day 70.

It was around the time of the publication of these novel Duroc pig HTS model papers that our lab became focused on developing a similar model for HTS. We began modeling with Duroc pigs to study partial thickness wounds in relation to donor site healing dynamics [152] and wound healing accelerating agents [153]. These wounds were created at a total dermatome setting of 0.06" and were 7.62 cm x 7.62 cm (3 inches x 3 inches) in size. These partial thickness wounds healed without the thick fibroproliferative nature of HTS; however, some hyper-pigmentation was observed. We then continued our investigation into the creation of full thickness wounds to generate HTS (**Figure 5**). During this project, where the primary goal was to study pressure delivery, HTSs were generated by full thickness wounding with a total dermatome setting of 0.09" and size of 10.16 cm by 10.16 cm (4 inches by 4 inches) [88, 154–158]. Throughout the course of this work, dyschromia, with regions of hyper- and hypo-pigmentation, was apparent [56].

3.2 Limitations to these models

3.2.1 Patient samples

Studying patient samples is most likely the best recapitulation of the disease process; however, this strategy has the drawback that it is a snapshot in time. These samples do not provide any information as to the natural history of HTS formation, as they must be taken after a scar is already formed. Additionally, HTS samples from patients are most likely at the severe end of the spectrum because the samples can most often only be collected during surgical HTS excisions.

3.2.2 Nude mice

While these models are useful, and they have shown retention of the HTS and pigmentation phenotype even 1-year post-xenografting, the etiology of HTS is not the same as the etiology of full thickness wounding or burn injury. Lastly, this model relies on the availability of large amounts of normal human skin, a resource that is not universally available.

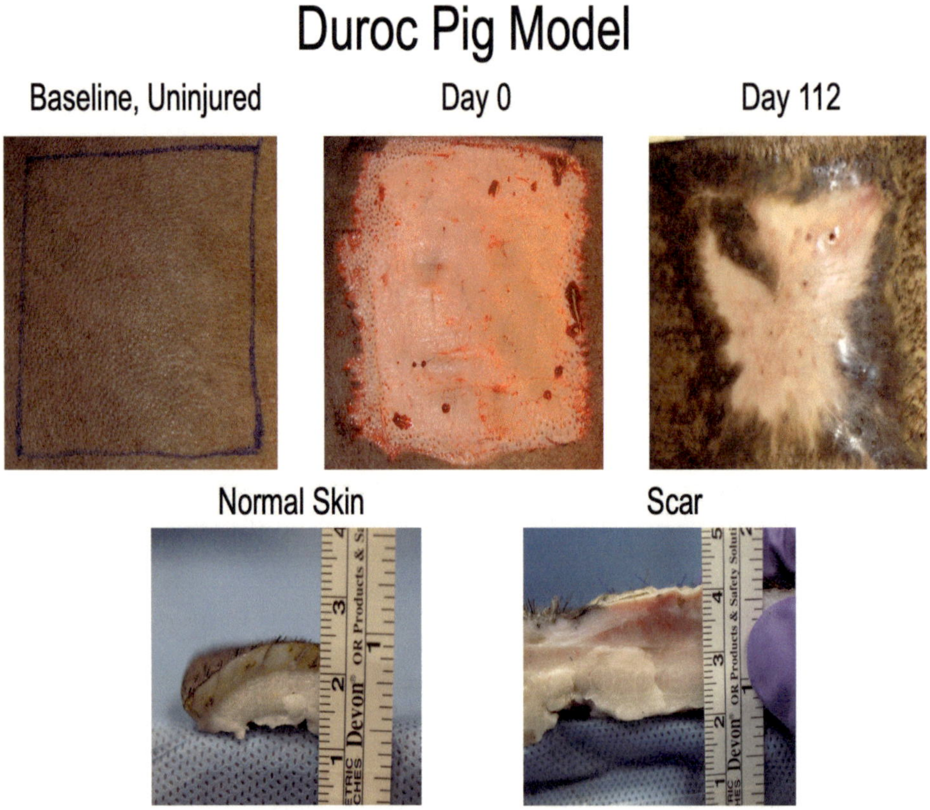

Figure 5.
Our lab's model of full-thickness excisional wounding to generate HTS in Red Duroc pigs. Baseline, un-injured Duroc skin has a red-brown phenotype. Full-thickness excisional wounds created by dermatome down to subcutaneous fat with no residual dermal appendages are created. Dyschromic, rigid, thick, HTS is generated 112 days post-wounding. This scar is thick compared to normal skin.

3.2.3 Rabbit ear

The model is affordable and has been used successfully to investigate a number of drug treatments; however, not many of these have made the leap to clinical treatments. This model does not acknowledge the potential local-regional effects of drug treatments on HTSs. Lastly, the overall skin structure of the rabbit ear is not similar to human skin because it sits upon a bed of avascular cartilage [138]. The model's main limitation is the size of the scars for study, which are small. In addition, dyschromia is not evident in these scars.

3.2.4 Yorkshire pig

In Yorkshire models of HTS, the resultant scars are not as thick as human HTS and they are not raised above the surrounding tissue. This phenomenon is most likely because fibroblasts derived from Yorkshire skin have an inherently less fibroproliferative phenotype compared to Duroc pig fibroblasts [159]. Fibroproliferation was demonstrated by Duroc pig fibroblasts to show increased actin stress fiber formation and adhesion complexes, decreased cell migration, increased cell contraction, and differential expression of HTS-related genes of interest (α-SMA, type I collagen, decorin, and TGFβ) compared to Yorkshire pig fibroblasts. Lastly, the

Yorkshire pig model for HTS is insufficient for certain research questions because there is no melanin-related dyschromia in this model.

3.2.5 Duroc pig

From 2012, when our lab began with this model, to present day, multiple labs have adopted the Duroc pig as a model for HTS formation. There is still no universal method for the creation of scars as some labs use excisional techniques at different depths and with different instruments [160–162], burn techniques [163–166], and burn, excision, and auto-grafting techniques [167–170]. Many scar models use small wound sizes that are not a significant wound burden on the animal. The full thickness nature of the injuries created in our model, as well as the large size, helps to closely mimic the HTS features that were observed in patients during the parallel timeline that experiments were taking place. Finally, the use of pigs, and specifically Duroc pigs, which are not a common animal breed, is expensive due to housing considerations and operative room time. This fact is often a limiting factor for their use.

3.3 Suggestions for topics of future research

3.3.1 Patient samples

Basic and translational scientists should work closely with physician-scientists to ensure that the questions they are trying to answer in basic or translational models are important for patients. As a community, we need to determine how improvements can be made to the implementation of translational work to the bedside. Too often, prevention or treatment techniques for HTS are developed in animal models only to stall out and never reach patient care settings despite their effectiveness.

3.3.2 All models

Often times, basic and translational science research lag behind current clinical findings such that patients receive treatments based on anecdotal evidence. This was the situation when fractional CO_2 ablative lasers were first used to treat HTS in patients. The cellular and molecular mechanisms behind this treatment had not been revealed even though patients continued to receive and benefit from this treatment. When questions arise in the clinical setting, it is useful to return back to the bench in order to test hypotheses. It is difficult, expensive, requires a large number of patients, and extensive regulatory review processes to conduct a clinical trial with patients. As an alternative, hypotheses that are early on in their development would benefit to be studied in animal models. The optimization of prevention or treatment effectiveness by testing different application techniques (systemic, injections, topical, laser channel drug delivery), dosing, and time-courses can all be studied in animals prior to testing in patients. Safety profiles are also critical to complete in translational work.

3.3.3 Pig models

Researchers using pig models for studying HTS debate which species produces the best model for study. Even when "definitive" papers are published declaring a model to be the most similar to human HTS, debate still follows. This was the case for the development of the Red Duroc pig model. Although the authors of the multiple papers characterizing this model never claimed that it was a perfect animal model, its development was still novel and important. Even so, researchers have been altering and optimizing this model ever since and rarely, if ever, use their original experimental methods to create HTS. The Duroc pig model, even in our laboratory, is admittedly not perfect. The resultant scars are not as raised above the surrounding skin compared to human scar. As such, they never truly become as thick as the most severe human scars. In addition, it is difficult to create a homogenous scar phenotype, specifically with regards to dyschromia, as the development of this symptom is still unclear in its etiology. In addition, full-thickness burning without excision and grafting, or the use of excisional wounding alone without burn is a controversial topic. Some researchers believe that including the burn, only to excise it after 2 days, may not be a judicious use of resources, and sometimes exclude the burn if the goal is to develop HTS for study. Some researchers emphasize the importance of including burn if the research question is mechanistic in nature. Models which incorporate healing by secondary intention or delayed excision and grafting more closely mimic burn-wound healing in low-income countries or in patients with very large TBSA injuries, two situations which are associated with some of the most severe HTS. In high income countries, early excision and autografting of full thickness or deep partial thickness burns is more common and accessible due to available resources. There are a few models that comprehensively include burn, excision, and autografting techniques in pigs, however, they often result in nicely healed wounds without extensive HTS. Patient factors that contribute to severe scarring even at autograft sites are not fully recapitulated in animal models. In addition, it is experimentally difficult to incorporate scarring across joints in animals. Frequently, wounds in pig models are situated on the flank, a site relatively shielded from tension with normal movement. Tension in healing wounds is an important topic for future study. Lastly, the use of pigs for scar research is extremely expensive. Low numbers of replicates can be incorporated onto each pig if systemic and local-regional contributions are being taken into account. The use of nude mouse models of scar or humanized mouse models, are thus a very intriguing concept. These models, which are substantially less expensive, will allow for large numbers of experimental replicates without systemic confounders. While current nude mouse models are useful, we should continue to report new techniques to create scars in these animals. For questions concerning the etiology of HTS, current models are inadequate.

4. Clinical research

4.1 Seminal findings

4.1.1 The development of hypertrophic scar

Incisional wound healing is well-described and typically marked by minimal inflammation and non-pathologic scar [171, 172]. Delayed wound closure or that which heals by secondary intention or contraction is, by contrast, marked by prolonged inflammatory events followed in many cases by degrees of fibrosis and ultimately HTS. Severity of scar after wounding of the skin is related to wound size, depth, anatomical location, tension, nature of injury, infection, environmental factors, and genetic predisposition [173]. HTSs have been succinctly summarized as an over-abundant synthesis of collagen and under-abundant or absent remodeling process. Despite this oversimplification, over the past several decades, there has been a large amount of research investigating the mechanism behind HTS

DOI: http://dx.doi.org/10.5772/intechopen.96943

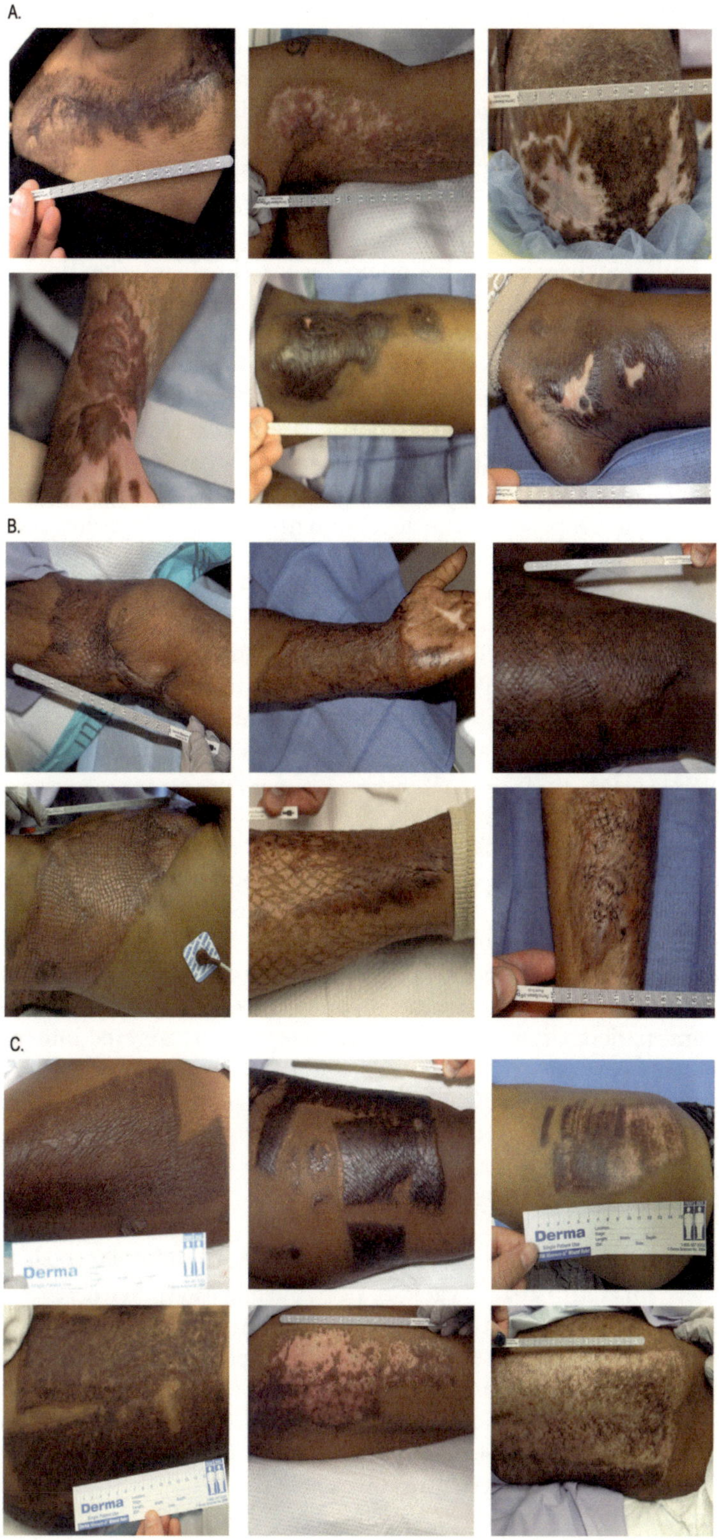

Figure 6.
HTS can result from a variety of injuries. HTS can result from wounds that are not treated with autologous skin grafting (A) treated with mSTSG (B) from donor sites (C). One of the main symptoms of HTS that can be observed is dyschromia. Patient photographs were collected under an IRB-approved protocol and shared with patient consent.

formation [100, 174]. The known severe inflammatory response that occurs after thermal injury has been suggested as an explanation for the greater incidence of HTS after burn injury than after other sources of injury [175]. A longer time to healing is associated with a greater risk of HTS, and in the case of burn injury, the most important prognostic indicators for HTS are the depth of original burn and corresponding time to wound closure [176, 177]. HTS can occur in wounds that were allowed to heal without mSTSG (**Figure 6A**), in wounds treated with mSTSG (**Figure 6B**), and in healed donor sites (**Figure 6C**) [178, 179]. Reliably, open wounds and full thickness burns that do not receive timely interventions to facilitate soft tissue coverage result in thickened, inflexible, pathologic HTS, though even wounds that do receive timely intervention may be susceptible.

Frequently, two to three weeks is used as a rule of thumb for time to wound closure for minimization of the development of HTS, with an understanding that a shorter time to healing is typically associated with a decrease in scar severity. It follows then that impairments to expedient wound healing are likely to contribute to the likelihood of HTS. Such impairments may include nutritional deficiencies (vitamin C, vitamin D, protein-calorie malnutrition), vasculopathy (peripheral arterial disease, diabetic microcirculatory disfunction, venous insufficiency), cigarette smoking, and infection among others [172]. It still occurs that patients with otherwise similar injury qualities and wound healing contributors develop varied severities of HTS, and this finding has been inadequately explained. There is evidence that certain genetic pre-dispositions put patients at risk for the development of HTS [180, 181]. Accordingly, patients of Asian, Hispanic, African American, or African descent are more likely to develop scar and exhibit increased scar severity [177, 181, 182].

The natural history of HTS generally predicts that a scar will be hypervascular, hypersensitive, dyschromic, and pruritic for the first few years after injury, typically accompanied by thickness and impaired flexibility. Some improvement in these qualities is to be expected over the following years, and some authors even suggest that HTS will revert to flat, asymptomatic scar [172]. In our own practice, however, patients with burn-related HTS may present decades after injury with persistent pain, itch, thickness, and range of motion limitations at sites of scar, suggesting that in at least some patients, these never truly resolve without targeted intervention. Due to the highly pervasive nature of HTS, and the fact that large total body surface area burn injuries are now survivable, a shift in focus has put HTS rehabilitation and recovery at the forefront of current research efforts by burn providers.

4.1.2 The evaluation of hypertrophic scar

Currently available scar evaluation tools include both subjective scales and objective mechanisms. In 2012, Tyack, *et al.* published a systematic review of eighteen different burn scar rating scales used in clinical and research settings [183]. The Vancouver Scar Scale (VSS) is most frequently cited and is a widely used, clinician-reported scale composed of four metrics: vascularity, pigmentation, pliability, and height. Scars with lower scores are characterized as "better" and more similar to normal skin [183, 184]. A number of modifications to the VSS have been made and applied in differing circumstances [183].

The Patient and Observer Scar Assessment Scale (POSAS) is also commonly used and is similar in its evaluation of the above metrics, but it provides additional levels of evaluation that quantify a patient's experience of pain and itch [185–191]. This scale was originally created for the evaluation of linear scars, but has been used in the evaluation of a much wider variety of scars [190]. Some criticism of the use of this scale in the context of HTS is that patients are asked to compare an area of scar to that of normal skin. This question prompts dissatisfying responses despite clinical interventions and improvements, as we know that there is no currently available method by which to convert HTS back to normal skin.

Other scar assessment scales noted in a 2010 systematic review by Brusselaers, *et al.* include the Seattle Scar Scale, Manchester Scar Scale, Hamilton Scar Scale, Inventory of Potential Reconstructive Needs, and the Stoney Brook Scar Evaluation [191]. The four original components of the VSS are commonly evaluated in most scar rating scales, but additional parameters beyond these do not share clear consensus in systematic reviews [183, 191].

A wide variety of objective scar measures have been developed and used to some degree, though without consistent or widespread adoption. A scar's height may be simply measured with a standard ruler, though this is an incomplete technique because it represents only scar thickness above the level of the surrounding skin and does not take into account variability in height within a given scar [192]. Planimetry improves upon this method by measuring the surface area of a scar, accounting for its variations in height, but still does not account for scar area deep to the visible surface [193]. Various three-dimensional imaging techniques are available, but these are not widely used due to their high costs [194, 195]. High frequency ultrasound may be used to more completely gauge scar thickness and is gaining some popularity for evaluation of the effects of HTS interventions [192, 196]. Elasticity or stiffness of scar can be measured by various methods including suction, pressure, torsion, and extension, all typically with a non-invasive probe [197]. Acoustic methods for scar assessment use sound waves to detect heterogeneity in scar tissue [198]. Transcutaneous oxygen tension can be measured with skin electrodes, as HTS have been noted to have a lower partial pressure of oxygen than healthy skin, however this technique has not been described frequently in the literature over the past 3 decades [199, 200]. Trans-epidermal water loss estimates the barrier function of scar related to the moisture content of skin [201]. Range of motion can be measured with a standard goniometer to estimate disability of movement due to scars in proximity to joints [197].

4.1.3 The treatment of hypertrophic scar

There are currently limited treatment options for HTS, and as such, prevention based on appropriate acute management of cutaneous injury is of paramount importance. When HTS develops despite good acute management, there are several treatment strategies that are employed. In decades past the main approach to the treatment of HTS was to "wait and see" and allow HTSs to regress over a period of years. While HTSs are known to get better over time, in contrast to their counter parts, keloid scars, which remain stagnant or worsen over time, HTSs almost never regress back to the structure or functionality of normal skin. This "wait and see" strategy often leaves patients with moribund scars that would benefit from additional treatments. Additionally, were interventions offered earlier on, patients have the potential to prevent multiple years of suffering. Early prevention strategies using our current multi-modal approach are critical to preventing severe scar. Common, longstanding treatments include compression, massage and stretch, silicone gel and sheeting, drug injection, and surgical tissue rearrangement, all of which have a role in prevention and treatment of HTS symptoms, but have drawbacks and can result in suboptimal outcomes when used in isolation [202–206].

Compression therapy is a widely used technique that has been considered standard of care for burn-related HTS for over 50 years. It is most commonly provided via elastic compression garments or plastic molded face masks for the first year following a burn injury. These are worn 23 hours per day and have been shown to improve scar height and erythema over time when custom fitted to a pressure of 20-30 mmHg [207]. Acceptance of this treatment modality is based mainly on anecdotal experience as the mechanism of action is not fully understood [208]. In a recent evidenced-based practice review by Sharp *et al.*, pressure therapy is recommended as a successful scar treatment which results in improved aesthetic outcomes by reducing scar height and erythema [203, 208–212]. Patient compliance and duration of treatment are important factors in the success of pressure therapy [213]. Our lab has studied the effect of compression on HTS extensively [55, 214] and revealed its mechanism of action to be primarily related to the induction of changes in collagen levels and types [157], elastin levels [156], and MMP levels [154]. Additionally, we have demonstrated that pressure therapy not only acts through mechanical forces, but induces changes in the HTS at the cellular and transcriptomic level that induce remodeling [155]. Despite pressure therapy's success in treating some symptoms of scar, patients often have sub-optimal functional and cosmetic outcomes even after treatment, which lead them to seek additional care.

Massage and stretch are routinely suggested for treatment of HTS despite mixed and limited evidence of their effectiveness [175, 215–218]. These techniques have minimal cost and can in many instances be self-administered with little to no risk, thus their use persists in the absence of convincing studies. A 2006 Cochrane review of silicone-based interventions for the prevention or treatment of HTS determined that there was only poor quality weak evidence of its benefit [219]. Since that time, more promising evidence for the benefit of silicone-based treatments have emerged. Proposed mechanisms of action include increased temperature, increased hydration, and bestowing a polarized charge to tissues, though none of these mechanisms have conclusively been shown [175]. It seems that the combination of silicone with compression therapy is advantageous compared to silicone or pressure therapy alone and provides benefits pertaining to pigmentation, vascularity, pliability, and itch [175, 220]. Intralesional injection of HTS may be with glucocorticoid (commonly triamcinolone, TAC) 5-fluorouracil (5-FU), or verapamil. Suggested mechanisms of action are suppression of the inflammatory response with TAC injection, reduction in the synthesis of ECM with verapamil injection, and inhibition of cell growth and induction of apoptosis with 5-FU injection [175]. The combination of 5-FU and TAC appears to have the greatest effect according to a recent systematic review [175, 221]. Surgical management of scar is a large topic in its own right and is not reviewed here; however, absent large scar excision with accompanied closure by grafts or flaps, zig-zag patterned incision, rearrangement, and suture approaches (z-plasty, w-plasty, and others) benefit linear HTS by a decrease in focal tension with accompanied histologic changes [222, 223].

Over the past 20 years, laser and light-based therapies have gained increasing popularity amongst clinicians who work to treat burn HTS [224–226]. Initially, the pulsed dye laser was most commonly used, and has now been supplemented in many centers by fractional ablative laser platforms [227–230]. Fractional photothermolysis was first described in 2004 [231]. This variation of laser treatment is based on the concept of creating multiple individual microscopic channels in a targeted treatment area. The laser causes small, limited zones of photothermolysis within tissue due to focal energy deposition at a wavelength absorbed by tissue water [232, 233]. The microinjuries are small enough that skin barrier function is preserved and healing is achieved without new scar formation [231, 234]. In addition to clinical improvements, histological and molecular evaluations of treated HTS reveal changes in inflammatory responses, matrix remodeling, and overall scar structure [168, 235]. This technology was initially created with the goal of aesthetic treatment of photo-damaged skin, but has shown increasing applicability for the treatment of various traumatic scars over the past decade [236].

4.2 Limitations to current clinical knowledge

4.2.1 The development of hypertrophic scar

Patients of similar age, health, and nutritional statuses with injury types and clinical managements in common may still develop different scar phenotypes. A trend toward worsened scar hypertrophy in skin of color has been observed [182, 237]. To further elucidate these basic genetic predispositions, various investigators have attempted to focus on genotypic variations associated with HTS. Carriers of some specific major histocompatibility complex alleles (HLA-DRB1*15, HLA-DQA1*0104, DQB1*0501, and DQB1*0503) show a genetic susceptibility to keloid disease, but these are not as clearly implicated in HTS [173]. The melanocortin 1 receptor single nucleotide polymorphism R163Q was associated with severe HTS in a study of 425 subjects in 2015 [182]. In 2016, the same group found that a missense variant of a mitogen-activated protein kinase pathway inhibitor PTPN5 was protective against HTS in a study of over 538 subjects [238]. Investigational studies such as that by Tsou, *et al.* have use cDNA microarray analysis to suggest that greater than 100 genes are differentially expressed between HTS and normal skin or non-pathologic scar. Implicated genes appear to be involved in collagen expression, growth factors, and MMPs and their inhibitors, however there was great variation between individual scars, and the total number of scars was small [239]. Given the expected high variability between individuals, large numbers of scars that will generate "big data" sets still need to be evaluated to discover reliable trends with respect to gene expression in HTS.

A less well-studied HTS feature is the dyspigmentation or dyschromia that occurs in the cells of the epidermis, namely the keratinocytes and melanocytes. In addition to the functional limitations of HTS, the aesthetic symptoms of HTS can also have severe psychosocial effects on patients which contribute to challenges with social reintegration and lead to decreased quality of life, and are, therefore, of importance to study [240–245]. In addition, dyspigmentation is difficult to predict, heterogeneous with regions of hyper- and hypo-pigmentation, can persist without improvement over time, and is pervasive amongst patients with baseline dark skin pigmentation [246].

4.2.2 The evaluation of hypertrophic scar

The various objective and subjective measures of hypertrophic scar have unique strengths and weaknesses [183, 191, 200]. The optimal combination of measures to evaluate scar severity and response to treatment has not been outlined. In a 2015 evaluation of the VSS, there was no consensus amongst 130 burn care providers as to what value on the scale constituted clinically significant HTS [247]. Lee *et al.* have recently attempted to delineate an optimal global scar evaluation protocol with the combination of a modified VSS and a panel of objective scar measurement tools [247]. While not yet validated or accepted widely, the intent of the work is valuable and a collaborative effort to this end will benefit both clinicians and researchers working with HTS.

4.2.3 The treatment of hypertrophic scar

As previously described, many current clinical interventions to prevent and treat HTS are used based on clinical experience with variable evidence. Proposed mechanisms exist for the use of silicone, compression, intralesional injection, and local tissue rearrangement, though these have not been explicitly outlined

[175]. The current treatments described above have varied effectiveness for relieving symptoms of HTS such as thickness, pliability, and pain, but are ineffective for the treatment of dyschromia. In fact, most research into HTS focuses on methods of targeting dermal remodeling, and does not focus on the epidermis. This focus is due to the fact that HTSs are often characterized by fibroblast cells and ECM that make up the dermis [99, 159]. These cells are the general focus of most research because they contribute to the thick, non-pliable, and contracted symptoms of HTS [248].

A consensus statement on laser treatment of burn scars was created in 2014 highlighting currently demonstrable benefits of **fractional ablative CO_2 (FCO_2) laser scar revision** (LSR). These include a small immediate increase in range of motion (ROM) as a result of photomechanical scar release, followed later by improvements in pliability, durability, texture, dyschromia, and further range of motion, all of which have been attributed to a collagen remodeling response [188]. Experience with FCO_2 LSR at our institution reflects these improvements in the evaluation of patients with burn HTS. The improvement in HTS after treatment with FCO_2 is well-documented [249, 250]. How and when these improvements occur has not been clearly defined. Existing studies frequently demonstrate changes in HTS in a bimodal fashion—only prior to and after multiple treatments in a course of LSR [225, 229, 230]. In practice, rarely does a patient undergo a single FCO_2 treatment for symptomatic HTS, however an adequate number of treatments, frequency of treatments, preferred settings, timing, and expected time course of outcomes is still undefined.

4.3 Suggestions for topics of future research

4.3.1 The development of hypertrophic scar

The incomplete understanding of genetic predisposition to scar is an area wide open for investigation. The patient-specific contributing factors leading to the development of HTS, as well as the degree to which a given individual responds to any clinical intervention, has not been elucidated with any practical clarity. If patient-specific information were to become available, targeted interventions for both the prevention and treatment of HTS could be developed for best outcomes. The work begun by Tsou, *et al.* as well as Sood, *et al.* could be continued, as the number of scar and skin samples needed to establish clear gene expression trends in HTS is overwhelming [182, 238, 239]. That said, banking results from skin and scar of varied patient ethnicities, ages, injury types, clinical interventions, and health backgrounds could yield enormous information pertaining to the prevention, development, and treatment of HTS. Once a genetic blueprint associated with or protective from HTS is more clearly outlined, the interplay of a specific patient's age, injury-specifics, and medical comorbidities will add further layers to the ability to develop targeted approaches to the prevention and treatment of severe HTS.

4.3.2 The evaluation of hypertrophic scar

Scar assessment tools have been evaluated largely in the context of burn HTS [200]. No clear standard exists and a clearly defined pathway to scar evaluation is yet to be determined. The standardization of these measures is needed in order to reliably evaluate the effectiveness of the clinical treatments for HTS. Many available tools are useful and promising; however, scales have not been established to define normal ranges nor expected values which represent clinically significant improvement. Likewise, devices have not been adopted similarly across multiple centers offering similar clinical managements. Work aimed at a standard set of metrics with accessible tools would benefit HTS-focused clinicians, researchers, and their patients. These metrics should incorporate patient-centered measures with a focus on symptoms affecting quality of life in the subjective realm; objectively, goals include a standard method to quantify scar size, thickness, vascularity, pigment, patterning, and flexibility with reproducibility and accessibility across healthcare delivery systems.

4.3.3 The treatment of hypertrophic scar

Many of the approaches for treatment of HTS has come from anecdotal use and experience. Future study of HTS may include validating any of these techniques. In any study of therapies for HTS intervention or prevention, there exists the challenge of developing and incorporation of appropriate controls. There is some expected improvement and remodeling of scars over time even without interventions, but the degree to which these occur is varied amongst different people and even within the same person. A valuable approach to this issue has often been through the design of interpatient controls by randomizing multiple distinct scars in a single patient or through split-scar studies, comparing treated and untreated portions of the same scar [251–253]. Separate scar interpatient controls are unable to account for the variability of scar physiology based on patient genetics, lesion location, or differences in original wound depth. Large scale trials, potentially with the assistance of multiple-center enrollment, would be most effective at minimizing these naturally-occurring confounding factors. In split-scar studies, the effect on an untreated portion of scar in direct proximity to a treated portion of scar is also not clear, and the systemic effect on areas untreated, however distant, deserves attention moving forward as various treatment approaches are studied.

Of course, the testing and validation of any scar treatment technique would require reliable, reproducible evaluation of treated and untreated HTS to speak to true efficacy. As noted above, current evaluation techniques carry wide potential, but have not been standardized in many cases with respect to normal ranges, multi-institutional adoption, timing of use, and expected values for scars of different ages, injury types, and locations. Clearly defining a suggested set of evaluation metrics for scars would contribute to the field by allowing researchers and clinicians to communicate consistently when testing various scar prevention and treatment strategies moving forward.

Laser scar revision is the most promising development for the treatment of HTS in the past decade. Variability in technology, frequency of treatment, power and density settings, and concomitant laser-assisted drug delivery all present potential targets of study to optimize this approach. The ideal laser depth of penetration has been suggested to be 50-75% of the thickness of a scar by Isler-Fischer, *et al.*, with depths of penetration outside this range offering little benefit [254]. Whether a difference exists between 50 and 75% depth of penetration is not known, nor whether these ranges are altered by various scar attributes, which may include scar age, patient age, scar vascularity, scar location, prior treatments, and more. Waibel, *et al.* introduced the use of optical coherence tomography (OCT) immediately prior to laser intervention to gauge the real time thickness of a given scar and optimization of power settings based on these results [255]. This approach holds promise for patient- and scar-specific interventions, though clarity is lacking on whether optimal power based on scar thickness changes in a linear or non-linear way. Laser-assisted drug delivery frequently includes the application of TAC or 5-FU to a scar treated with fractional ablative laser resurfacing. A 2019 study did not show a clear advantage of one medication over the other, and continuing to optimize this technique is an area still available for future study [256]. The inherent variability in the administration of laser and light based technologies with and without the concomitant application of medications is a target for study in a clinical trial proposed out of UNC in 2018 [257]. The authors offer a flowsheet with proposed combinations of the above with the goal of highlighting efficacy of different treatments and combinations thereof. Study designs such as these are sophisticated and are likely to assist in defining treatment guidelines from a large pool of differing approaches to laser scar revision.

5. Conclusion

The development of HTS is widespread after cutaneous traumatic injury and has profound effects on the quality of life of the patients who suffer from it. The variability between patients' injury etiologies, wound locations, acute and long-term treatment approaches, medical comorbidities, and ethnicities makes research into the pathophysiology and treatment of HTS complex and multilayered. The combination of optimal modeling and broad patient representation in research is likely to afford improved translatability of future scientific discovery related to HTS.

Author details

Bonnie C. Carney[1,2,4*], Jeffrey W. Shupp[1,2,3,4] and Taryn E. Travis[2,3,4]

1 Department of Biochemistry and Molecular and Cellular Biology, Georgetown University School of Medicine, Washington, DC, United States

2 Firefighters' Burn and Surgical Research Laboratory, MedStar Health Research Institute, Washington, DC, United States

3 Department of Surgery, The Burn Center, MedStar Washington Hospital Center, Washington, DC, United States

4 Department of Surgery, Georgetown University School of Medicine, Washington, DC, United States

*Address all correspondence to: bonnie.c.carney@medstar.net

References

[1] Limandjaja, G.C., et al., *Increased epidermal thickness and abnormal epidermal differentiation in keloid scars.* Br J Dermatol, 2017. **176**(1): p. 116-126.

[2] Yang, S., et al., *Abnormalities in the basement membrane structure promote basal keratinocytes in the epidermis of hypertrophic scars to adopt a proliferative phenotype.* Int J Mol Med, 2016. **37**(5): p. 1263-1273.

[3] Kischer, C.W., A.C. Thies, and M. Chvapil, *Perivascular myofibroblasts and microvascular occlusion in hypertrophic scars and keloids.* Hum Pathol, 1982. **13**(9): p. 819-824.

[4] Kischer, C.W. and M.R. Shetlar, *Microvasculature in hypertrophic scars and the effects of pressure.* J Trauma, 1979. **19**(10): p. 757-764.

[5] Ehrlich, H.P., et al., *Morphological and immunochemical differences between keloid and hypertrophic scar.* Am J Pathol, 1994. **145**(1): p. 105-113.

[6] Linares, H.A., et al., *On the origin of the hypertrophic scar.* J Trauma, 1973. **13**(1): p. 70-75.

[7] Linares, H.A., et al., *The histiotypic organization of the hypertrophic scar in humans.* J Invest Dermatol, 1972. **59**(4): p. 323-331.

[8] Nedelec, B., et al., *Myofibroblasts and apoptosis in human hypertrophic scars: the effect of interferon-alpha2b.* Surgery, 2001. **130**(5): p. 798-808.

[9] Santucci, M., et al., *Keloids and hypertrophic scars of Caucasians show distinctive morphologic and immunophenotypic profiles.* Virchows Arch, 2001. **438**(5): p. 457-463.

[10] Aarabi, S., et al., *Mechanical load initiates hypertrophic scar formation through decreased cellular apoptosis.* FASEB J, 2007. **21**(12): p. 3250-3261.

[11] Hayakawa, T., et al., *Changes in type of collagen during the development of human post-burn hypertrophic scars.* Clin Chim Acta, 1979. **93**(1): p. 119-125.

[12] Bailey, A.J., et al., *Characterization of the collagen of human hypertrophic and normal scars.* Biochim Biophys Acta, 1975. **405**(2): p. 412-421.

[13] Kischer, C.W. and M.J. Hendrix, *Fibronectin (FN) in hypertrophic scars and keloids.* Cell Tissue Res, 1983. **231**(1): p. 29-37.

[14] Sorrell, J.M. and A.I. Caplan, *Fibroblast heterogeneity: more than skin deep.* J Cell Sci, 2004. **117**(Pt 5): p. 667-675.

[15] Dunkin, C.S., et al., *Scarring occurs at a critical depth of skin injury: precise measurement in a graduated dermal scratch in human volunteers.* Plast Reconstr Surg, 2007. **119**(6): p. 1722-1732; discussion 1733-4.

[16] Wang, J., et al., *Deep dermal fibroblasts contribute to hypertrophic scarring.* Lab Invest, 2008. **88**(12): p. 1278-1290.

[17] Desmouliere, A., et al., *Transforming growth factor-beta 1 induces alpha-smooth muscle actin expression in granulation tissue myofibroblasts and in quiescent and growing cultured fibroblasts.* J Cell Biol, 1993. **122**(1): p. 103-111.

[18] Kuang, R., et al., *Exposure to Varying Strain Magnitudes Influences the Conversion of Normal Skin Fibroblasts Into Hypertrophic Scar Cells.* Ann Plast Surg, 2016. **76**(4): p. 388-393.

[19] Sorrell, J.M., M.A. Baber, and A.I. Caplan, *Human dermal fibroblast subpopulations; differential interactions*

with vascular endothelial cells in coculture: nonsoluble factors in the extracellular matrix influence interactions. Wound Repair Regen, 2008. **16**(2): p. 300-309.

[20] Rennekampff, H.O. and M. Tenenhaus, *Theoretical basis for optimal surgical incision planning to reduce hypertrophic scar formation.* Med Hypotheses, 2020. **140**: p. 109672.

[21] Li-Tsang, C.W., et al., *A histological study on the effect of pressure therapy on the activities of myofibroblasts and keratinocytes in hypertrophic scar tissues after burn.* Burns, 2015. **41**(5): p. 1008-1016.

[22] Russo, B., N.C. Brembilla, and C. Chizzolini, *Interplay Between Keratinocytes and Fibroblasts: A Systematic Review Providing a New Angle for Understanding Skin Fibrotic Disorders.* Front Immunol, 2020. **11**: p. 648.

[23] SF., G., *Developmental Biology.* The Epidermis and the Origin of Cutaneous Structures. Vol. 6th edition. 2000, Sunderland (MA): Sinauer Associates.

[24] Houben, E., K. De Paepe, and V. Rogiers, *A keratinocyte's course of life.* Skin Pharmacol Physiol, 2007. **20**(3): p. 122-132.

[25] Hakvoort, T., et al., *Transforming growth factor-beta(1), -beta(2), -beta(3), basic fibroblast growth factor and vascular endothelial growth factor expression in keratinocytes of burn scars.* Eur Cytokine Netw, 2000. **11**(2): p. 233-239.

[26] Bellemare, J., et al., *Epidermis promotes dermal fibrosis: role in the pathogenesis of hypertrophic scars.* J Pathol, 2005. **206**(1): p. 1-8.

[27] Wang, Z., Q. Song, and H. Li, *Suppressive effects of human fetal keratinocytes on the proliferation, differentiation and extracellular matrix synthesis of human hypertrophic scar fibroblasts in vitro.* Mol Med Rep, 2017. **16**(4): p. 5377-5385.

[28] Machesney, M., et al., *Activated keratinocytes in the epidermis of hypertrophic scars.* Am J Pathol, 1998. **152**(5): p. 1133-41.

[29] Paladini, R.D., et al., *Onset of re-epithelialization after skin injury correlates with a reorganization of keratin filaments in wound edge keratinocytes: defining a potential role for keratin 16.* J Cell Biol, 1996. **132**(3): p. 381-97.

[30] Hakvoort, T.E., et al., *Epidermal participation in post-burn hypertrophic scar development.* Virchows Arch, 1999. **434**(3): p. 221-6.

[31] Andriessen, M.P., et al., *Hypertrophic scarring is associated with epidermal abnormalities: an immunohistochemical study.* J Pathol, 1998. **186**(2): p. 192-200.

[32] Depianto, D., et al., *Keratin 17 promotes epithelial proliferation and tumor growth by polarizing the immune response in skin.* Nat Genet, 2010. **42**(10): p. 910-4.

[33] Nithya, S., T. Radhika, and N. Jeddy, *Loricrin - an overview.* J Oral Maxillofac Pathol, 2015. **19**(1): p. 64-8.

[34] Edriss, A.S. and J. Mestak, *Epidermal Keratinocytes May Have an Important role in Hypertrophic Scarring Pathogenesis: an Immunohistochemical Study (Using P63 and Ki-67 Staining).* Ann Burns Fire Disasters, 2005. **18**(3): p. 133-9.

[35] Wang, F., A. Zieman, and P.A. Coulombe, *Skin Keratins.* Methods Enzymol, 2016. **568**: p. 303-350.

[36] Fitzpatrick, T.B. and G. Szabo, *The melanocyte: cytology and cytochemistry.* J Invest Dermatol, 1959. **32**(2, Part 2): p. 197-209.

[37] Rawles, M.E., *Origin of pigment cells from the neural crest in the mouse embryo.* Physiol Zool, 1947. **20**(3): p. 248-266.

[38] Staricco, R.J. and H. Pinkus, *Quantitative and qualitative data on the pigment cells of adult human epidermis.* J Invest Dermatol, 1957. **28**(1): p. 33-45.

[39] Jimbow, K., et al., *Some aspects of melanin biology: 1950-1975.* J Invest Dermatol, 1976. **67**(1): p. 72-89.

[40] Dessinioti, C., et al., *A review of genetic disorders of hypopigmentation: lessons learned from the biology of melanocytes.* Exp Dermatol, 2009. **18**(9): p. 741-9.

[41] Taki, T., et al., *Surgical treatment of skin depigmentation caused by burn injuries.* J Dermatol Surg Oncol, 1985. **11**(12): p. 1218-1221.

[42] Onur Erol, O. and K. Atabay, *The treatment of burn scar hypopigmentation and surface irregularity by dermabrasion and thin skin grafting.* Plast Reconstr Surg, 1990. **85**(5): p. 754-758.

[43] Kahn, A.M., M.J. Cohen, and L. Kaplan, *Treatment for depigmentation resulting from burn injuries.* J Burn Care Rehabil, 1991. **12**(5): p. 468-473.

[44] Kahn, A.M. and M.J. Cohen, *Treatment for depigmentation following burn injuries.* Burns, 1996. **22**(7): p. 552-554.

[45] Acikel, C., E. Ulkur, and M.M. Guler, *Treatment of burn scar depigmentation by carbon dioxide laser-assisted dermabrasion and thin skin grafting.* Plast Reconstr Surg, 2000. **105**(6): p. 1973-1978.

[46] Burm, J.S., S.C. Rhee, and Y.W. Kim, *Superficial dermabrasion and suction blister epidermal grafting for postburn dyspigmentation in Asian skin.* Dermatol Surg, 2007. **33**(3): p. 326-332.

[47] Al-Qattan, M.M., *Surgical management of post-burn skin dyspigmentation of the upper limb.* Burns, 2000. **26**(6): p. 581-6.

[48] Grover, R. and B.D. Morgan, *Management of hypopigmentation following burn injury.* Burns, 1996. **22**(8): p. 627-630.

[49] Tyack, Z.F., S. Pegg, and J. Ziviani, *Postburn dyspigmentation: its assessment, management, and relationship to scarring--a review of the literature.* J Burn Care Rehabil, 1997. **18**(5): p. 435-440.

[50] Brandt, M.G., et al., *A pilot randomized control trial of scar repigmentation with UV light and dry tattooing.* Otolaryngol Head Neck Surg, 2008. **139**(6): p. 769-774.

[51] Guyuron, B. and C. Vaughan, *Medical-grade tattooing to camouflage depigmented scars.* Plast Reconstr Surg, 1995. **95**(3): p. 575-579.

[52] van der Velden, E.M., et al., *Dermatography: a method for permanent repigmentation of achromic burn scars.* Burns, 1995. **21**(4): p. 304-307.

[53] Rayner, V.L., *Camouflage therapy.* Dermatol Clin, 1995. **13**(2): p. 467-472.

[54] Driscoll, D.N., A.N. Levy, and A.R. Gama, *Dermabrasion and Thin Epidermal Grafting for Treatment of Large and Small Areas of Postburn Leukoderma: A Case Series and Review of the Literature.* J Burn Care Res, 2016. **37**(4): p. e387-e393.

[55] Alkhalil, A., et al., *A Translational Animal Model for Scar Compression Therapy Using an Automated Pressure Delivery System.* Eplasty, 2015. **15**: p. e29.

[56] Travis, T.E., et al., *A multimodal assessment of melanin and melanocyte activity in abnormally pigmented hypertrophic scar.* J Burn Care Res, 2015. **36**(1): p. 77-86.

[57] Carney, B.C., et al., *Pigmentation Diathesis of Hypertrophic Scar: An Examination of Known Signaling Pathways to Elucidate the Molecular Pathophysiology of Injury-Related Dyschromia.* J Burn Care Res, 2019. **40**(1): p. 58-71.

[58] Alkhalil, A., et al., *Dyspigmented hypertrophic scars: Beyond skin color.* Pigment Cell Melanoma Res, 2019. **32**(5): p. 643-656.

[59] Carney, B.C., et al., *Treatment Strategies for Hypopigmentation in the Context of Burn Hypertrophic Scars.* Plast Reconstr Surg Glob Open, 2018. **6**(1): p. e1642.

[60] Dutta, S., et al., *Hypopigmentation in burns is associated with alterations in the architecture of the skin and the dendricity of the melanocytes.* Burns, 2020. **46**(4): p. 906-917.

[61] Gonzalez Rodriguez, E., et al., *Syndecan-1: A Quantitative Marker for the Endotheliopathy of Trauma.* J Am Coll Surg, 2017. **225**(3): p. 419-427.

[62] Puskarich, M.A., et al., *Plasma syndecan-1 levels identify a cohort of patients with severe sepsis at high risk for intubation after large-volume intravenous fluid resuscitation.* J Crit Care, 2016. **36**: p. 125-129.

[63] Welling, H., et al., *Endothelial glycocalyx shedding in patients with burns.* Burns, 2020. **46**(2): p. 386-393.

[64] Weinbaum, S., J.M. Tarbell, and E.R. Damiano, *The structure and function of the endothelial glycocalyx layer.* Annu Rev Biomed Eng, 2007. **9**: p. 121-167.

[65] Vigiola Cruz, M., et al., *Plasma Ameliorates Endothelial Dysfunction in Burn Injury.* J Surg Res, 2019. **233**: p. 459-466.

[66] Osuka, A., et al., *Glycocalyx Shedding is Enhanced by Age and Correlates with Increased Fluid Requirement in Patients with Major Burns.* Shock, 2018. **50**(1): p. 60-65.

[67] Page, R.E., G.A. Robertson, and N.M. Pettigrew, *Microcirculation in hypertrophic burn scars.* Burns Incl Therm Inj, 1983. **10**(1): p. 64-70.

[68] Xie, Y., et al., *The microvasculature in cutaneous wound healing in the female red Duroc pig is similar to that in human hypertrophic scars and different from that in the female Yorkshire pig.* J Burn Care Res, 2007. **28**(3): p. 500-506.

[69] Van-Buendia, L.B., et al., *What's behind the mask? A look at blood flow changes with prolonged facial pressure and expression using laser Doppler imaging.* J Burn Care Res, 2010. **31**(3): p. 441-447.

[70] Ribatti, D. and R. Tamma, *A revisited concept. Tumors: Wounds that do not heal.* Crit Rev Oncol Hematol, 2018. **128**: p. 65-69.

[71] Ogawa, R. and S. Akaishi, *Endothelial dysfunction may play a key role in keloid and hypertrophic scar pathogenesis - Keloids and hypertrophic scars may be vascular disorders.* Med Hypotheses, 2016. **96**: p. 51-60.

[72] Huang, C. and R. Ogawa, *The link between hypertension and pathological scarring: does hypertension cause or promote keloid and hypertrophic scar pathogenesis?* Wound Repair Regen, 2014. **22**(4): p. 462-466.

[73] Zhang, J., et al., *Amentoflavone inhibits angiogenesis of endothelial cells and stimulates apoptosis in hypertrophic scar fibroblasts.* Burns, 2014. **40**(5): p. 922-929.

[74] Kwak, D.H., et al., *Anti-Vascular Endothelial Growth Factor (Bevacizumab) Therapy Reduces Hypertrophic Scar Formation in a Rabbit Ear Wounding Model.* Arch Plast Surg, 2016. **43**(6): p. 491-497.

[75] Jia, S., et al., *Local Application of Statins Significantly Reduced Hypertrophic Scarring in a Rabbit Ear Model.* Plast Reconstr Surg Glob Open, 2017. **5**(6): p. e1294.

[76] Ren, H.T., et al., *Endostatin inhibits hypertrophic scarring in a rabbit ear model.* J Zhejiang Univ Sci B, 2013. **14**(3): p. 224-230.

[77] Li, Y. and H.T. Ren, *Endostatin inhibits fibrosis by modulating the PDGFR/ERK signal pathway: an in vitro study.* J Zhejiang Univ Sci B, 2017. **18**(11): p. 994-1001.

[78] Gong, Y.F., et al., *Effect of recombinant human endostatin on hypertrophic scar fibroblast apoptosis in a rabbit ear model.* Biomed Pharmacother, 2017. **91**: p. 680-686.

[79] Lim, K.H., et al., *Stem Cells in Keloid Lesions: A Review.* Plast Reconstr Surg Glob Open, 2019. **7**(5): p. e2228.

[80] Lee, W.J., et al., *Endothelial-to-mesenchymal transition induced by Wnt 3a in keloid pathogenesis.* Wound Repair Regen, 2015. **23**(3): p. 435-442.

[81] Bucala, R., et al., *Circulating fibrocytes define a new leukocyte subpopulation that mediates tissue repair.* Mol Med, 1994. **1**(1): p. 71-81.

[82] Metz, C.N., *Fibrocytes: a unique cell population implicated in wound healing.* Cell Mol Life Sci, 2003. **60**(7): p. 1342-1350.

[83] Blakaj, A. and R. Bucala, *Fibrocytes in health and disease.* Fibrogenesis Tissue Repair, 2012. **5**(Suppl 1): p. S6.

[84] Bellini, A. and S. Mattoli, *The role of the fibrocyte, a bone marrow-derived mesenchymal progenitor, in reactive and reparative fibroses.* Lab Invest, 2007. **87**(9): p. 858-870.

[85] Yang, L., et al., *Identification of fibrocytes in postburn hypertrophic scar.* Wound Repair Regen, 2005. **13**(4): p. 398-404.

[86] Wang, J.F., et al., *Fibrocytes from burn patients regulate the activities of fibroblasts.* Wound Repair Regen, 2007. **15**(1): p. 113-121.

[87] Yang, L., et al., *Peripheral blood fibrocytes from burn patients: identification and quantification of fibrocytes in adherent cells cultured from peripheral blood mononuclear cells.* Lab Invest, 2002. **82**(9): p. 1183-1192.

[88] Travis, T.E., et al., *Biphasic presence of fibrocytes in a porcine hypertrophic scar model.* J Burn Care Res, 2015. **36**(3): p. e125-e135.

[89] Wang, J., et al., *Improvement in postburn hypertrophic scar after treatment with IFN-alpha2b is associated with decreased fibrocytes.* J Interferon Cytokine Res, 2007. **27**(11): p. 921-930.

[90] Liu, H., et al., *A novel subpopulation of peripheral blood mononuclear cells presents in major burn patients.* Burns, 2015. **41**(5): p. 998-1007.

[91] Zhang, K., et al., *Increased types I and III collagen and transforming growth factor-beta 1 mRNA and protein in hypertrophic burn scar.* J Invest Dermatol, 1995. **104**(5): p. 750-754.

[92] Wang, R., et al., *Hypertrophic scar tissues and fibroblasts produce more transforming growth factor-beta1 mRNA and protein than normal skin and cells.* Wound Repair Regen, 2000. **8**(2): p. 128-137.

[93] Ghahary, A., et al., *Expression and localization of insulin-like growth factor-1 in normal and post-burn hypertrophic scar tissue in human.* Mol Cell Biochem, 1998. **183**(1-2): p. 1-9.

[94] Mori, T., et al., *Role and interaction of connective tissue growth factor with transforming growth factor-beta in*

persistent fibrosis: A mouse fibrosis model. J Cell Physiol, 1999. **181**(1): p. 153-159.

[95] Younai, S., et al., *Role of growth factors in scar contraction: an in vitro analysis.* Ann Plast Surg, 1996. **36**(5): p. 495-501.

[96] Zhang, Q., et al., *Elevated expression of pleiotrophin in human hypertrophic scars.* J Mol Histol, 2013. **44**(1): p. 91-96.

[97] Scott, P.G., et al., *Chemical characterization and quantification of proteoglycans in human post-burn hypertrophic and mature scars.* Clin Sci (Lond), 1996. **90**(5): p. 417-425.

[98] Tredget, E.E., et al., *Regulation of collagen synthesis and messenger RNA levels in normal and hypertrophic scar fibroblasts in vitro by interferon alfa-2b.* Wound Repair Regen, 1993. **1**(3): p. 156-165.

[99] Lian, N. and T. Li, *Growth factor pathways in hypertrophic scars: Molecular pathogenesis and therapeutic implications.* Biomed Pharmacother, 2016. **84**: p. 42-50.

[100] Kwan, P.O. and E.E. Tredget, *Biological Principles of Scar and Contracture.* Hand Clin, 2017. **33**(2): p. 277-292.

[101] Armour, A., P.G. Scott, and E.E. Tredget, *Cellular and molecular pathology of HTS: basis for treatment.* Wound Repair Regen, 2007. **15 Suppl 1**: p. S6-17.

[102] Zhu, Z., et al., *The molecular mechanism of hypertrophic scar.* J Cell Commun Signal, 2013. 7(4): p. 239-252.

[103] Scott, P.G., et al., *Immuno histochemical localization of the proteoglycans decorin, biglycan and versican and transforming growth factor-beta in human post-burn hypertrophic and mature scars.* Histopathology, 1995. **26**(5): p. 423-431.

[104] Zhu, H.Y., et al., *MicroRNA-21 regulates hTERT via PTEN in hypertrophic scar fibroblasts.* PLoS One, 2014. **9**(5): p. e97114.

[105] Zhang, J., et al., *MicroRNA-130a has pro-fibroproliferative potential in hypertrophic scar by targeting CYLD.* Arch Biochem Biophys, 2019. **671**: p. 152-161.

[106] Wu, X., et al., *miR-155 inhibits the formation of hypertrophic scar fibroblasts by targeting HIF-1alpha via PI3K/AKT pathway.* J Mol Histol, 2018. **49**(4): p. 377-387.

[107] Li, Y., et al., *MicroRNA-192 regulates hypertrophic scar fibrosis by targeting SIP1.* J Mol Histol, 2017. **48**(5-6): p. 357-366.

[108] He, T., et al., *MicroRNA-494 targets PTEN and suppresses PI3K/AKT pathway to alleviate hypertrophic scar formation.* J Mol Histol, 2019. **50**(4): p. 315-323.

[109] Zhou, R., et al., *Aberrant miR-21 and miR-200b expression and its pro-fibrotic potential in hypertrophic scars.* Exp Cell Res, 2015. **339**(2): p. 360-366.

[110] Li, G., et al., *Fibroproliferative effect of microRNA-21 in hypertrophic scar derived fibroblasts.* Exp Cell Res, 2016. **345**(1): p. 93-99.

[111] Wang, S., et al., *Decreased expression of microRNA-145 promotes the biological functions of fibroblasts in hypertrophic scar tissues by upregulating the expression of transcription factor SOX-9.* Exp Ther Med, 2019. **18**(5): p. 3450-3460.

[112] Shen, W., et al., *miR-145-5p attenuates hypertrophic scar via reducing Smad2/Smad3 expression.* Biochem Biophys Res Commun, 2020. **521**(4): p. 1042-1048.

[113] Kwan, P., J. Ding, and E.E. Tredget, *MicroRNA 181b regulates decorin production by dermal fibroblasts and may*

be a potential therapy for hypertrophic scar. PLoS One, 2015. **10**(4): p. e0123054.

[114] Dong, S. and Y. Sun, *MicroRNA-22 may promote apoptosis and inhibit the proliferation of hypertrophic scar fibroblasts by regulating the mitogen-activated protein kinase kinase/ extracellular signal-regulated kinase/p21 pathway.* Exp Ther Med, 2017. **14**(4): p. 3841-3845.

[115] Mu, S., et al., *MicroRNA-143-3p inhibits hyperplastic scar formation by targeting connective tissue growth factor CTGF/CCN2 via the Akt/mTOR pathway.* Mol Cell Biochem, 2016. **416**(1-2): p. 99-108.

[116] Bi, S., et al., *Regulatory mechanism of miR-29 over TGF-beta1 and COL1 in scar cells.* Eur Rev Med Pharmacol Sci, 2017. **21**(10): p. 2512-2517.

[117] Zhang, Q., et al., *miR-137 Inhibits Proliferation and Metastasis of Hypertrophic Scar Fibroblasts via Targeting Pleiotrophin.* Cell Physiol Biochem, 2018. **49**(3): p. 985-995.

[118] Li, M., et al., *Highthroughput sequencing reveals differentially expressed lncRNAs and circRNAs, and their associated functional network, in human hypertrophic scars.* Mol Med Rep, 2018. **18**(6): p. 5669-5682.

[119] Tu, L., et al., *Aberrantly expressed long noncoding RNAs in hypertrophic scar fibroblasts in vitro: A microarray study.* Int J Mol Med, 2018. **41**(4): p. 1917-1930.

[120] Nong, Q., et al., *LncRNA COL1A2-AS1 inhibits the scar fibroblasts proliferation via regulating miR-21/ Smad7 pathway.* Biochem Biophys Res Commun, 2018. **495**(1): p. 319-324.

[121] Zhao, J., et al., *Epidermal HMGB1 Activates Dermal Fibroblasts and Causes Hypertrophic Scar Formation in Reduced Hydration.* J Invest Dermatol, 2018. **138**(11): p. 2322-2332.

[122] Zhong, A., et al., *S100A8 and S100A9 Are Induced by Decreased Hydration in the Epidermis and Promote Fibroblast Activation and Fibrosis in the Dermis.* Am J Pathol, 2016. **186**(1): p. 109-122.

[123] Harrison, C.A., et al., *Investigation of keratinocyte regulation of collagen I synthesis by dermal fibroblasts in a simple in vitro model.* Br J Dermatol, 2006. **154**(3): p. 401-410.

[124] Niessen, F.B., et al., *Keratinocyte-derived growth factors play a role in the formation of hypertrophic scars.* J Pathol, 2001. **194**(2): p. 207-216.

[125] Wang, X.Q., et al., *Isolation, culture and characterization of endothelial cells from human hypertrophic scar.* Endothelium, 2008. **15**(3): p. 113-119.

[126] Good, R.B., et al., *A high content, phenotypic 'scar-in-a-jar' assay for rapid quantification of collagen fibrillogenesis using disease-derived pulmonary fibroblasts.* BMC Biomed Eng, 2019. **1**: p. 14.

[127] Fan, C., et al., *In Vitro Model of Human Cutaneous Hypertrophic Scarring using Macromolecular Crowding.* J Vis Exp, 2020(159).

[128] Graupp, M., et al., *Towards an in vitro fibrogenesis model of human vocal fold scarring.* Eur Arch Otorhinolaryngol, 2018. **275**(5): p. 1211-1218.

[129] Zhang, Y., et al., *tRNAderived small RNAs: A novel class of small RNAs in human hypertrophic scar fibroblasts.* Int J Mol Med, 2020. **45**(1): p. 115-130.

[130] Ramos, M.L., A. Gragnani, and L.M. Ferreira, *Is there an ideal animal model to study hypertrophic scarring?* J Burn Care Res, 2008. **29**(2): p. 363-368.

[131] Domergue, S., C. Jorgensen, and D. Noel, *Advances in Research in Animal Models of Burn-Related Hypertrophic Scarring.* J Burn Care Res, 2015. **36**(5): p. e259-e266.

[132] Abdullahi, A., S. Amini-Nik, and M.G. Jeschke, *Animal models in burn research.* Cell Mol Life Sci, 2014. **71**(17): p. 3241-3255.

[133] Ud-Din, S. and A. Bayat, *Non-animal models of wound healing in cutaneous repair: In silico, in vitro, ex vivo, and in vivo models of wounds and scars in human skin.* Wound Repair Regen, 2017. **25**(2): p. 164-176.

[134] Wang, J., et al., *Human hypertrophic scar-like nude mouse model: characterization of the molecular and cellular biology of the scar process.* Wound Repair Regen, 2011. **19**(2): p. 274-285.

[135] Honardoust, D., et al., *Novel methods for the investigation of human hypertrophic scarring and other dermal fibrosis.* Methods Mol Biol, 2013. **1037**: p. 203-231.

[136] Momtazi, M., et al., *A nude mouse model of hypertrophic scar shows morphologic and histologic characteristics of human hypertrophic scar.* Wound Repair Regen, 2013. **21**(1): p. 77-87.

[137] Alrobaiea, S.M., et al., *A Novel Nude Mouse Model of Hypertrophic Scarring Using Scratched Full Thickness Human Skin Grafts.* Adv Wound Care (New Rochelle), 2016. **5**(7): p. 299-313.

[138] Nabai, L. and A. Ghahary, *Hypertrophic Scarring in the Rabbit Ear: A Practical Model for Studying Dermal Fibrosis.* Methods Mol Biol, 2017. **1627**: p. 81-89.

[139] Singer, A.J., et al., *Validation of a vertical progression porcine burn model.* J Burn Care Res, 2011. **32**(6): p. 638-646.

[140] Cuttle, L., et al., *A porcine deep dermal partial thickness burn model with hypertrophic scarring.* Burns, 2006. **32**(7): p. 806-820.

[141] Rapp, S.J., et al., *Establishing a Reproducible Hypertrophic Scar following Thermal Injury: A Porcine Model.* Plast Reconstr Surg Glob Open, 2015. **3**(2): p. e309.

[142] Chan, Q.E., et al., *The correlation between time to skin grafting and hypertrophic scarring following an acute contact burn in a porcine model.* J Burn Care Res, 2012. **33**(2): p. e43-e48.

[143] Rapp, S.J., et al., *Effects of Autologous Fat and ASCs on Swine Hypertrophic Burn Scars: A Multimodal Quantitative Analysis.* Plast Reconstr Surg Glob Open, 2017. **5**(11): p. e1547.

[144] Ulrich, M.M., et al., *Expression profile of proteins involved in scar formation in the healing process of full-thickness excisional wounds in the porcine model.* Wound Repair Regen, 2007. **15**(4): p. 482-490.

[145] Zhu, K.Q., et al., *The female, red Duroc pig as an animal model of hypertrophic scarring and the potential role of the cones of skin.* Burns, 2003. **29**(7): p. 649-664.

[146] Liang, Z., et al., *Nerve quantification in female red Duroc pig (FRDP) scar compared to human hypertrophic scar.* Burns, 2004. **30**(1): p. 57-64.

[147] Harunari, N., et al., *Histology of the thick scar on the female, red Duroc pig: final similarities to human hypertrophic scar.* Burns, 2006. **32**(6): p. 669-677.

[148] Zhu, K.Q., et al., *Further similarities between cutaneous scarring in the female, red Duroc pig and human hypertrophic scarring.* Burns, 2004. **30**(6): p. 518-530.

[149] Zhu, K.Q., et al., *Changes in VEGF and nitric oxide after deep dermal injury in the female, red Duroc pig-further similarities between female, Duroc scar and human hypertrophic scar.* Burns, 2005. **31**(1): p. 5-10.

[150] Gallant, C.L., M.E. Olson, and D.A. Hart, *Molecular, histologic, and gross phenotype of skin wound healing in red Duroc pigs reveals an abnormal healing phenotype of hypercontracted, hyperpigmented scarring.* Wound Repair Regen, 2004. **12**(3): p. 305-319.

[151] Gallant-Behm, C.L., M.E. Olson, and D.A. Hart, *Cytokine and growth factor mRNA expression patterns associated with the hypercontracted, hyperpigmented healing phenotype of red duroc pigs: a model of abnormal human scar development?* J Cutan Med Surg, 2005. **9**(4): p. 165-177.

[152] Mauskar, N.A., et al., *Donor site healing dynamics: molecular, histological, and noninvasive imaging assessment in a porcine model.* J Burn Care Res, 2013. **34**(5): p. 549-562.

[153] Travis, T.E., et al., *Commercially Available Topical Platelet-Derived Growth Factor as a Novel Agent to Accelerate Burn-Related Wound Healing.* J Burn Care Res, 2014.

[154] Travis, T.E., et al., *Matrix Metalloproteinases Are Differentially Regulated and Responsive to Compression Therapy in a Red Duroc Model of Hypertrophic Scar.* Eplasty, 2018. **18**: p. e1.

[155] Alkhalil, A., et al., *Key Cell Functions are Modulated by Compression in an Animal Model of Hypertrophic Scar.* Wounds, 2018. **30**(12): p. 353-362.

[156] Carney, B.C., et al., *Elastin Is Differentially Regulated by Pressure Therapy in a Porcine Model of Hypertrophic Scar.* J Burn Care Res, 2017. **38**(1): p. 28-35.

[157] Tejiram, S., et al., *Compression therapy affects collagen type balance in hypertrophic scar.* J Surg Res, 2016. **201**(2): p. 299-305.

[158] Ghassemi, P., et al., *A portable automatic pressure delivery system for scar compression therapy in large animals.* Rev Sci Instrum, 2015. **86**(1): p. 015101.

[159] Sood, R.F., et al., *Dermal Fibroblasts from the Red Duroc Pig Have an Inherently Fibrogenic Phenotype: An In Vitro Model of Fibroproliferative Scarring.* Plast Reconstr Surg, 2015. **136**(5): p. 990-1000.

[160] Foubert, P., et al., *Autologous adipose-derived regenerative cell therapy modulates development of hypertrophic scarring in a red Duroc porcine model.* Stem Cell Res Ther, 2017. **8**(1): p. 261.

[161] Gurtner, G.C., et al., *Improving cutaneous scar formation by controlling the mechanical environment: large animal and phase I studies.* Ann Surg, 2011. **254**(2): p. 217-225.

[162] Liang, Z., et al., *[Pathomorphological observation of the hypertrophic scar induced by injury to conical structure in female red Duroc pig].* Zhonghua Shao Shang Za Zhi, 2006. **22**(1): p. 29-32.

[163] Blackstone, B.N., et al., *Scar formation following excisional and burn injuries in a red Duroc pig model.* Wound Repair Regen, 2017. **25**(4): p. 618-631.

[164] Kim, J.Y., et al., *Burn Scar Biomechanics after Pressure Garment Therapy.* Plast Reconstr Surg, 2015. **136**(3): p. 572-581.

[165] Rodriguez-Menocal, L., et al., *Assessment of Ablative Fractional CO2 Laser and Er:YAG Laser to Treat Hypertrophic Scars in a Red Duroc Pig Model.* J Burn Care Res, 2018. **39**(6): p. 954-962.

[166] Xie, H., et al., *Treatment of Burn and Surgical Wounds With Recombinant Human Tropoelastin Produces New Elastin Fibers in Scars.* J Burn Care Res, 2017. **38**(5): p. e859-e867.

[167] Bailey, J.K., et al., *Effects of early combinatorial treatment of autologous split-thickness skin grafts in red duroc pig model using pulsed dye laser and fractional CO2 laser.* Lasers Surg Med, 2018. **50**(1): p. 78-87.

[168] DeBruler, D.M., et al., *Inflammatory responses, matrix remodeling, and re-epithelialization after fractional CO2 laser treatment of scars.* Lasers Surg Med, 2017. **49**(7): p. 675-685.

[169] DeBruler, D.M., et al., *Early cessation of pressure garment therapy results in scar contraction and thickening.* PLoS One, 2018. **13**(6): p. e0197558.

[170] DeBruler, D.M., et al., *Effect of skin graft thickness on scar development in a porcine burn model.* Burns, 2018. **44**(4): p. 917-930.

[171] Ross, R., *Wound healing.* Sci Am, 1969. **220**(6): p. 40-50.

[172] Hawkins, H.K., Jay, J., Finnerty, C.C., *Pathophysiology of Burn Scar*, in *Total Burn Care*, D.N. Herndon, Editor. 2018, Elsevier. p. 466-475.

[173] Brown, J.J. and A. Bayat, *Genetic susceptibility to raised dermal scarring.* Br J Dermatol, 2009. **161**(1): p. 8-18.

[174] Aarabi, S., M.T. Longaker, and G.C. Gurtner, *Hypertrophic scar formation following burns and trauma: new approaches to treatment.* PLoS Med, 2007. **4**(9): p. e234.

[175] Nischwitz, S.P., et al., *Evidence-based therapy in hypertrophic scars: An update of a systematic review.* Wound Repair Regen, 2020.

[176] Cubison, T.C., S.A. Pape, and N. Parkhouse, *Evidence for the link between healing time and the development of hypertrophic scars (HTS) in paediatric burns due to scald injury.* Burns, 2006. **32**(8): p. 992-999.

[177] Deitch, E.A., et al., *Hypertrophic burn scars: analysis of variables.* J Trauma, 1983. **23**(10): p. 895-898.

[178] Otene, C.I., et al., *Donor Site Morbidity Following Harvest of Split-Thickness Skin Grafts in South Eastern Nigeria.* J West Afr Coll Surg, 2011. **1**(2): p. 86-96.

[179] Karlsson, M., et al., *Scarring At Donor Sites After Split-Thickness Skin Graft: A Prospective, Longitudinal, Randomized Trial.* Adv Skin Wound Care, 2018. **31**(4): p. 183-188.

[180] Sood, R.F., et al., *Genome-wide Association Study of Postburn Scarring Identifies a Novel Protective Variant.* Ann Surg, 2015. **262**(4): p. 563-569.

[181] Lewis, W.H. and K.K. Sun, *Hypertrophic scar: a genetic hypothesis.* Burns, 1990. **16**(3): p. 176-178.

[182] Sood, R.F., et al., *Race and Melanocortin 1 Receptor Polymorphism R163Q Are Associated with Post-Burn Hypertrophic Scarring: A Prospective Cohort Study.* J Invest Dermatol, 2015. **135**(10): p. 2394-2401.

[183] Tyack, Z., et al., *A systematic review of the quality of burn scar rating scales for clinical and research use.* Burns, 2012. **38**(1): p. 6-18.

[184] Baryza, M.J. and G.A. Baryza, *The Vancouver Scar Scale: an administration tool and its interrater reliability.* J Burn Care Rehabil, 1995. **16**(5): p. 535-538.

[185] Draaijers, L.J., et al., *The patient and observer scar assessment scale: a reliable and feasible tool for scar*

evaluation. Plast Reconstr Surg, 2004. **113**(7): p. 1960-1965; discussion 1966-7.

[186] Lin, J.Y., et al., *A prospective, randomized controlled trial on the efficacy of fractional photothermolysis on scar remodeling.* Lasers Surg Med, 2011. **43**(4): p. 265-272.

[187] Qu, L., et al., *Clinical and molecular effects on mature burn scars after treatment with a fractional CO(2) laser.* Lasers Surg Med, 2012. **44**(7): p. 517-524.

[188] Anderson, R.R., et al., *Laser treatment of traumatic scars with an emphasis on ablative fractional laser resurfacing: consensus report.* JAMA Dermatol, 2014. **150**(2): p. 187-193.

[189] Patel, S.P., et al., *Fractional CO2 Laser Treatment Outcomes for Pediatric Hypertrophic Burn Scars.* J Burn Care Res, 2019. **40**(4): p. 386-391.

[190] van de Kar, A.L., et al., *Reliable and feasible evaluation of linear scars by the Patient and Observer Scar Assessment Scale.* Plast Reconstr Surg, 2005. **116**(2): p. 514-522.

[191] Brusselaers, N., et al., *Burn scar assessment: a systematic review of different scar scales.* J Surg Res, 2010. **164**(1): p. e115-e123.

[192] Hambleton, J., P.G. Shakespeare, and B.J. Pratt, *The progress of hypertrophic scars monitored by ultrasound measurements of thickness.* Burns, 1992. **18**(4): p. 301-307.

[193] Oliveira, G.V., et al., *Objective assessment of burn scar vascularity, erythema, pliability, thickness, and planimetry.* Dermatol Surg, 2005. **31**(1): p. 48-58.

[194] Taylor, B., D.A. McGrouther, and A. Bayat, *Use of a non-contact 3D digitiser to measure the volume of keloid scars: a useful tool for scar assessment.* J Plast Reconstr Aesthet Surg, 2007. **60**(1): p. 87-94.

[195] Ardehali, B., et al., *Objective assessment of keloid scars with three-dimensional imaging: quantifying response to intralesional steroid therapy.* Plast Reconstr Surg, 2007. **119**(2): p. 556-561.

[196] Du, Y.C., et al., *Implementation of a burn scar assessment system by ultrasound techniques.* Conf Proc IEEE Eng Med Biol Soc, 2006. **2006**: p. 2328-2331.

[197] van Zuijlen, P.P., et al., *Scar assessment tools: implications for current research.* Plast Reconstr Surg, 2002. **109**(3): p. 1108-1122.

[198] McHugh, A.A., et al., *Biomechanical alterations in normal skin and hypertrophic scar after thermal injury.* J Burn Care Rehabil, 1997. **18**(2): p. 104-108.

[199] Sloan, D.F., et al., *Tissue gases in human hypertrophic burn scars.* Plast Reconstr Surg, 1978. **61**(3): p. 431-436.

[200] Brusselaers, N., et al., *Burn scar assessment: A systematic review of objective scar assessment tools.* Burns, 2010. **36**(8): p. 1157-1164.

[201] Kim, Y.J., et al., *Evaluation of natural change of skin function in split-thickness skin grafts by noninvasive bioengineering methods.* Dermatol Surg, 2006. **32**(11): p. 1358-1363.

[202] Tredget, E.E., J.W. Shupp, and J.C. Schneider, *Scar Management Following Burn Injury.* J Burn Care Res, 2017. **38**(3): p. 146-147.

[203] Bloemen, M.C., et al., *Prevention and curative management of hypertrophic scar formation.* Burns, 2009. **35**(4): p. 463-475.

[204] Anthonissen, M., et al., *The effects of conservative treatments on burn scars: A*

systematic review. Burns, 2016. **42**(3): p. 508-518.

[205] Friedstat, J.S. and C.S. Hultman, *Hypertrophic burn scar management: what does the evidence show? A systematic review of randomized controlled trials.* Ann Plast Surg, 2014. **72**(6): p. S198-S201.

[206] Robson, M.C., et al., *Prevention and treatment of postburn scars and contracture.* World J Surg, 1992. **16**(1): p. 87-96.

[207] Sharp, P.A., et al., *Development of a Best Evidence Statement for the Use of Pressure Therapy for Management of Hypertrophic Scarring.* J Burn Care Res, 2016. **37**(4): p. 255-264.

[208] Sharp, P.A., et al., *Development of a Best Evidence Statement for the Use of Pressure Therapy for Management of Hypertrophic Scarring.* J Burn Care Res, 2015.

[209] Van den Kerckhove, E., et al., *The assessment of erythema and thickness on burn related scars during pressure garment therapy as a preventive measure for hypertrophic scarring.* Burns, 2005. **31**(6): p. 696-702.

[210] Cheng, W., et al., *Ultrasound assessment of scald scars in Asian children receiving pressure garment therapy.* J Pediatr Surg, 2001. **36**(3): p. 466-469.

[211] Candy, L.H., L.T. Cecilia, and Z.Y. Ping, *Effect of different pressure magnitudes on hypertrophic scar in a Chinese population.* Burns, 2010. **36**(8): p. 1234-1241.

[212] Garcia-Velasco, M., et al., *Compression treatment of hypertrophic scars in burned children.* Can J Surg, 1978. **21**(5): p. 450-452.

[213] Chang, L.W., et al., *Pressure effects on the growth of human scar fibroblasts.* J Burn Care Res, 2008. **29**(5): p. 835-841.

[214] Travis, T., Mino, MJ, Mauskar, NA, Jo, DY, Ghassemi, P, Moffatt, LT, Jordan, MH, Ramella-Roman, JC, Shupp, JW. *A novel and reproducible porcine scar model for testing the effects of pressure therapy while correlating non-invasive imaging metrics to molecular and histological changes.* in *45th Annual Meeting of the American Burn Association*. 2013. Palm Springs, CA.

[215] Anthonissen, M., et al., *Influence on clinical parameters of depressomassage (part I): The effects of depressomassage on color and transepidermal water loss rate in burn scars: A pilot comparative controlled study.* Burns, 2018. **44**(4): p. 877-885.

[216] Ault, P., A. Plaza, and J. Paratz, *Scar massage for hypertrophic burns scarring-A systematic review.* Burns, 2018. **44**(1): p. 24-38.

[217] Nedelec, B., et al., *Randomized controlled trial of the immediate and long-term effect of massage on adult postburn scar.* Burns, 2019. **45**(1): p. 128-139.

[218] Zhang, Y.T., C.W.P. Li-Tsang, and R.K.C. Au, *A Systematic Review on the Effect of Mechanical Stretch on Hypertrophic Scars after Burn Injuries.* Hong Kong J Occup Ther, 2017. **29**(1): p. 1-9.

[219] O'Brien, L. and A. Pandit, *Silicon gel sheeting for preventing and treating hypertrophic and keloid scars.* Cochrane Database Syst Rev, 2006(1): p. CD003826.

[220] Momeni, M., et al., *Effects of silicone gel on burn scars.* Burns, 2009. **35**(1): p. 70-74.

[221] Khan, M.A., M.M. Bashir, and F.A. Khan, *Intralesional triamcinolone alone and in combination with 5-fluorouracil for the treatment of keloid and hypertrophic scars.* J Pak Med Assoc, 2014. **64**(9): p. 1003-1007.

[222] Longacre, J.J., et al., *The effects of Z plasty on hypertrophic scars.* Scand J Plast Reconstr Surg, 1976. **10**(2): p. 113-128.

[223] Ogawa, R., *Surgery for scar revision and reduction: from primary closure to flap surgery.* Burns Trauma, 2019. 7: p. 7.

[224] Willows, B.M., M. Ilyas, and A. Sharma, *Laser in the management of burn scars.* Burns, 2017. **43**(7): p. 1379-1389.

[225] El-Hoshy, K., et al., *Efficacy of Fractional Carbon Dioxide Laser in the Treatment of Mature Burn Scars: A Clinical, Histopathological, and Histochemical Study.* J Clin Aesthet Dermatol, 2017. **10**(12): p. 36-43.

[226] Miletta, N.R., M.B. Donelan, and C.M. Hivnor, *Management of trauma and burn scars: the dermatologist's role in expanding patient access to care.* Cutis, 2017. **100**(1): p. 18-20.

[227] Kono, T., et al., *Treatment of hypertrophic scars using a long-pulsed dye laser with cryogen-spray cooling.* Ann Plast Surg, 2005. **54**(5): p. 487-493.

[228] Peprah, K. and S. McCormack, *Fractionated CO2 Laser for Scar Improvement: A Review of Clinical Effectiveness and Cost-Effectiveness*, in *Fractionated CO2 Laser for Scar Improvement: A Review of Clinical Effectiveness and Cost-Effectiveness*. 2019: Ottawa (ON).

[229] Lee, S.J., et al., *Dermal Remodeling of Burn Scar by Fractional CO2 Laser.* Aesthetic Plast Surg, 2016. **40**(5): p. 761-768.

[230] Douglas, H., et al., *Carbon dioxide laser treatment in burn-related scarring: A prospective randomised controlled trial.* J Plast Reconstr Aesthet Surg, 2019. **72**(6): p. 863-870.

[231] Manstein, D., et al., *Fractional photothermolysis: a new concept for cutaneous remodeling using microscopic patterns of thermal injury.* Lasers Surg Med, 2004. **34**(5): p. 426-438.

[232] Bogdan Allemann, I. and J. Kaufman, *Fractional photothermolysis--an update.* Lasers Med Sci, 2010. **25**(1): p. 137-144.

[233] Bogdan Allemann, I. and J. Kaufman, *Fractional photothermolysis.* Curr Probl Dermatol, 2011. **42**: p. 56-66.

[234] Tierney, E.P., D.J. Kouba, and C.W. Hanke, *Review of fractional photothermolysis: treatment indications and efficacy.* Dermatol Surg, 2009. **35**(10): p. 1445-1461.

[235] Ozog, D.M., et al., *Evaluation of clinical results, histological architecture, and collagen expression following treatment of mature burn scars with a fractional carbon dioxide laser.* JAMA Dermatol, 2013. **149**(1): p. 50-57.

[236] Seago, M., et al., *Laser Treatment of Traumatic Scars and Contractures: 2020 International Consensus Recommendations.* Lasers Surg Med, 2020. **52**(2): p. 96-116.

[237] Thompson, C.M., et al., *Genetic risk factors for hypertrophic scar development.* J Burn Care Res, 2013. **34**(5): p. 477-482.

[238] Sood, R.F., et al., *Missense Variant in MAPK Inactivator PTPN5 Is Associated with Decreased Severity of Post-Burn Hypertrophic Scarring.* PLoS One, 2016. **11**(2): p. e0149206.

[239] Tsou, R., et al., *Analysis of hypertrophic and normal scar gene expression with cDNA microarrays.* J Burn Care Rehabil, 2000. **21**(6): p. 541-550.

[240] Stoddard, F.J., Jr., C.M. Ryan, and J.C. Schneider, *Physical and psychiatric recovery from burns.* Surg Clin North Am, 2014. **94**(4): p. 863-878.

[241] Wisely, J.A., et al., *Where to start? Attempting to meet the psychological needs of burned patients.* Burns, 2007. **33**(6): p. 736-746.

[242] Zeitlin, R.E., *Long-term psychosocial sequelae of paediatric burns.* Burns, 1997. **23**(6): p. 467-472.

[243] Taal, L. and A.W. Faber, *Posttraumatic stress and maladjustment among adult burn survivors 1 to 2 years postburn. Part II: the interview data.* Burns, 1998. **24**(5): p. 399-405.

[244] Goverman, J., et al., *The Presence of Scarring and Associated Morbidity in the Burn Model System National Database.* Ann Plast Surg, 2019. **82**(3 Suppl 2): p. S162-S168.

[245] Robert, R., et al., *Disfiguring burn scars and adolescent self-esteem.* Burns, 1999. **25**(7): p. 581-585.

[246] de Chalain, T.M., C. Tang, and H.G. Thomson, *Burn area color changes after superficial burns in childhood: can they be predicted?* J Burn Care Rehabil, 1998. **19**(1 Pt 1): p. 39-49.

[247] Thompson, C.M., et al., *What score on the Vancouver Scar Scale constitutes a hypertrophic scar? Results from a survey of North American burn-care providers.* Burns, 2015. **41**(7): p. 1442-1448.

[248] Ghazawi, F.M., et al., *Insights into the Pathophysiology of Hypertrophic Scars and Keloids: How Do They Differ?* Adv Skin Wound Care, 2018. **31**(1): p. 582-595.

[249] Miletta, N., et al., *Fractional Ablative Laser Therapy is an Effective Treatment for Hypertrophic Burn Scars: A Prospective Study of Objective and Subjective Outcomes.* Ann Surg, 2019.

[250] Daoud, A.A., et al., *Efficacy of Combined Intense Pulsed Light (IPL) With Fractional CO2 -Laser Ablation in the Treatment of Large Hypertrophic Scars: A Prospective, Randomized Control Trial.* Lasers Surg Med, 2019. **51**(8): p. 678-685.

[251] Bailey, J.K., et al., *Multimodal quantitative analysis of early pulsed-dye laser treatment of scars at a pediatric burn hospital.* Dermatol Surg, 2012. **38**(9): p. 1490-1496.

[252] Tidwell, W.J., et al., *Fractionated Er:YAG laser versus fully ablative Er:YAG laser for scar revision: Results of a split scar, double blinded, prospective trial.* Lasers Surg Med, 2016. **48**(9): p. 837-843.

[253] Alster, T.S., A.B. Lewis, and A. Rosenbach, *Laser scar revision: comparison of CO2 laser vaporization with and without simultaneous pulsed dye laser treatment.* Dermatol Surg, 1998. **24**(12): p. 1299-1302.

[254] Issler-Fisher, A.C., et al., *Ablative fractional resurfacing with laser-facilitated steroid delivery for burn scar management: Does the depth of laser penetration matter?* Lasers Surg Med, 2020. **52**(2): p. 149-158.

[255] Waibel, J.S., et al., *The Diagnostic Role of Optical Coherence Tomography (OCT) in Measuring the Depth of Burn and Traumatic Scars for More Accurate Laser Dosimetry: Pilot Study.* J Drugs Dermatol, 2016. **15**(11): p. 1375-1380.

[256] Waibel, J.S., et al., *Treatment of Hypertrophic Scars Using Laser-Assisted Corticosteroid Versus Laser-Assisted 5-Fluorouracil Delivery.* Dermatol Surg, 2019. **45**(3): p. 423-430.

[257] Hibbard, J.C., et al., *LIBERTI: A SMART study in plastic surgery.* Clin Trials, 2018. **15**(3): p. 286-293.

Section 2

Chronic Ulcers

Chapter 3

Pharyngocutaneous Fistulas Following Total Laryngectomy

Alexandru Nicolaescu, Șerban V.G. Berteșteanu, Raluca Grigore, Mihnea Cojocărița-Condeescu, Bogdan Popescu, Catrinel Simion-Antonie, Paula Bejenaru and Simona Gloria Munteanu

Abstract

Total laryngectomy is still the final therapeutic solution in cases of locally advanced laryngeal cancer, as well as in cases of therapeutic failure of organ-sparing surgery or radiation therapy. Following excision of the larynx, the remaining pharynx is reconstructed to obtain continuity of the upper digestive tract. One of the most common complications in these patients, despite constant refinement of the procedure, is the development of a pharyngo-cutaneous fistula. These fistulas prolong hospital stay and often require a second surgical procedure, increasing morbidity and cost for the patient, while diminishing his quality of life. Some risk-factors have been identified, but only some may be corrected before surgery to lower this risk. Managing the fistula once present depends on multiple factors, essential being the size of the fistula as well as the position and concomitant factors, with options ranging from conservative measures to aggressive reconstructive surgery with local miocutaneous flaps. Modern vocal rehabilitation with T.E.P. (tracheo-esophageal puncture) and vocal prosthesis placement presents a new challenge – because of the risk of developing a tracheo-esophageal fistula, with an even higher risk for the patient because of tracheal aspiration. Understanding healing mechanisms of these structures is key to proper management of this complication.

Keywords: fistula, laryngectomy, TEP, vocal rehabilitation, Head & Neck surgery, Wound healing

1. Introduction

Although a well-known technique, having been around from 1873 when Prof. Billroth of Vienna recorded the first procedure, total laryngectomy was constantly refined seeking to improve surgical outcome. Today, narrow-field and wide-field total laryngectomy are combined with partial pharyngectomy and neck dissection to obtain good results following surgery – regarding disease-free survival of patients as well as a good quality-of-life (especially when it comes to speech and swallowing) [1–3].

After the larynx is removed, in the anterior part of the hypopharynx, there is always a resulting defect. This lack of substance is caused by the shared anatomy of the larynx and pharynx. Because most laryngeal neoplasia that warrants a total laryngectomy is usually a locally advanced disease, and the glottis and supraglottic regions are the most frequent regions involved in the disease process, there is often an extension of the neoplasia to the adjacent hypopharynx. This requires an extended resection of the diseased pharynx – a total laryngectomy with a partial pharyngectomy.

After completing the resection, reconstruction of the area uses the principle of separation of the respiratory and digestive tracts. Thus, a permanent tracheostomy is performed by anchoring the subglottic tracheal end to the skin in the suprasternal notch and the remaining pharynx is sutured around a naso-gastric feeding tube and usually covered with the prelaryngeal muscle layers (when available). This is called a three-layer closure – with the pharynx being the first layer, the prelaryngeal strap muscles the second layer and the cervical skin the third [4]. Depending on the size and shape of the resulting pharyngeal defect, primary closure by suturing of the pharyngeal margins may be done in a horizontal pattern or by a T shape pattern (**Figure 1**). The horizontal closure, when feasible, offers the best healing chance and has the lowest risk of development of a pharyngeal fistula. The T shape closure has more stitching, and the tips of the 2 vertical pharyngeal tranches which form the upper part of the T have the least vascularization, which make them more susceptible to necrosis and therefore a salivary leak, which may progress towards fistula formation.

There are multiple types of suturing techniques used to close the pharynx. Choosing a closure type often depends on the size of the defect to be closed, as well as the surgeon's personal preference. The only recommendation, which every student in Otorhinolaryngology learns from compulsory surgery textbooks is that an inverting suture should be used, similar to sutures used in digestive surgery [4].

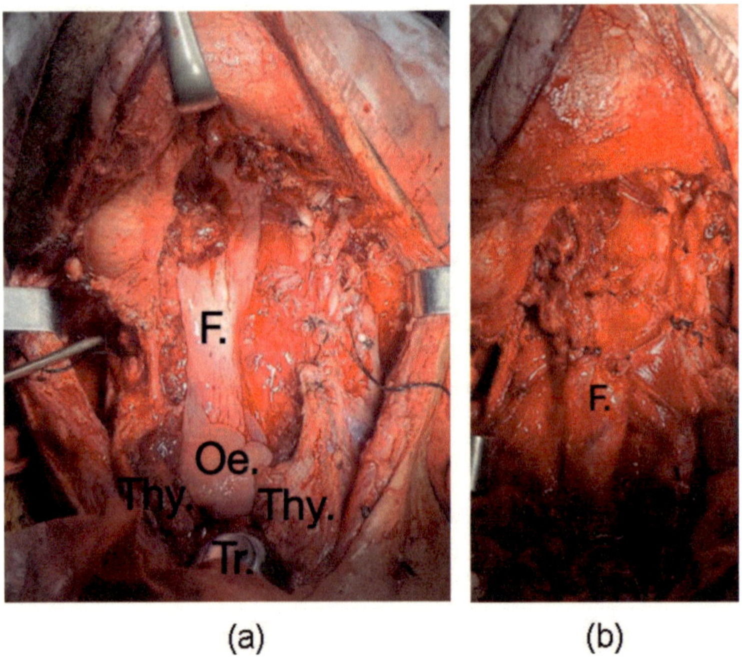

Figure 1.
Pharyngeal closure following total laryngectomy – Left (a): before suturing; Right (b): T-shaped pharyngoraphy on a naso-gastric feeding tube. Legend: F – pharynx, Tr. – trachea, Thy. – thyroid lobes, Oe – Oesophagus.

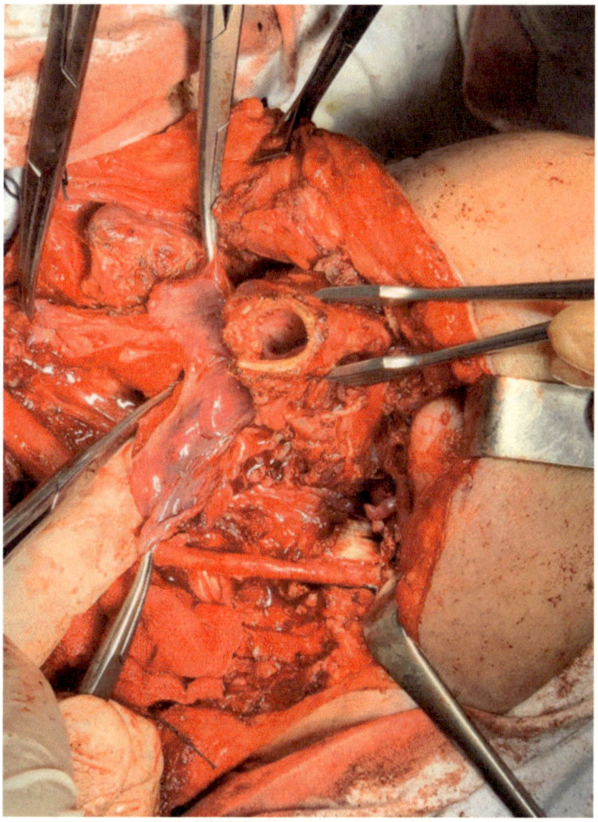

Figure 2.
Resulting defect following total laryngectomy "en bloc" with right thyroid lobe, large segment of pharynx as well as right side prelaryngeal muscle and skin. The resulting defect made primary reconstruction impossible – a local pedicled miocutaneous flap was used.

The most frequent type of suture used is the Connell suture, which is a continuous (running) inverting suture. The needle is passed parallel to the incision line, through all the layers of the pharynx, and out on the same side, after which it runs perpendicular to the incision line to the opposite side, where it passes in similar fashion. Some authors use variations of this suture, but there is not a consensus yet on a superior technique of suturing [5].

In cases of locally advanced tumours, where surgical excision extends to the pharynx, the resulting pharyngeal defect often makes primary closure impossible (**Figure 2**). Such cases warrant a second, reconstructive step to obtain surgical healing, such as using a local miocutaneous pedicled flap (pectoralis major or latissimus dorsi).

After wound healing – deglution is possible by oral intake, and respiration will always remain through the tracheostomy. Advances in speech rehabilitation made tracheoesophageal fistulisation with vocal prosthesis placement the gold-standard for vocal rehabilitation after total laryngectomy, assuring the possibility for adequate communication even without the larynx.

2. Surgical healing mechanism

As with most tissue injuries, after sectioning the pharyngeal wall through all three layers and then reapproximating them to close the resulting pharyngostoma, the healing mechanism is activated by way of inflammation, angiogenesis, migration and proliferation of fibroblasts, scar formation and subsequent connective tissue remodelling [6]. Following the surgeon's cut, the surface of the resected pharynx forms blood clots. These contain trapped red blood cells, as well as fibrin, fibronectin and complement components. Clots not only act a bleeding preventing mechanism, but also as a matrix for cells that are attracted by cytokines, chemokines and growth factors released in the area. Release of VEGF (vascular endothelial growth factor) permits increased blood vessel permeability – with subsequent inflammation and oedema. Within 24 hours from the injury, neutrophils migrate to the area and enter the local injury site by way of the blood clot matrix, to contribute to healing by releasing proteolytic enzymes. These enzymes clear debris and destroy bacteria. Between 24 and 72 hours after injury, granulation tissue is formed, by proliferating fibroblasts and vascular endothelial cells. This type of tissue has special properties, because of the high vascular permeability of new endothelial cells. This granulation tissue progressively fills all the injury space, and by 5 to 7 days the entire wound area is filled by this new tissue and neovascularization is maximal [7, 8]. Chemokines and different growth factors that are released by macrophages and neutrophils attract fibroblasts, which usually colonize the wound area in the first two days after injury. Macrophages stimulate the fibroblasts to produce IL-6 as well as epithelial growth factors, which in turn leads to epithelial cell proliferation and subsequent epithelization of the wound. During the second week after injury, the oedema, vascularity and lymphocytic infiltrate subside, and the granulation tissue scaffolding is replaced by dense collagen fibres, spindle-cell fibroblasts and other extracellular matrix components [6]. These collagen fibres are responsible for the tensile strength of the repaired wound. Shear resistance is only about 10% of normal tissue at 7 days following injury. It increases at a fast pace during the following 4 weeks, only to plateau around 70-80% of the normal tissue strength. It is of great importance to note that a repaired wound never acquires the same resistance as normal tissue [6].

3. Fistula formation – predisposing factors

One of the most important aspects in pharyngocutaneous fistulas is the lack of understanding on how the different risk factors affect and potentially cause this complications. Several factors are widely accepted as risk factors in developing a pharyngocutaneous fistula like concomitant or preexisting radiotherapy or chemotherapy, the extension and localization of the tumor – which invariably affects how large the resulting pharyngeal excision will be, the surgical technique (if a deficient surgical closure is performed – either by incorrect approximation of the tissues or improper suturing) used or septic complications of the wound (rarely encountered currently due to antibiotic therapy preoperatively as well as postoperatively) (**Figure 3**). Other lesser-known risk factors include preexisting comorbidities like diabetes, low hemoglobin and albumin levels, liver conditions and malnutrition as well as GERD (gastro-esophageal reflux disease).

What is highly specific about the pharyngeal segment following total laryngectomy is that it is permanently, since day 1 of surgery, in contact with saliva as well as the microbiota of the oral cavity. The chemical composition of saliva is known for its antibacterial and mucosal protection properties, however the mucin content as well as proteases in its composition are often inefficient to prevent even dental plaque formation. Modern studies aimed to use saliva as a diagnostic tool showed however that the proteases are very active and protein cleaving is a dynamic and fast-paced process, with protein degradation being a challenge for developing

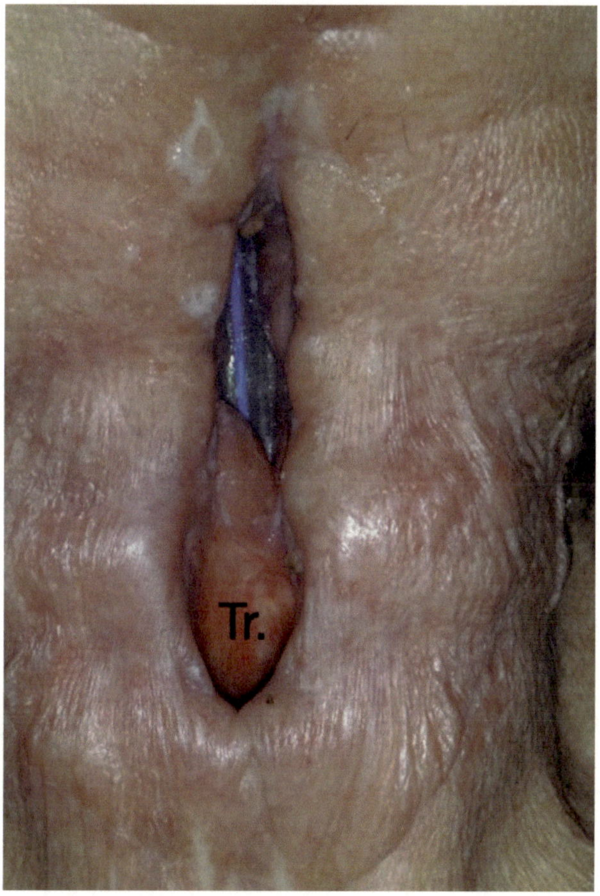

Figure 3.
Large midline pharyngocutaneous and pharyngotracheal fistula following total laryngectomy and radiation therapy. A nasogastric feeding tube is visibile through the fistula orifice, just above the tracheostomy (Tr.)

reliable diagnostic tests [9]. This may factor in the decision to use a salivary bypass tube after total laryngectomy (a Montgomery tube). Some authors reported favorable results using this method [10] – but the small sample size of the study groups, as well as a lack of uniform inclusion criteria and patient distribution resulted in results that were not statistically significant [11, 12].

GERD is another factor which is demonstrated to elevate the risk of fistula formation. Studies have shown that after total laryngectomy, because of upper oesophageal sphincter impairment, patients have elevated acidity and pepsin levels at this level [13, 14]. This affects pharyngeal wound healing – with a higher incidence of fistula formation. Studies showed that postoperative antisecretory and antiacid medication lower the risk for fistula formation after total laryngectomy [15, 16].

The extent of pharyngeal resection – and consequent pharyngeal tissue remaining for pharyngeal closure is one of the factors influencing the rate of postoperative fistula formation. This is probably due to tension around the suture lines, as well as postoperative tension generated by swallowing when resuming oral feeding [17]. Another factor, this time linked to the quality of remaining pharyngeal tissues, is radiation therapy. Salvage surgery, a term coined to describe surgery following other therapies of curative intent that failed (in cases of larynx cancer usually radiation therapy and conservative surgery), has a much higher rate of postoperative complications, including pharyngocutaneous fistulas [18]. In this aspect, radiation

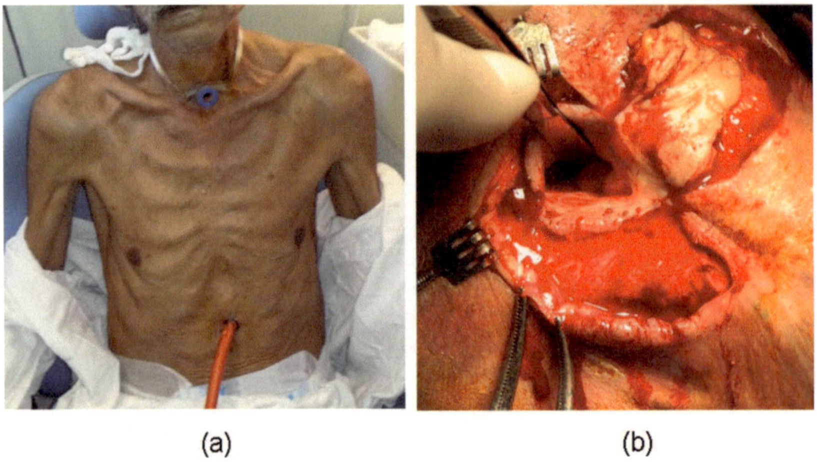

Figure 4.
Malnourished patient suffering from neoplasia of the larynx and hypopharynx. Left (a): Tracheostomy and gastrostomy – before surgical treatment. Right (b): Postoperative lateral cervical fistula – intraoperative aspect showing the diameter of the fistula, as well as the metaplasia of the epithelium of the fistula tract.

therapy is considered the main risk factor for complications because of the changes it produces in the irradiated tissues, and as important is the interval between radiation therapy and salvage surgery. Surgery in the first year after radiation therapy presents a significant higher risk for fistula formation, risk that decreases yearly after the first one [19]. Also demonstrated to present a higher risk of pharyngocutaneous fistula formation is concomitant bilateral neck dissection [20].

Systemic factors that influence wound healing, with regard to pharyngocutaneous fistula formation following total laryngectomy are linked to malnutrition and protein deficit (**Figure 4**). Studies showed that laryngeal cancer in itself negatively influences the nutritional status of patients, oftentimes patients presenting with malnutrition on diagnosis of laryngeal or pharyngo-laryngeal neoplasia [21]. Regarding pharyngocutaneous fistula formation after total laryngectomy, available data demonstrates that malnutrition (**Figure 6**) and protein deficiency (measured by albumin and prealbumin levels), is an independent risk factor. Current medical thought process encourages correcting malnutrition in the perioperative period to lower the risk of fistula formation [22].

4. Management of pharyngocutaneous fistulas

If present, managing pharyngo-cutaneous fistulas is important because their persistence can lead to increased hospital visits, a longer hospital stay and increased time for the surgical wound to heal and can prolong the time from surgery to oncological treatment. It can also have severe complication like aspiration pneumonia or carotid blowout. Although self limiting in most cases, it poses some important complications and sequelae like vessel ruptures or aspirative pneumonia if it is not resolved [23].

4.1 Conservative treatment

Conservative treatment is usually considered the first option for pharyngocutaneous fistulas. The first step in assuring a chance for spontaneous healing of the fistula is to bypass the fistula by ceasing oral feeding. This is done by either placing a naso-gastric feeding tube (which is usually kept for a limited time) or by parenteral feeding. Conservative measures consist of medical therapy with antibiotics and anti-inflammatory drugs. Daily wound care is also an important aspect with the need for fluid drainage from the fistula, local cleaning and the removal of necrotic tissues if they are present. In the same time the comorbidities of the patient must be addressed for example diabetes and hemodynamic parameters of the patient must be optimized [3] especially hemoglobin and albumin levels [4]. Applying pressure dressing above the fistula has also been seen traditionally as an important routine for daily management of the pharyngocutaneous fistula. However, traditional simple dressings are not suited for fistulas due to high output of saliva and exudate. They act more as a stopgap, so that the saliva and exudate does not come out, rather it stagnates along the fistula canal. The current concept is to move away from the simple wound dressing and use modern dressings like hydrocolloid, hydrogel or silver coated dressings [24, 25]. Sterilizing the fistula from within has also been used by different authors with substances like 0,25% acetic acid by mouth [26]. Another important aspect is the nutritional status of the patient prior and after surgery. Usually head and neck cancer patient are malnourished long time before surgery is even considered and this nutritional status is seen as a risk factor for developing complications like fistulas. Immunonutrition is a process that can modulate the immune system with certain nutrients like arginine, glutamine, omega 3 fatty acids and nucleotides, that can lead to an improvement of protein synthesis. Although not universally accepted, there is evidence that preoperative immunonutrition may lower the risk of developing fistulas [27]. Literature reviews demonstrated decreased hospital stay by an average of at least 3.5 days, but the mechanism by which this was achieved is still unclear [28]. Casas-Rodero et al. demonstrated that immunonutrition by itself did not improve fistula rate, but in the group where nutritional support was administered concomitant with immunoenhanced products the best results were obtained [29].

4.2 Negative pressure wound therapy

Negative pressure wound therapy represents a dressing process in which subatmospheric pressure is applied to the wound in a continuous or intermittent way. By decreasing local tissue swelling, improving blood flow and removing excess fluid it can trigger intracellular signals that may increase the rate of cell division and promotes the formation of granulation tissue transforming the wound into a closed controlled environment with a better management of secretions [30]. In recent years this method of wound dressing has been increasingly used by head and neck surgeons to manage pharyngocutaneous fistulas with good results. It can be used even on large size fistulas and can reduce the size and even heal the fistula. It comes with some contraindications like the presence of necrotic tissues and important wound infection that cannot be controlled. Another important aspect is the cost of this system and the accessibility of it for the patient that develop fistulas [31].

Despite being a complicated site with the presence of the tracheostomy tube which can make it difficult to maintain everything airtight negative wound pressure therapy has proven to be an effective alternative treatment for pharyngocutaneous fistula as a first line or in cases where fistulas persist after surgical revisions [32].

4.3 Hyperbaric oxygen therapy

Hyperbaric oxygen therapy involves breathing 100% oxygen in a pressurized environment with increased atmospheric pressure. Initially used for treating decompression sickness and carbon monoxide poisoning it has proven to be also effective in treating gangrene and wounds. This therapy promotes angiogenesis and cellular synthesis. The literature available on the use of hyperbaric oxygen therapy consists mostly of studies on chronic wounds such as diabetic ulcers and venous ulcers. A Cochrane database literature review demonstrated that a large part of studies had bias issues, but most had similar results, positive short-term impact on wound healing, with statistically non-significant long-term improvement [33] Published data regarding its use in treating pharyncocutaneous fistulas is scarce. Some results look promising ranging from 87,5% -100% fistula closure [34]. The drawbacks of this therapy despite the promising results are the high cost and the availability of such pressurized rooms.

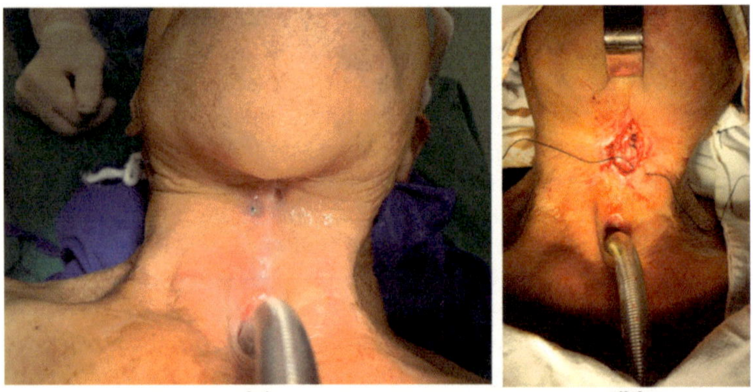

(a) (b)

Figure 5.
(Up - a) Midline submandibular fistula following total laryngectomy. (Right - b) Closure of the fistula after resections of margins and 3 plane suturing – pharyngeal mucosa, platysma muscle, skin.

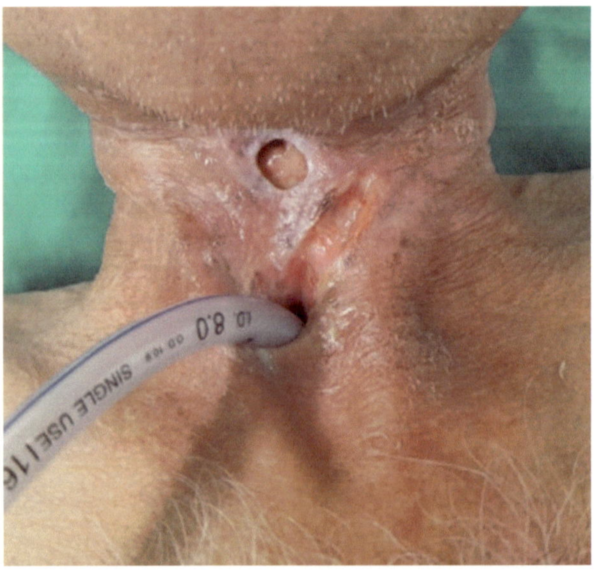

Figure 6.
Midline medium diameter (12 mm) pharyngocutaneous fistula following total laryngectomy and radiation therapy.

4.4 Surgical management

All pharyngo-cutaneous fistulas should be promptly treated, but the urgency as well as aggressiveness of the therapeutic response should be adapted to the size of the fistula, the potential for complications (e.g.: carotid blowout by salivary erosion), the underlying conditions of the patient, and the impact the fistula has on the patient's quality of life. For example: a small, midline fistula orifice, with little to no exudate that appeared during or immediately after radiation therapy in an otherwise healthy individual poses no immediate risk for complications and is easily tolerated by the patient with little to no impact on his quality of life, and has a large

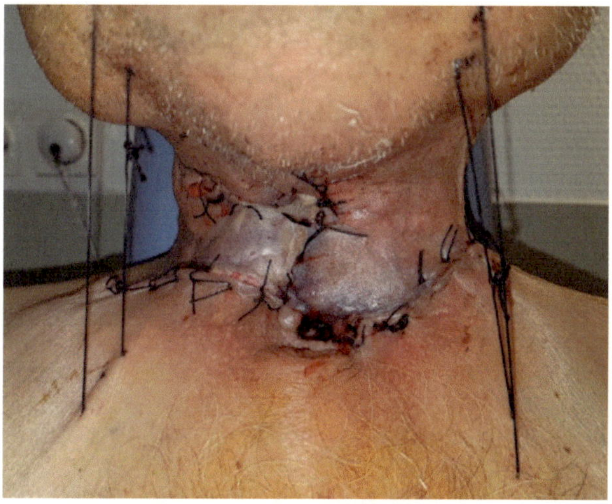

Figure 7.
Surgical closure using two opposing miocutaneous rotation flaps from the sternocleidomastoid muscle and overlying skin. 2 safety sutures placed to prevent head extension and tensioning of the wound.

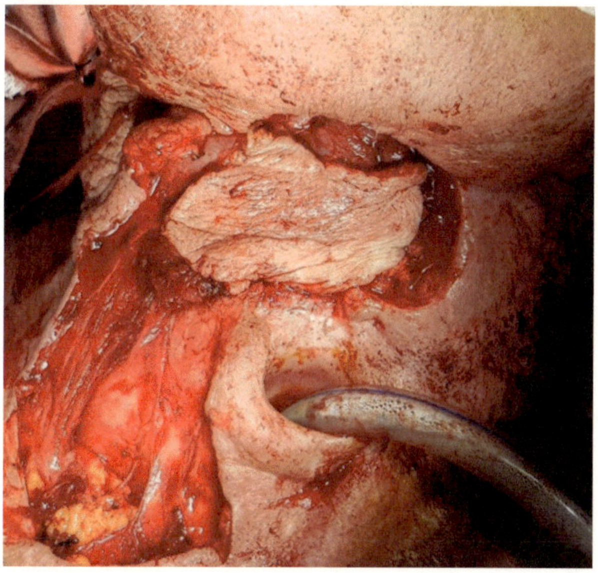

Figure 8.
Closure of a large midline pharyngocutaneous fistula after total laryngectomy. Translation of a miocutaneous pectoralis major flap to cover de defect.

chance for spontaneous healing, which makes it ideal for conservative treatment. Unfortunately, in head and neck cancer surgery most cases of fistulas developing after laryngectomy are not so straightforward to treat and require surgical interventions. A universal set of recommendations does not exist, but basic surgical principles should be tailored and applied to each case depending on each patient's characteristics and the surgeon's preference and experience. These principles state that for small diameter orifices, closure by margin resection and two plane suturing is usually sufficient (**Figure 5**).

Larger defects require interposition of a muscle layer – usually from a local source by way of a pedicled flap. One of the closest available flaps is the sternocleidomastoid muscle, however oftentimes the skin or even the muscle has modifications following neck dissection or/and radiation, which make it not ideal for dissection and manipulation. When available, the SCM pedicled flap is an ideal solution to close small to medium midline or paramedian fistulas (**Figures 6** and 7).

The workhorse of cervical defect reconstructions, therefore including pharyngocutaneous fistula closure, is the pectoralis major miocutaneous pedicled flap. Because of the size of the muscle, the arterial supply (the pectoral artery is situated in the upper-lateral quadrant of the muscle, ideal for translation towards superior and medial) as well as the subcutaneous fatty tissue, this is ideal for closing large and deep fistulas or pharyngostomas [35] (**Figure 8**). Unbiased data regarding surgical closure methods is hard to obtain, because there is a great deal of variation between surgeons and centres, however some studies shown that use of the pectoralis major flap is the most morbidity prone technique, with a high rate of complications (bleeding, flap dehiscence, recurrent fistula, carotid blowout), but it remains the most used method (**Figures 9** and **10**) [36].

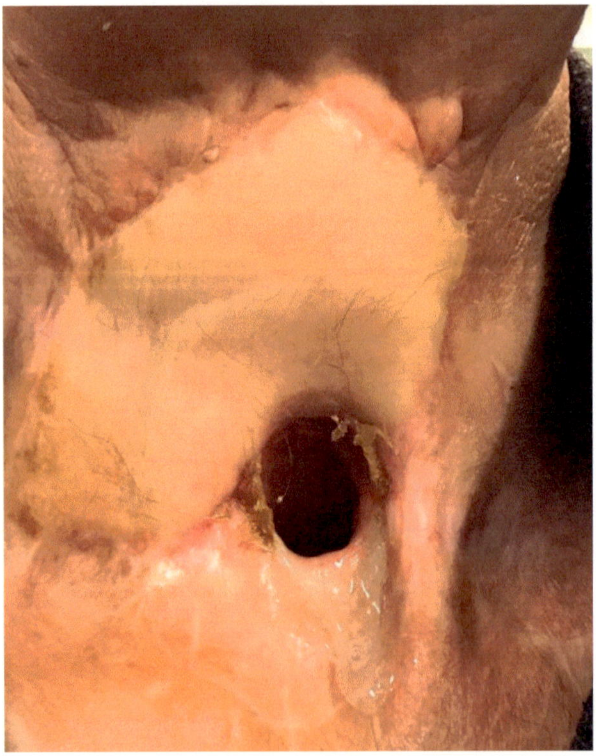

Figure 9.
Final postoperative aspect of closure of an anterior pharyngocutaneous fistula using a pectoral miocutaneous flap. Notice the hair follicules on the flap skin – different from normal cervical skin.

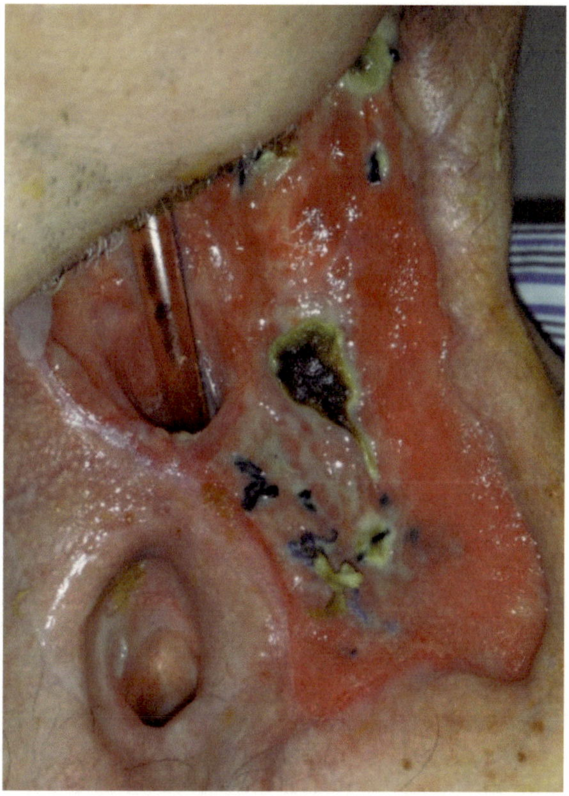

Figure 10.
Postoperative aspect of patient with necrosis of the miocutaneous pectoral flap. After muscle tissue necrosis – large pharyngostomy, with abundant salivary leakage, as well as exposure of the underlying carotid vessels (whitish contour parallel to the NG feeding tube) with great risk of carotid blowout.

Temporoparietal fascia flap is a new addition to the increasing techniques of fistula repair and is based on the temporoparietal branch of the superficial temporalis artery. One advantage of this flap is that the pedicle is safe from radiotherapy damage but its disadvantages of pedicle length and size of flap can limit its use [37].

In recent years the need for minimal invasive surgeries has grown and endoscopic techniques have been developed to lower comorbidities, complications and try to lower hospital stay. Endoscopic techniques for fistula repair have been developed but have some limitations depending on the size of the fistula and the condition of the surrounding tissues (like the platysma muscle and the accessibility of the fistula transorally) [38].

4.5 Free flaps

Free flaps are used when proximal tissues are unavailable or cannot offer epithelial surface for the repair of the fistula. The advantages of free flaps are that the donor site is far from the primary wound and therefore safe from infection and have not been irradiated. The important limitation of using free flaps is the availability of neck vessels for anastomosis (especially in cases of previous radical neck dissection with ligation of internal jugular vein) [39]. The most common free flap used is the radial forearm flap and anterior thigh flap. Other free flaps that can be used are jejunal flap and latissimus dorsi flap. Another relative disadvantage of using free flaps is the significant longer operating time needed – with harvesting and implantation taking longer than using local pedicled flaps, as well as sometimes requiring two surgical teams [39].

5. Particular case: tracheoesophageal puncture vocal rehabilitation – fistula enlargement and management

One particular situation of fistula formation is in cases of vocal rehabilitation using tracheo-esophageal fistulization with vocal prosthesis implant. In these cases, a fistula is made by the surgeon, between the trachea and the upper cervical esophagus through the posterior tracheal wall right at the level of the tracheostomy. In this iatrogenic fistula the surgeon inserts a vocal prosthesis – basically a two-flanged device with a lumen that has a unidirectional valve. This is placed so as to permit air from the trachea to pass through towards the pharynx, but not so as to allow food and liquids to pass from the pharynx. This method permits a higher quality esophageal speech and is currently the gold-standard method for vocal rehabilitation following total laryngectomy and has been for the last 30 years [40]. However, long term studies showed that a number of complications may arise in these patients. The hardest to treat is enlargement of the fistula. This is currently linked to local factors, such as acid reflux in the upper esophageal and pharyngeal areas [41], as well as inflammation of the tissues surrounding the prosthesis – inflammation which in turn is caused by the biofilm that forms on the body and flanges of the device [42]. Once enlargement begins (**Figure 11**), one of the first signs will be leakage around the prosthesis, with coughing especially during drinking. Salivary leakage and micro aspiration are potentially very harmful, because of the risk of aspiration pneumonia, which may endanger the patient's life. Methods to treat fistula enlargement vary from using larger and larger diameter flanges, to surgically closing the fistula using a local muscle flap (usually sternocleidomastoid) and after surgical healing refistulization in a different site. Some patients however after such complications abandon this technique of vocal rehabilitation altogether and opt for other methods of communication (esophageal speech or an electric larynx) [43, 44].

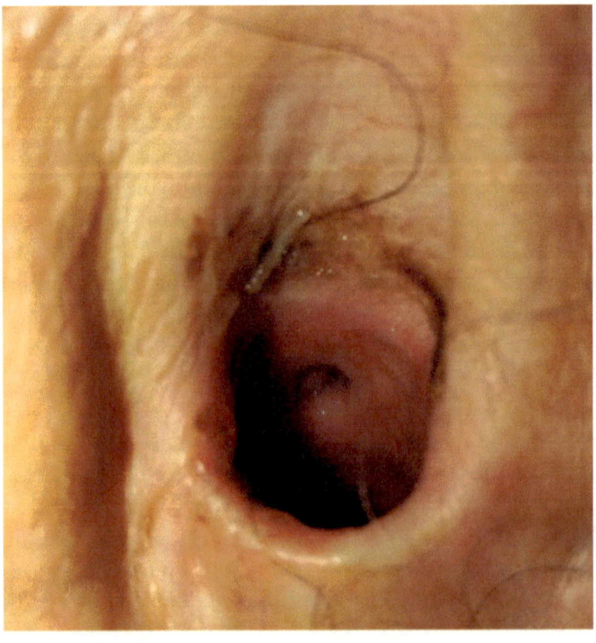

Figure 11.
Tracheoesophageal puncture orifice – enlarged, with spontaneous expulsion of vocal prosthesis. Small granulation tissue visible through opening.

6. Conclusions

Following total laryngectomy, some anatomical and functional modifications of the cervical region and especially of the pharynx and upper cervical esophagus are important for the consequent evolution of the laryngectomee. Wound healing follows the same basic principles as everywhere else in the human body, but this region presents a series of particular elements. Understanding the importance of not just the quantity of the remaining pharyngeal tissue and the pharyngeal closure technique but equally the quality of said tissues (affected by recent previous radiation therapy and malnutrition) and the intrinsic factors that influence local healing (bacterial colonization, gastro-esophageal acid reflux) – is paramount to micro-managing each total laryngectomy case, in order to decrease the risk of developing a pharyngo-cutaneous fistula. Once formed, fistulas are treated by a multitude of techniques, from conservative to radical surgical plastic reconstructions using local or distant free miocutaneous flaps. Either way, treatment of fistulas is always a more expensive and higher-risk procedure than preventing fistula formation. A particular case is vocal rehabilitation of the laryngectomees, by way of iatrogenic tracheo-esophageal fistula formation with vocal prosthesis placement. In this case, managing the fistula orifice presents another set of challenges, the goal being to maintain fistula patency without granulation tissue formation and without orifice enlargement, so as to maintain patency and prevent leakage or expulsion/aspiration of the prosthesis. The same intrinsic factors – biofilm formation and GERD have been established as risk factors for complications regarding the size of the fistula orifice.

Conflict of interest - disclosure

The authors declare that there are no conflicts of interests among them. All authors have contributed equally and would like to thank their colleagues for the considerable work and support.

Author details

Alexandru Nicolaescu[1,2*†], Şerban V.G. Berteşteanu[3,4†], Raluca Grigore[3,4†], Mihnea Cojocăriţa-Condeescu[1,4†], Bogdan Popescu[3,4†], Catrinel Simion-Antonie[1,4†], Paula Bejenaru[1,4†] and Simona Gloria Munteanu[1,5†]

1 "Carol Davila" University of Medicine and Pharmacy, Bucharest, Romania

2 ENT Head and Neck Surgery Compartment, "Prof. Dimitrie Gerota" Emergency Hospital of the Ministry of Internal Affairs, Bucharest, Romania

3 ENT Head and Neck Surgery, "Carol Davila" University of Medicine and Pharmacy, Bucharest, Romania

4 ENT Head and Neck Surgery Clinic, "Colţea" Clinical Hospital, Bucharest, Romania

5 ENT Head and Neck Surgery Clinic, "Dr. Carol Davila" Central Military Hospital, Bucharest, Romania

*Address all correspondence to: alexandru87nicolaescu@gmail.com

† All authors have contributed equally.

References

[1] Donegan WL. An early history of total laryngectomy. Surgery. 1965;57(6): 902-5.

[2] Ceachir O, Hainarosie R, Zainea V. Total laryngectomy - past, present, future. Mædica [Internet]. 2014;9(2): 210-6. Available from: http://www.ncbi.nlm.nih.gov/pubmed/25705281%5Cnhttp://www.pubmedcentral.nih.gov/articlerender.fcgi?artid=PMC4296768

[3] KAZI R, SALAMA H, ALMUTAIRY A, DECORDOVA J, CLARKE P, NUTTING C, et al. Quality of Life after Total Laryngectomy. Otolaryngology - Head and Neck Surgery. 2005;133(2): P205-6.

[4] Theissing J, Rettinger G, Werner JA. ENT - Head and Neck Surgery: Essential Procedures. Thieme; 2012.

[5] Haksever M, Akduman D, Aslan S, Solmaz F, Ozmen S. Modified continuous mucosal connell suture for the pharyngeal closure after total laryngectomy: Zipper suture. Clinical and Experimental Otorhino laryngology. 2015;

[6] Kumar V, Abbas AK, Fausto N, Aster JK. Robbins and Cotran Pathologic Basis of Disease, 8/E. 8th ed. Philadelphia, PA: Saunders-Elsevier; 2010.

[7] Molteni G, Sacchetto A, Sacchetto L, Marchioni D. Optimal Management of Post-Laryngectomy Pharyngo-Cutaneous Fistula. Open Access Surgery. 2020;

[8] Khanh NT, Iyer NG. Management of post-operative fistula in head and neck surgery: Sweeping it under the carpet? World Journal of Otorhino laryngology. 2015;

[9] Helmerhorst EJ, Oppenheim FG. Saliva: A dynamic proteome. Journal of Dental Research. 2007.

[10] Punthakee X, Zaghi S, Nabili V, Knott PD, Blackwell KE. Effects of salivary bypass tubes on fistula and stricture formation. JAMA Facial Plastic Surgery. 2013;

[11] Kamhieh Y, Fox H, Hallett E, Berry S. Routine use of salivary bypass tubes in laryngectomy patients: Systematic review. Journal of Laryngology and Otology. 2018.

[12] Hone RWA, Rahman E, Wong G, Annan Y, Alexander V, Al-Lami A, et al. Do salivary bypass tubes lower the incidence of pharyngocutaneous fistula following total laryngectomy? A retrospective analysis of predictive factors using multivariate analysis. European Archives of Oto-Rhino-Laryngology. 2017;

[13] Hadzibegovic AD, Danic D, Prgomet D, Ticac R, Kozmar A. Analysis of Saliva Pepsin Level in Patients with Tracheoesophageal Fistula and Voice Prosthesis Complications. COLLEGIUM ANTROPOLOGICUM. 2012;36(2):93-7.

[14] Smit CF, Tan J, Mathus-Vliegen LMH, Devriese PP, Brandsen M, Grolman W, et al. High incidence of gastropharyngeal and gastroesophageal reflux after total laryngectomy. Head and Neck. 1998;20(7):619-22.

[15] Mannelli G, Santoro R, Segala F, Surrenti E, Gallo O. Gastro-pharyngeal reflux and total laryngectomy. Increasing knowledge about its management. American Journal of Otolaryngology - Head and Neck Medicine and Surgery. 2018 Mar 1;39(2):127-32.

[16] Seikaly H, Park P. Gastroesophageal reflux prophylaxis decreases the incidence of pharyngocutaneous fistula after total laryngectomy. Laryngoscope. 1995;105(11):1220-2.

[17] Dedivitis RA, Aires FT, Cernea CR, Brandão LG. Pharyngocutaneous fistula after total laryngectomy: Systematic review of risk factors. Vol. 37, Head and Neck. 2015.

[18] Ganly I, Patel S, Matsuo J, Singh B, Kraus D, Boyle J, et al. Postoperative complications of salvage total laryngectomy. Cancer. 2005;

[19] Basheeth N, O'Leary G, Sheahan P. Pharyngocutaneous fistula after salvage laryngectomy: IMPACT of interval between radiotherapy and surgery, and performance of bilateral neck dissection. Head and Neck. 2014;

[20] Kwong DLW, Nicholls J, Wei WI, Chua DTT, Sham JST, Yuen PW, et al. The incidence and etiology of postlaryngectomy pharyngocutaneous fistulae. Head and Neck. 2001;

[21] Flórez Almonacid CI, Jurado Ramos A, Rodríguez Borrego MA. Evaluation of the nutritional profile of patients with total laryngectomy. e-SPEN Journal. 2013.

[22] Mattioli F, Bettini M, Molteni G, Piccinini A, Valoriani F, Gabriele S, et al. Analysis of risk factors for pharyngocutaneous fistula after total laryngectomy with particular focus on nutritional status. Acta otorhino laryngologica Italica : organo ufficiale della Societa italiana di otorino laringologia e chirurgia cervico-facciale. 2015;

[23] DALE BA, WRIGHT DH. Say Goodbye to Wet-to-Dry Wound Care Dressings. Home Healthcare Nurse: The Journal for the Home Care and Hospice Professional. 2011;

[24] Kayano K, Okamoto K, Shimada T, Bamba H. Experience with wound dressings for surgical wound dehiscence and oropharyngeal fistulae after excision of head and neck cancer. Practica Oto-Rhino-Laryngologica. 2009;

[25] Parry GW, Juma A, Dussek JE. Broncho-oesophageal fistula treated effectively without surgical resection. Thorax. 1993;

[26] Howes N, Atkinson C, Thomas S, Lewis SJ. Immunonutrition for patients undergoing surgery for head and neck cancer. Cochrane Database of Systematic Reviews. 2018.

[27] Stableforth WD, Thomas S, Lewis SJ. A systematic review of the role of immunonutrition in patients undergoing surgery for head and neck cancer. International Journal of Oral and Maxillofacial Surgery. 2009.

[28] Casas Rodera P, de Luis DA, Gómez Candela C, Culebras JM. Immunoenhanced enteral nutrition formulas in head and neck cancer surgery; A systematic review. Nutrición hospitalaria: Organo oficial de la Sociedad española de nutrición parenteral y enteral. 2012;

[29] Huang C, Leavitt T, Bayer LR, Orgill DP. Effect of negative pressure wound therapy on wound healing. Current Problems in Surgery. 2014;

[30] Loaec E, Vaillant PY, Bonne L, Marianowski R. Negative-pressure wound therapy for the treatment of pharyngocutaneous fistula. European Annals of Otorhinolaryngology, Head and Neck Diseases. 2014;

[31] Teixeira S, Costa J, Bartosch I, Correia B, Silva Á. Management of Pharyngocutaneous Fistula with Negative-Pressure Wound Therapy. Journal of Craniofacial Surgery. 2017;

[32] Kranke P, Bennett MH, Martyn-St James M, Schnabel A, Debus SE, Weibel S. Hyperbaric oxygen therapy for chronic wounds. Cochrane Database of Systematic Reviews. 2015.

[33] Abu Eta R, Eviatar E, Gavriel H. Hyperbaric oxygen therapy as an alternative to surgery for non-healing pharyngocutaneous fistula. European Archives of Oto-Rhino-Laryngology. 2016;

[34] Magdy EA. Surgical closure of postlaryngectomy pharyngocutaneous fistula: A defect based approach. European Archives of Oto-Rhino-Laryngology. 2008;

[35] Mclean JN, Nicholas C, Duggal P, Chen A, Grist WG, Losken A, et al. Surgical management of pharyngocutaneous fistula after total laryngectomy. In: Annals of Plastic Surgery. 2012.

[36] Fabrizio T, Donati V, Nava M. Repair of the pharyngocutaneous fistula with a fasciocutaneous island flap pedicled on the superficial temporalis artery. Plastic and Reconstructive Surgery. 2000;

[37] Fink DS, Peña S, Hanby D, Kunduk M, McWhorter AJ. Repair of pharyngocutaneous fistula after total laryngectomy: A novel endoscopic approach. Head and Neck. 2015;

[38] Bohannon IA, Carroll WR, Magnuson JS, Rosenthal EL. Closure of post-laryngectomy pharyngocutaneous fistulae. Head and Neck Oncology. 2011;

[39] Horn D, Jonas R, Engel M, Freier K, Hoffmann J, Freudlsperger C. A comparison of free anterolateral thigh and latissimus dorsi flaps in soft tissue reconstruction of extensive defects in the head and neck region. Journal of Cranio-Maxillofacial Surgery. 2014;

[40] HILGERS FJM, BALM AJM. Long-term results of vocal rehabilitation after total laryngectomy with the low-resistance, indwelling Provox TM Voice prosthesis system. Clinical Otolaryngology [Internet]. 1993 Dec;18(6):517-23. Available from: http://doi.wiley.com/10.1111/j.1365-2273.1993.tb00627.x

[41] Nicolaescu A, Berteşteanu Ş., Grigore R, Popescu B, Hainăroşie R, Zainea V. GASTRO-ESOPHAGEAL REFLUX DISEASE AND ITS IMPACT ON TRACHEO-ESOPHAGEAL SPEAKING VALVE REHABILITATION AFTER TOTAL LARYNGECTOMY. Journal of Surgical Sciences. 2019;

[42] Leonhard M, Schneider-Stickler B. Voice prostheses, microbial colonization and biofilm formation. In: Advances in Experimental Medicine and Biology. 2015. p. 123-36.

[43] Frowen J, Perry a. Reasons for success or failure in surgical voice restoration after total laryngectomy: an Australian study. The Journal of laryngology and otology. 2001;115(5):393-9.

[44] Gates GA, Ryan W, Cantu E, Hearne E. Current status of laryngectomee rehabilitation: II. Causes of failure. American Journal of Otolaryngology--Head and Neck Medicine and Surgery. 1982;3(1):8-14.

Chapter 4

Combined Administration of Stem Cells and Photobiomodulation on Wound Healing in Diabetes

Mohammad Bayat and Sufan Chien

Abstract

Wound healing is an active and compound biological course which can be divided into four steps: hemostasis, inflammation, proliferation, and remodeling. Diabetes mellitus induces weakened wound healing by disturbing one or more of the biological functions of these steps. Diabetic foot ulcers result from the simultaneous action of multiple disturbing causes. Mesenchymal stem cells, especially autologous ones, are easily accessible with noninvasive methods and have been shown to provide a regenerative microenvironment at wound sites. Despite current knowledge, major hurdles remain to be overcome in order to achieve effective therapeutic effects. Photobiomodulation is the use of light to reduce pain and inflammation and stimulate healing and the proliferation of stem cells, which would be very useful in increasing stem cell function and in regenerative medicine. The current study analyzes the results of studies using separate and combined administrations of stem cells and photobiomodulation on diabetic wound healing in patients and animal models. We hypothesize that the combined application of photobiomodulation and stem cells will accelerate the repair process and assist the healing of foot ulcers in diabetes mellitus patients.

Keywords: wound healing, diabetes mellitus, diabetic foot ulcers, mesenchymal stem cells, adipose tissue-derived stem cells, photobiomodulation

1. Introduction

Diabetes mellitus (DM) is the most important cause of illness and death, affecting 422 million adults worldwide [1]. Epidemiological studies of DM in the U.S. have shown that almost one out of every three people in the U.S. is prone to preDM or suffering from DM. The Centers for Disease Control and Prevention (CDC) recently reported that more than 100 million adults in the U.S. have DM or pre-DM. In 2015, a total of 30.3 million people of all ages, or 9.4% of the U.S. populace, were reported to have DM. Moreover, a total of 33.9% of the U.S. adults aged 18 years or older (84.1 million people) had pre-DM in 2015. Almost half (48.3%) of adults aged 65 years or older have pre-DM which, if left untreated, will develop into Type 2 DM within 5 years [2]. Of the entire population of the U.S., 33% are predicted to be afflicted by DM by the year 2050 [3]. Diabetic foot ulcer (DFU) is still the predominant cause of hospitalization for patients with DM,

IntechOpen

and DM is the chief reason for more than 50% of nontraumatic leg amputations. Obviously, these operations increase the death ratio [3].

In this chapter notes are provided about the following subjects: 2, acute wound healing in healthy subjects; 3, a mechanistic approach to wound healing in DM; 4, DFU;5, administration of stem cells in DFUs; 6, adipose tissue-derived stem cells (ADSC); 7, regenerative potential of ADSC; 8, PBM and its effects on cells and stem cells; 9, how the combined application of photobiomodulation (PBM) and ADSCs accelerates healing in DFU; and 10, finally we will deliver our conclusions in section 10.

2. Acute normal skin injury repair course in healthy subjects

The acute normal skin injury repair course can be separated into four overlying steps: 1. coagulation; 2. inflammation; 3. proliferation; and 4. remodeling. During the first step, blood-clotting actions preclude extreme hemorrhage and deliver temporary protection to the injured area. The development of inflammation directs the use of leukocytes, neutrophils, and macrophages; the creation of growth factors; and the stimulation of fibroblasts, keratinocytes, and angiogenesis. Achievement of the proliferation step in wound repair directs the creation of extracellular matrix (ECM), i.e. rich, vascularized granulation tissue. Lastly, ECM maturation and cell apoptosis direct the creation of scar tissue with physical features that are similar to unwounded skin [4]. The repair of an acute skin injury comprises synchronized cellular and molecular responses. First, immune cells migrate to the injury site, then they initiate pathogen clearance, while also participating in the repair course. Cut epidermal borders upregulate wound-related genes, thereby allowing mutual cell migration. Local and blood-borne fibroblasts increase and migrate to produce wound granulation tissue, provide organization and signaling clues, and deliver new ECM. Some fibroblasts differentiate into myofibroblasts to help wound closure. The wound bed is perfused with oxygen and nutrients through new blood vessels derived by angiogenesis [5].

3. A mechanistic approach to wound healing in DM

DM causes the repair course directed to a non-healing wound (chronic wound or ulcer) to lag, resulting in practical restrictions, gait trouble, and contamination. The weakening of repair in DM patients is well-known, but the connection between pathophysiology and weakened skin injury repair in DM is still an unidentified etiology. The repair course requires cooperation between inflammatory cells and biochemical mediators encouraged by many elements. Nevertheless, alterations in the cellular and biochemical elements and accomplishments are concerns associated with wound healing failure in DM patients. Neutrophils, monocytes, macrophages, keratinocytes, fibroblasts, T and B cells, mast cells, and endothelial cells all contribute to wound repair and dynamically to the creation and regulation of various cytokines and growth factors. Monocytes, which later transform into macrophages, are the principal manufacturers of pro-inflammatory cytokines, including interleukin-1 (IL) -1β, tumor necrosis factor (TNF)-α, IL-6 and cytokines, and growth factors such as vascular endothelial growth factor (VEGF), insulin-like growth factor (IGF)-1, and transforming growth factor (TGF) - β in both healthy and diabetic subjects. Neutrophils, such as T and B cells, are also important producers of TNF-α and IL-10 cells among others, keratinocytes, fibroblasts, mast cells, and endothelial cells which participate in the production of VEGF, IGF-1, and TGF-β.

Macrophages are fundamental providers in healing. Hyperglycemia and oxidative stress alter the epigenetic code that results in alterations to the polarization and plastination of macrophages. Dysregulated macrophage polarization is one of the key hindrances to wound repair. Investigations have revealed that in DM, a compound function is included at the molecular level which is accountable for hindered wound repair. Actions like the continued production of pro-inflammatory cytokines, weakened angiogenic response and microvascular difficulties, weakened macrophage and neutrophils function, weakened keratinocytes and fibroblast migration, and increased and weakened creation of healing-associated elements like decreased growth factor creation have been reported in animal simulations of DM. The steps of the remedial course in diabetic sufferers are also delayed (in the inflammatory stage) by other elements as well as specific metabolic insufficiencies, weakened functional responses like hypoxia due to glycation of hemoglobin, and changes in red blood cell membranes and the tapering of blood vessels. Hypoxia reduces the oxygen stream to wounds because of tapering blood vessels. Hemoglobin glycation causes a lack of nutrients and oxygen to tissue, which further interrupts the repair course. Diabetic wounds continuously stimulate the unfolded protein response (UPR) and increase expression of pro-inflammatory chemokine in comparison with normal wounds. Native ischemia because of microvascular problems in DM significantly delays the repair course [6].

Reduced IGF-1 and TGF-β values at sites of tissue injury have been described in both diabetic animals and human (h) s with DM and are accountable for delayed repair to skin injuries. TGF-β employs and encourages the motivation of inflammatory cells, including neutrophils, macrophages, and lymphocytes, as well as keratinocytes, fibroblasts, and the creation of growth factors, which hasten neovascular formation, and the creation and delayed deterioration of ECMs. The decreased attentiveness of TGF-β has been described in skin injury repair in diabetic subjects. Many studies have proven that matrix metalloproteinase (MMP)-encoding genes have a TGF-β1-dependent preventative component in the promoter region, which down-regulates expression of the gene. Reduced TGF-β values and improved expression of MMPs induce the extreme deterioration of growth factors. Accompanied by MMP-encoding genes, transcription factors like Smad-2, Smad-3, and Smad-4 also trigger and suppress TGF-β target genes. TGF-β1 triggers Smad-2 and 3 for the creation of collagen. Reductions in TGF-β1 values augment the use of triggered inflammatory cells to hinder progression from the inflammatory step to the proliferation step in the repair course of diabetic wounds. Elevated TGF-β3 values are supposed to reduce TGF-β1 values in diabetic subjects, which leads to augmented macrophage action and reduced collagen creation. In DM, elevated glucose levels increase macrophage action, directing more reactive oxygen species (ROS) to extend the inflammatory step. Reduced values and expression of these growth factors weaken and extend the skin injury repair course in DM [6].

4. DFU

Disturbances in the coordination of glucose homeostasis induce hyperglycemic prominence and result in the initiation of certain metabolic pathways that, in their unusual situation, lead to the progression of vascular deficiency, nerve damage caused by ulcerations in inferior limbs because of changed patterns of plantar pressure, and consequently foot abnormalities. Abuse to the foot produced by trauma to the affected area remains hidden to the patient because of damage to afferent sensory nerves [7]. Diabetic neuropathy results in foot muscular inequality, inadequate feeling in the skin, and ultimately foot irregularities that lead to augmented force applied to the skin when walking. Collectively, the above-mentioned occurrences are accompanied by foot ischemia [8] and DFU formation.

When a foot ulcer develops, the foot is at increased risk for aggressive infection, and as soon as it is combined with a peripheral artery occlusive disease, the sufferer will have dangerous foot ischemia [8]. Thus, the etiology for DFU is composite. Disruption of harmony in glucose homeostasis causes hyperglycemic status, results in activation of certain metabolic pathways which in their abnormal state subsequently leads to development of vascular insufficiency, nerve damages headed by ulceration in lower extremity due to plantar pressures and foot deformity. Staphylococcus is the most common infectious bacterium [9]. A diabetic foot infection may be a warning limb complaint. Infection is identified by the occurrence or augmented ratio of inflammation markers. Frequently, these markers are less noticeable than anticipated. Imaging investigations can identify or better define profound, soft tissue-infected areas and are regularly required to detect pathological results in bone. The primary bactericidal cure as well as the length of cure are observational. There is a considerable delay in DFU injury repair that has been correlated to many irregularities [9]. Today, DM is the chief origin of non-traumatic amputations in the U.S. Generally, around 5% of DM patients develop DFUs, and 1% of them wind up with an amputation. Around 60% of diabetic patients will develop neuropathy, ultimately leading to a DFU. The danger of a DFU is augmented in people with flatfoot, as they apply uneven pressure across the foot, leading to local inflammation in risky areas of the foot. The yearly occurrence of DFU ranges from 9.1 to 26.1 million cases globally, and about 15% to 25% of DM patients will develop a DFU sometime during their lifespan.

As the number of newly identified DM cases rises annually, the occurrence of DFU is also destined to rise. DFUs are accountable for higher medical charges than any other diabetic difficulty. The usual cost of curing one DFU is $8,000, that of an infected DFU is $17,000, and that of a chief amputation is $45,000. Over 80,000 amputations are done yearly on diabetic patients in the U.S., and approximately 50% of patients with amputations will develop ulcers and infections in the other foot within 1.5 years. Sadly, 58% of people with DM will experience a second amputation 3–5 years after the first one. Furthermore, the prevalence of death occurring 3 years after a first amputation has been estimated to be as high as 20%–50%, and these statistics have not altered considerably in the past 30 years despite major developments in the medicinal and surgical management of DM patients [10]. Management of DFUs is mainly based on severity (score), blood vessel status, and the existence of contamination. Inhibiting the reappearance of DFUs remains a chief medical objective [11]. Numerous novel cures correlated to these aberrations have been discovered in wound repair with differing achievements [9].

5. Administration of mesenchymal stem cells (MSC) in DFUs

As previously described, DFUs are one of the more frequent and severe difficulties of DM, as wound repair is weakened in the diabetic foot. Investigations concentrated on comprehensively understanding these functions could allow for a precisely directed cure for DFUs. The main treatments for DFUs are currently wound debridement, weight off-loading, neovascularization, and contamination treatment. Nevertheless, some DFUs are extremely impervious to routine cures, and the development of wound repair remains to be the goal of numerous cure policies. Novel cure choices such as bioengineered skin substitutes, ECM proteins, cytokines, and negative pressure wound therapy, have been developed as supplementary remedies for DFUs [12]. Stem cell therapies have appeared as top-notch cure methods with the possibility of returning tissue to its pre-injury state.

The use of cellular therapy in the treatment of skin injuries is presently a dynamic field of research. Multi-potent adult stem cells are an attractive option for cell therapy, as they have a high possibility of proliferation and the capability of differentiating into diverse cell types and creating a range of cytokines and growth factors essential to wound repair. This study concentrated on the involvement of three types of adult stem cell populations through a skin injury repair course and their beneficial possibilities for use in cell therapy.

Endothelial progenitor cells (EPCs) are endothelial precursors involved in the revascularization of injured tissue and tissue repair. Their vascular repairing potentials have been described in a range of translational and human investigations into ischemic illnesses, together with myocardial infarction, stroke, and peripheral arterial illness. Furthermore, numerous articles have stated that EPC engraftment can enhance wound repair by improving new blood vessel formation in granulation tissue. It has been reported that the administrated EPCs released a variety of wound repair-related growth factors and cytokines, thus encouraging the implementation of monocyte/macrophage and exciting endogenous new blood vessel formation during the course of skin injury repair. Another study showed that the transplantation of human cluster of differentiation (CD) 133^+ progenitor cells into streptozotocin-induced diabetic mice amplified the wound closure rate and capillary density in granulation tissues. These results suggest that EPC engraftment would be favorable for the cure of skin wounds, specifically chronic wounds which are often connected with reduced peripheral blood flow and continue to be tough to heal using existing beneficial tactics [13].

Bone marrow-derived mesenchymal stem cells (BM-MSCs), comprise another talented nominee for the reparation or substitution of injured tissue. BM-MSCs have the ability to differentiate into numerous lineages, such as endothelial cells, neural cells, and hepatocytes, among others. Furthermore, research has shown that BM-MSCs participate in wound repair by differentiating into numerous cutaneous cell types. It has further been reported that BM-MSCs differentiate into keratinocytes, endothelial cells, pericytes, and monocytes. One study reported that BM-MSCs significantly improved wound repair in both diabetic and nondiabetic mice; BM-MSC-treated wounds displayed augmented wound contraction by discharging proangiogenic elements including VEGF and angiopoietin-1. Analysis of paracrine elements released from BM-MSCs with real-time polymerase chain reaction (PCR) and of BM-MSC-CM by enzyme-linked immunosorbent assay (ELISA) showed that BM-MSCs secreted VEGF, IGF-1, epidermal growth factor (EGF), keratinocyte growth factor (KGF), angiopoietin-1, and stromal derived factor (SDF)-1. These paracrine elements from MSC-condition media (CM) displayed a pronounced influence in utilizing $CD14^+$ monocytes, keratinocytes, and endothelial cells in injured tissue, thus encouraging the skin injury repair course [13].

6. Adipose tissue-derived stem cells (ADSCs)

ADSCs are placed inside the stromal vascular fraction of adipose tissue. They have the ability to differentiate into adipogenic, osteogenic, chondrogenic, and myogenic cells when they are cultivated in particular culture circumstances. New information has shown the possible effects of ADSCs on new blood vessel formation in ischemic illness animal simulation. ADSCs discharge numerous powerful antigenic elements and were also shown to collaborate in angiogenesis by differentiating into endothelial cells in an *in vivo* study. The engraftment of ADSCs is reported to encourage wound contraction and enhance blood perfusion in injured skin. When ADSCs were cultivated in hypoxic circumstances, they released VEGF 5-time more than in normoxic circumstances [13].

In regenerative medicine, adult stem cells are the greatest encouraging cell types for cell-based therapies. Human adipose tissue has been presented as a novel origin for multipotent stem cells. These so-named ADSCs are considered perfect for use in regenerative therapies. Their chief benefit over MSC extracted from other origins, e.g., from bone marrow, is that they can be simply and repeatable collected using negligibly aggressive methods with little injury. ADSCs are multipotent and can differentiate into numerous cell types. Interestingly, ADSCs are categorized by immunosuppressive properties and have little immunogenicity. Their discharge of trophic elements make compulsory the healing and regenerative results in an extensive variety of administrations. Generally, these specific characteristics of ADSCs make them very much applicable for medical uses. Therefore, the beneficial probability of ADSCs is huge [13].

7. Regenerative potential of adipose tissue-derived stem cells

The beneficial impacts of ADSCs have been determined to be valuable in regenerative therapies for many illnesses. Specifically, ADSCs can be collected, handled, and cultured in a nominally aggressive, yet calm and persuasive method, and they have the great probability of differentiating into mature cells along the mesodermal, ectodermal, and endodermal lineages. Throughout recent years, crucial advancements have been made concerning the separation, morphological features, molecular biology, and in vitro differentiation potential of stem cells, and it has become clear that ADSCs might facilitate beneficial effects. Not only do they act as tissue-specific progenitor cells, but they also participate in a number of chief functions, e.g., paracrine-mediated signaling of angiogenesis, inflammation, cell homing, and cell survival. The above-mentioned essential results have assisted us in gradually closing the hole between basic knowledge and clinical application; meanwhile, ADSCs have been used in clinical trials all over the globe, presenting as harmless and realistic options in a range of simulations.

Nevertheless, before ADSCs can be used in conventional medical administrations, numerous obvious queries associated with ADSCs must be resolved. With the intention of fully appreciating the fundamental functions which control ADSCs, future experimentations should, for example, concentrate on additional accurate markers for the improved and source-precise classification of ADSCs. Moreover, the genetic alteration of ex vivo-cultivated cells should not be ignored, and the controllers concerning differentiation, migration, and cell viability after in vivo engraftment must be clarified. Furthermore, as the scientific comprehension of the regenerative capabilities and, therefore, the potential uses of ADSCs increases, the possible dangerous threats must be addressed, and the supervisory outline that directs their medical usage must be established. Presently, precise supervisory instructions are set by the country in which treatment occurs. Clearly, the worldwide standardization of rules of use is crucial. In conclusion, scientific advancements, supervisory rules, and a commercial substructure are all vital factors in the development and conversion of this talented MSC origin [14].

Conversely, there are some methodological questions for the application of MSCs and ADSCs for skin regeneration in DM patients, as discussed below.

1. The elevated extracellular glucose density in diabetic wounds leads to the collection of advanced glycosylation end products (AGEs). The creation

of AGEs prevents proliferation, leads to hADSCs apoptosis, prevents the differentiation, proliferation, and homeostasis of ADSCs into endothelial cells, and also prevents the production of collagen protein, ultimately hindering wound repair [15].

2. Despite the rising usage of MSCs in medicinal human research, the curative benefit continues to be insignificant [16]. This is partially related to the normal, limited disease-modifying ability of MSCs [16]. At the same time, tissue destruction and the remedial response lead to the excretion of interior danger signals [17], comprising Toll-like receptors (TLRs) and interleukin-1 receptors, type 1 (IL-1R1) ligands, that alter the immune microenvironment [18]. TLRs and IL-1R1 unfavorably impress the cure of numerous injured organs [19]. IL-1R1/myeloid differentiation primary response 88 (MYD88) signaling unfavorably regulates bone repair in mice by injuring the regenerative abilities of murine MSCs. Furthermore, IL-1b that is released at bone injury areas inhibits the regenerative abilities of MSCs [20]. Thus, new approaches to increasing the strength of MSCs is an active area of life science research with medical importance [16]. MSCs have been one of the profoundly investigated options for cell therapy. As the homing ability of MSCs is a key influential element of effective MSC-based cures, the progress of homing effectiveness is important for creating faultless, positive outcomes. Therefore, tactics to stimulate and reinforce the function, mobilization, and homing of MSCs have advanced a key option in regenerative medicine [21].

3. Stem cell numbers have been reduced in some animal simulations of skin damage. Wu et al. observed a significant rise in the survival of stem cells 7 days after inducing skin damage and a quick reduction in cell viability 14 days after damage [22]. Muhammad et al. presented that the engraftment of ADSCs hastens the course of acid burn skin injury repair [23].

8. PBM and its effect on cells and stem cells

The term "LASER" originated as an acronym for "light amplification by stimulated emission of radiation." Laser radiation could encourage a photobiomodulatory impact on cells and tissues, participating in a concentrating inflection of cell behaviors, increasing the courses of tissue repair. PBM, also recognized by its former term low-level laser therapy (LLLT), is a safe technique that participates in pain reduction and decreases inflammation, along with improving cure and tissue healing. It also encourages cell propagation and increases stem cell differentiation [24]. PBM is a fast-developing technology applied many medical situations where stimulus of repair, decrease in pain and inflammation, and renovation of action are needed. While skin is obviously exposed to light more than any other organ, it still reacts fine to red and near-infrared wavelengths. The photons are absorbed by mitochondrial chromophores in skin cells. Therefore, electron transport, adenosine triphosphate nitric oxide release, blood flow, ROS increase, and various signaling paths are triggered. Stem cells can be activated, permitting augmented tissue repair and healing [25]. PBM, with its above-mentioned properties, can mediate numerous illnesses and circumstances, such as DM, brain damage, spinal cord injury, dermatological circumstances, oral annoyance, and diverse fields in dentistry. Most studies have reported a rise in the propagation ratio of radiated cells [24]. PBM definitely controlled the in vitro propagation of the ADSC examined, and new in vitro documents have been presented where PBM meaningfully augmented hADSCs cell survival in comparison to control and PBM-treated hBM-MSC groups [26].

9. How the combined application of PBM and ADSCs can accelerate DFU healing

Concerning the low viability ratio of ADSCs transplanted onto a wound, the application of some superior pretreatment agents not only makes available a good biological circumstance for the transplanted ADSC, but also encourages their propagation, differentiation, and paracrine capabilities and causes them to discharge more cytokines and growth factors [27]. Because PBM can augment the proliferation ratio of cultivated ADSCs [26], it can be considered as an effective approach for the preconditioning of ADSCs in in vitro situations preceding ADSC transplantation. In Zare et al. study [26] both in vitro human bone marrow-derived mesenchymal stem cells (hBM-MSCs) and h adipose-derived stem cells (hADSCs) were irradiated with 36 protocols using two different laser types (helium-neon [He-Ne] and diodes), four different laser wavelengths (HeNe laser, 630 nm, 810 nm, 630 + 810 nm); three different energy densities (0.6 J/cm^2, 1.2 J/cm^2, 2.4 J/cm^2); and three different PBM times (1, 2, and 3). A total of 1×10^4 MSCs were seeded in each well of a 24 well-plate. Next, the He–Ne laser at 632.8 nm, (IR-2000; IAEA, Tehran, Iran), red laser at 630 nm, NIR laser at 810 nm, and 630 nm +810 nm (NILTVIR202 Noura Instruments, Tehran, Iran) were applied. It should be mentioned that immediately after switched on the laser machine, it was ready for PBM therapy. In order to ensure exposure of the entire well (15.6 mm well) to PBM, the He–Ne laser emission was expanded by an optic culminator and the spot size of the red and NIR lasers were increased by a cone shaped pine hole culminator. Control MSCs did not receive PBM. **Table 1** lists the PBM protocol specifications.

Zare et al. study [26] demonstrated that PBM with the combined 630 + 810 nm lasers significantly stimulated 3-(4,5-dimethylthiazol-2-yl)-2,5-diphenyltetrazolium bromide (MTT) assay which was measured the effects of PBM on MSC viability, and significantly decreased population doubling time (PDT) and apoptosis rate of hBM-MSCs and hASDCs in vitro. There were no pharmacological side effects of PBM on MSC as evidenced by measuring apoptosis rate of MSCs. Zare et al. reported new in vitro evidence where PBM administered at 630 nm (one and two times, 0.6 and 1.2 J/cm^2) and 630 + 810 nm (three times, 2.4 J/cm^2) significantly increased hADSC cell viability compared to its control and the PBM-treated hBM-MSC groups. PBM-based medical trials and experiments will display new uses for PBM and MSC remedies [28].

Laser type	Wavelength (nm)	Power (W)	Duration of each session (s)	Energy density (J/cm^2)	Laser beam diameter (cm)	Laser beam area (cm^2)	Power density (W/cm^2)
He-Ne	632.8	0.005	229, 458, 917	0.6, 1.2, 2.4	1.56	1.91	0.00261
Red	630	0.05	23, 46, 92	0.6, 1.2, 2.4	1.56	1.91	0.0261
Near infrared (NIR)	810	0.05	23, 46, 92	0.6, 1.2, 2.4	1.56	1.91	0.0261

Table 1.
Specifications of the photobiomodulation (PBM) protocol.

Accordingly, Ahmadi et al. examined the efficiency of several preconditioned ADSCs and PBM regimes on healing an infected ischemic delayed-healing wound in type 1 diabetic rats. Their study included five groups of rats: (1) control, (2) control ADSCs [diabetic ADSCs were engrafted into the wound bed], (3) ADSCs + PBM in vivo (diabetic ADSCs were transplanted into the wound, followed by in vivo PBM therapy), (4) ADSCs + PBM in vitro, and (5) ADSCs + PBM in vitro + in vivo.

Ahmadi et al. for in vitro study seeded a total of 1×10^4 passage-4 ADSCs in each well of a 24-well plate for each of three groups: healthy control ADSC, diabetic control ADSC, and experimental diabetic ADSC. Here, red laser alone plus infrared laser alone (NILTVIR202 Noura Instruments, Tehran, Iran) at two energy densities (1.2 J/cm^2 and 2.4 J/cm^2) were used to irradiate the ADSC every other day for three sessions according to a previously published protocol. Ahmadi et al. found that diabetic ADSCs preconditioned with PBM had significantly increased the MSC viability, and significantly decreased PDT, and apoptotic rate of ADSCs in comparison with diabetic ADSCs. **Table 2** lists the in vitro, and in vivo PBM parameters. The control ADS did not receive PBM. The wounds of the rats in groups 3 and 5 were subjected to PBM in vivo (**Figure 1**).

Specifications of in vitro photobiomodulation							
Laser type	**Wavelength (nm)**	**Power (W)**	**Time of each session (s)**	**Energy density (J/cm^2)**	**Laser beam diameter (cm)**	**Laser beam area (cm^2)**	**Power density (W/cm^2)**
Red	630	0.05	46	1.2	1.56	1.91	0.0261
Near infrared	810	0.05	46	1.2	1.56	1.91	0.0261

Specifications of in vivo photobiomodulation	
Parameters	**Dose and unit**
Peak power output	75 W
Average power	0.001 W
Power density	0.001 W/cm^2
Wavelength	890 nm
Wavelength range of the device	890 ± 10 nm
Pulse frequency	80 Hz
Spot size	1 cm^2
Diameter	1.12 cm
Pulsed duration	180 ns
Duration of exposure for each point	200 s
Energy density	0.2 J/cm^2
Number of laser shootings in each session	9
Energy densities for one session and for the total sessions	1.8 and 25.2 J/cm^2
PBM radiation scheduling	Immediately after surgery, 6 days per week, for 16 consecutive days
Probe	L07
Company	MUSTANG 2000, Technica Co., Russia

Table 2.
Specifications of in vitro and in vivo photobiomodulation parameters.

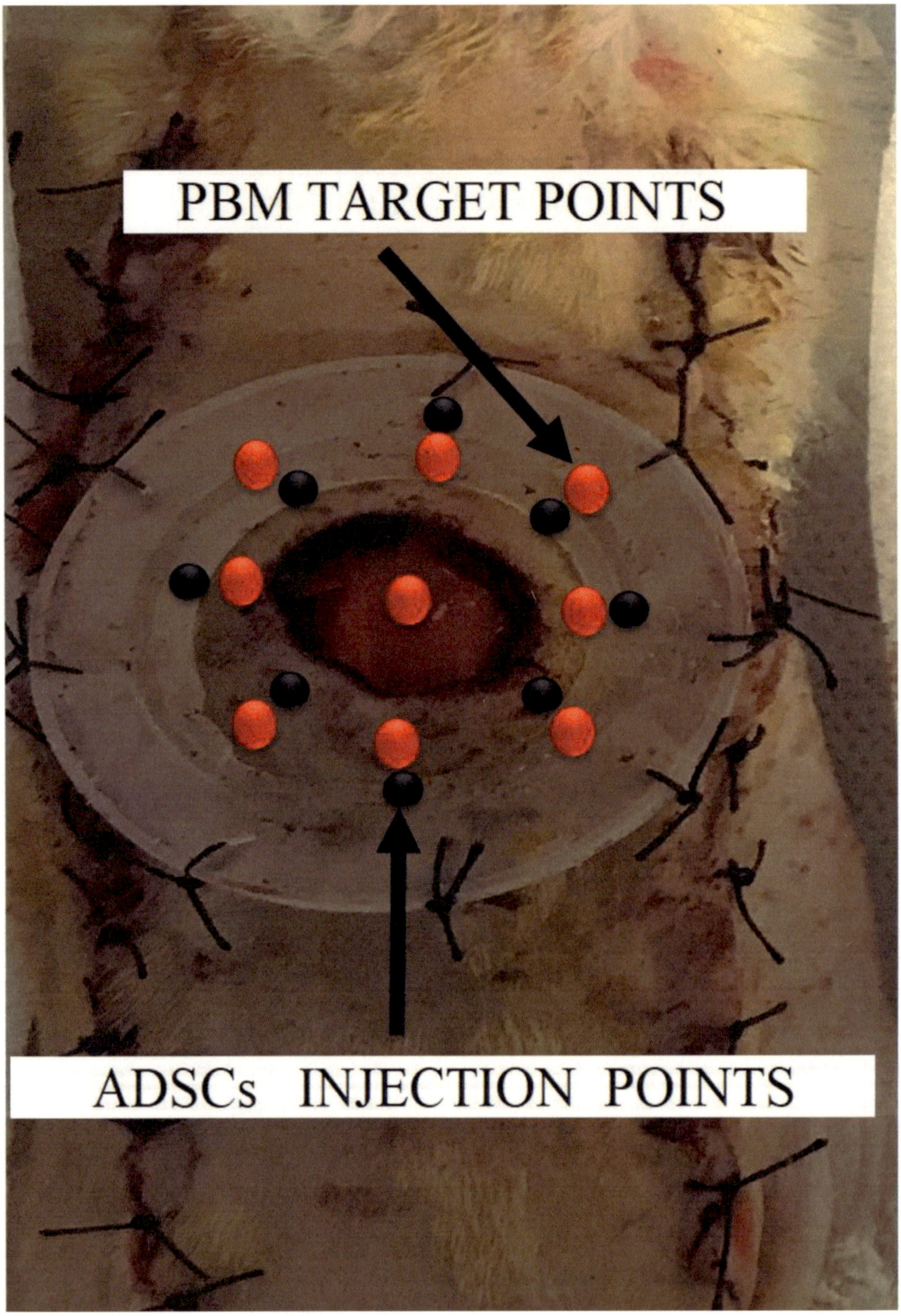

Figure 1.
A photo of the wound, photobiomodulation (PBM) target points, and adipose tissue -derived stem cell (ADSCs) injection points.

Table 2 lists the complete specifications of the PBM protocols for invitro and in vivo studies. There were no pharmacological side effects of PBM on MSC in Ahmadi et al. study as evidenced by histological examination of wounds.

Groups 3 and 5 showed significant reductions in bacterial contamination compared to groups 1 and 2. Groups 2, 3, 4, and 5 showed significantly enhanced wound contraction ratios in comparison with group 1. Groups 2–5 displayed significantly increased wound strength compared to group 1.In most cases, group 5 had significantly better results than groups 2, 3, and 4. Ahmadi et al. concluded that preconditioning diabetic ADSCs with PBM in vitro plus PBM in vivo significantly accelerated healing in the diabetic rat model of an ischemic infected delayed-healing wound [29]. In other related studies, the same results were reported. Khosravi et al. reported that the in vitro preconditioning of hADSCs with PBM significantly amplified bone repair in a rat model of critical size femoral defect in vivo [30]. Liao et al. explored the therapeutic potential of hADSCs preconditioned with PBM. Cultured ADSCs were treated with PBM. In addition, a mouse photoaged skin simulation was proven by UVB radiation. Liao et al. concluded that PBM is a persuasive bioenhancer of ADSCs and may improve the healing possibility of ADSCs for medical use [31]. While few studies give some evidence for the positive effects of PBM alone for wounds in diabetic patients [32], or PBM plus skin grafts for burn ulcers in diabetic patients [33, 34], there have been no clinical trials using human models to show stem cells plus PBM as an effective agent in wound care regimes to date. Further well designed clinical trials are necessary to determine the true value of ADSCs plus PBM in routine wound care regimes for patients with DM.

10. Conclusions

Present knowledge dictates that when an organ is healthy, the inflammatory phase of wound healing is well orchestrated, lasting only a few days, and the steps of tissue repair proceed normally. However, when an organ is hyperglycemic, as with DM, the inflammatory process is extended, the integrity of the skin is not restored, and DFU occurs. DFUs are a serious clinical problem and affect millions of people around the world. They need repetitious cures, impose extensive medical expenses, and create a major economic burden on healthcare systems worldwide. Thus, much work has been concentrated on evolving new healing approaches for wound treatment. Preclinical studies have shown that preconditioning diabetic ADSCs with PBM in vitro significantly increases ADSC function over that of diabetic ADSCs. Preconditioning diabetic ADSC with PBM significantly hastened healing in ischemic MRSA–infected, delayed-healing wounds in rats with type one DM compared to the control, ADSC alone, and ADSC plus PBM-in vivo rats. The combined administration of preconditioned diabetic-ADSC with PBM plus PBM therapy in vivo demonstrated a significantly superior effect compared to other treatment protocols [29].

Whereas our hypothesis (combined application of PBM and stem cells can accelerate repairing process and assist healing DFU in animal models and patients) was confirmed through preclinical studies [29, 30, 31], we suggest further animal and clinical trial investigations be conducted in order to provide more documentation. Hopefully these outcomes would help the use of ADSCs plus PBM as a routine treatment protocol for the healing of severe DFU in patients with DM.

We confirm there were no conflicts of interest.

Author details

Mohammad Bayat[1,2*] and Sufan Chien[2]

1 Department of Biology and Anatomical Sciences, School of Medicine, Shahid Beheshti University of Medical Sciences, Tehran, Iran

2 Price Institute of Surgical Research, University of Louisville, and Noveratech LLC of Louisville, United States

*Address all correspondence to: bayat_m@yahoo.com

References

[1] W.H. Organization, Global report on diabetes, (2016).

[2] C. New, report: more than 100 million Americans have diabetes or prediabetes, Centers for Disease Control and Prevention 2017Available from: https:// www. cdc. gov/media/releases/2017/ p0718-diabetes-report. html (2017).

[3] L. Yazdanpanah, H. Shahbazian, I. Nazari, H.R. Arti, F. Ahmadi, S.E. Mohammadianinejad, B. Cheraghian, S. Hesam, Incidence and risk factors of diabetic foot ulcer: a population-based diabetic foot cohort (ADFC study)—two-year follow-up study, International journal of endocrinology, 2018:7631659. doi: 10.1155/2018/7631659.

[4] T.N. Demidova-Rice, M.R. Hamblin, I.M. Herman, Acute and impaired wound healing: pathophysiology and current methods for drug delivery, part 1: normal and chronic wounds: biology, causes, and approaches to care, Advances in skin & wound care 2015;25:304. DOI: 10.1097/01. ASW.0000416006.55218.d0

[5] P. Martin, R. Nunan, Cellular and molecular mechanisms of repair in acute and chronic wound healing, British Journal of Dermatology.2015; 173:2015: 370-378. DOI: 10.1111/bjd.13954

[6] S. Patel, S. Srivastava, M.R. Singh, D. Singh, Mechanistic insight into diabetic wounds: Pathogenesis, molecular targets and treatment strategies to pace wound healing. Biomedicine & Pharmacotherapy.2019; 112: 108615. DOI: 10.1016/j.biopha.2019.108615

[7] S. Noor, M. Zubair, J. Ahmad, Diabetic foot ulcer—a review on pathophysiology, classification and microbial etiology, Diabetes & Metabolic Syndrome: Clinical Research & Reviews. 2015; 9: 192-199. DOI: 10.1016/j.dsx.2015.04.007

[8] M.E. Levin, L. O'Neal, The diabetic foot: pathophysiology, evaluation, and treatment, The diabetic foot. 1988, 1-50.

[9] T.I. Oliver, M. Mutluoglu, Diabetic foot ulcer, StatPearls [Internet], StatPearls Publishing, 2019.

[10] I. Kruse, S. Edelman, Evaluation and treatment of diabetic foot ulcers, Clinical diabetes. 2006;24 : 91-93. DOI: 10.1177/014572179902500408

[11] R.G. Frykberg, J. Banks, Management of diabetic foot ulcers: a review, Federal Practitioner. 2016; 33: 16. PMCID: PMC6368931.

[12] D. Baltzis, I. Eleftheriadou, A. Veves, Pathogenesis and treatment of impaired wound healing in diabetes mellitus: new insights, Advances in therapy. 2014; 31: 817-836. DOI: 10.1007/ s12325-014-0140-x

[13] J.Y. Kim, W. Suh, Stem cell therapy for dermal wound healing, International journal of stem cells. 2010; 3: 29. DOI: 10.15283/ijsc.2010.3.1.29

[14] L. Frese, P.E. Dijkman, S.P. Hoerstrup, Adipose tissue-derived stem cells in regenerative medicine, Transfusion Medicine and Hemotherapy.2016; 43: 268-274. doi: 10.1159/ 000448180.

[15] J.-H. Gong, J.-Y. Dong, T. Xie, S.-L. Lu, The influence of AGEs environment on proliferation, apoptosis, homeostasis, and endothelial cell differentiation of human adipose stem cells, The International Journal of Lower Extremity Wounds. 2017; 16: 94-103. DOI: 10.1177/1534734617701575

[16] J. Abdi, I. Rashedi, A. Keating, Concise Review: TLR pathway-miRNA interplay in mesenchymal stromal cells: regulatory roles and therapeutic directions, Stem cells 36 (2018) 1655-1662. DOI: 10.1002/stem.2902

[17] J. Pugin, How tissue injury alarms the immune system and causes a systemic inflammatory response syndrome, Annals of intensive care. 2012; 2: 27. DOI: 10.1186/2110-5820-2-27

[18] S. Basith, B. Manavalan, T.H. Yoo, S.G. Kim, S. Choi, Roles of toll-like receptors in cancer: a double-edged sword for defense and offense, Archives of pharmacal research. 2012; 35: 1297-1316. 10.1007/s12272-012-0802-7

[19] Z. Julier, A.J. Park, P.S. Briquez, M.M. Martino, Promoting tissue regeneration by modulating the immune system, Acta biomaterialia.2017; 53; 13-28. DOI: 10.1016/j.actbio.2017.01.056

[20] M.M. Martino, K. Maruyama, G.A. Kuhn, T. Satoh, O. Takeuchi, R. Müller, S. Akira, Inhibition of IL-1R1/MyD88 signalling promotes mesenchymal stem cell-driven tissue regeneration, Nature communications. 2016; 7: 11051. DOI: 10.1038/ncomms11051

[21] W. Lin, L. Xu, S. Zwingenberger, E. Gibon, S.B. Goodman, G. Li, Mesenchymal stem cells homing to improve bone healing, Journal of orthopaedic translation. 2017; 9: 19-27. DOI: 10.1016/j.jot.2017.03.002

[22] Y. Wu, L. Chen, P.G. Scott, E.E. Tredget, Mesenchymal stem cells enhance wound healing through differentiation and angiogenesis, Stem cells. 2007; 25: 2648-2659. DOI: 10.1634/stemcells.2007-0226

[23] G. Muhammad, J. Xu, J.W. Bulte, A. Jablonska, P. Walczak, M. Janowski, Transplanted adipose-derived stem cells can be short-lived yet accelerate healing of acid-burn skin wounds: a multimodal imaging study, Scientific reports. 2017; 7: 1-11. DOI: 10.1038/s41598-017-04484-0

[24] C. Dompe, L. Moncrieff, J. Matys, K. Grzech-Leśniak, I. Kocherova, A. Bryja, M. Bruska, M. Dominiak, P. Mozdziak, T.H.I. Skiba, Photobiomodulation—Underlying Mechanism and Clinical Applications, Journal of Clinical Medicine. 2020; 9: 1724. DOI: 10.3390/jcm9061724

[25] P. Avci, A. Gupta, M. Sadasivam, D. Vecchio, Z. Pam, N. Pam, M.R. Hamblin, Low-level laser (light) therapy (LLLT) in skin: stimulating, healing, restoring, Seminars in cutaneous medicine and surgery, NIH Public Access., 2013: 41. PMID: 24049929.

[26] F. Zare, A. Moradi, S. Fallahnezhad, S.K. Ghoreishi, A. Amini, S. Chien, M. Bayat, Photobiomodulation with 630 plus 810 nm wavelengths induce more in vitro cell viability of human adipose stem cells than human bone marrow-derived stem cells, J Photochem Photobiol B. 2019;201: 111658. DOI: 10.1016/j.jphotobiol.2019.111658

[27] P. Li, X. Guo, A review: therapeutic potential of adipose-derived stem cells in cutaneous wound healing and regeneration, Stem Cell Research & Therapy. 2018; 9:) 302. doi: 10.1186/s13287-018-1044-5.

[28] T. Kushibiki, T. Hirasawa, S. Okawa, M. Ishihara, Low reactive level laser therapy for mesenchymal stromal cells therapies, Stem cells international. 2015;2015:974864. doi: 10.1155/2015/974864.

[29] H. Ahmadi, A. Amini, F. Fadaei Fathabady, A. Mostafavinia, F. Zare, R. Ebrahimpour-Malekshah, M.N. Ghalibaf, M. Abrisham, F. Rezaei, R. Albright, S.K. Ghoreishi, S. Chien, M. Bayat, Transplantation of photobiomodulation-preconditioned diabetic stem cells accelerates ischemic wound healing in diabetic rats, Stem Cell Res Ther. 2010; 11: 494. doi: 10.1186/s13287-020-01967-2

[30] A. Khosravipour, A. Amini, R. Masteri Farahani, F. Zare, A. Mostafavinia, S. Fallahnezhad, S. Akbarzade, P. Ava, M. Asgari, A.

Mohammadbeigi, F. Rezaei, S.K. Ghoreishi, S. Chien, M. Bayat, Preconditioning adipose-derived stem cells with photobiomodulation significantly increased bone healing in a critical size femoral defect in rats, Biochem Biophys Res Commun. 2020; 531 : 105-111. 10.1016/j.bbrc.2020.07.048.

[31] X. Liao, S.H. Li, G.H. Xie, S. Xie, L.L. Xiao, J.X. Song, H.W. Liu, Preconditioning With Low-Level Laser Irradiation Enhances the Therapeutic Potential of Human Adipose-derived Stem Cells in a Mouse Model of Photoaged Skin, Photochemistry and photobiology 94 (2018) 780-790. doi: 10.1111/php.12912.

[32] M.C. Feitosa, A.F. Carvalho, V.C. Feitosa, I.M. Coelho, R.A. Oliveira, E. Arisawa, Effects of the Low-Level Laser Therapy (LLLT) in the process of healing diabetic foot ulcers, Acta Cir Bras. 2015; 30: 852-857. doi: 10.1590/S0102-865020150120000010.

[33] M. Dahmardehei, N. Kazemikhoo, R. Vaghardoost, S. Mokmeli, M. Momeni, M.A. Nilforoushzadeh, F. Ansari, A. Amirkhani, Effects of low level laser therapy on the prognosis of split-thickness skin graft in type 3 burn of diabetic patients: a case series, Lasers Med Sci. 2016; 31: 497-502. doi: 10.1007/s10103-016-1896-9.

[34] R. Vaghardoost, M. Momeni, N. Kazemikhoo, S. Mokmeli, M. Dahmardehei, F. Ansari, M.A. Nilforoushzadeh, P. Sabr Joo, S. Mey Abadi, S. Naderi Gharagheshlagh, S. Sassani, Effect of low-level laser therapy on the healing process of donor site in patients with grade 3 burn ulcer after skin graft surgery (a randomized clinical trial), Lasers Med Sci.2018; 33: 603-607. doi: 10.1007/s10103-017-2430-4.

Chapter 5

Chronic Venous Ulcer

Walid A.M. Ganod

Abstract

This chapter sheds light on the cause and effect of chronic venous ulcers (CVUs) and the therapeutic procedures used to treat them. In the last two decades, many changes have occurred in the strategy of wound management through the development of adjunctive therapy that supports wound healing. Eventually, the latest development in platelet concentration technology produced platelet-rich fibrin (PRF). It was categorized as the second-generation platelet concentration family after platelet-rich plasma (PRP). Venous leg ulcers (VLUs) account for 70% of all leg ulcers and are estimated to affect 1% of the population; prevalence increases with age. The chronicity and refractory nature of venous ulcers have a great effect on the quality of life (QoL) and work productivity of patients, in addition to the expenditure of significant medical resources and efforts. Therefore, the goal of VLU management is to induce rapid healing without recurrence, which mainly helps to improve QoL. The first therapeutic procedure used in the treatment of VLU was compression therapy, in which the application of effective graduated compression decreased the overload in the venous system and venous reflux. Furthermore, it accelerated the capillary blood flow and decreased capillary fluid leakage, which alleviated limb edema.

Keywords: venous ulcer, ambulatory venous hypertension, chronic venous insufficiency, compression therapy, platelet-rich fibrin

1. Introduction

Chronic leg ulcers (CLUs) are chronic wounds that do not show a tendency to heal within a reasonable period. This period can determine the state of a chronic wound; if there is no tendency to heal after 3 months or if the wound does not fully heal after 12 months, the ulcer is determined to be chronic [1]. The aforementioned period is not a fixed number; it is governed by other factors, such as ulcer ethology, size, and so on [2].

In general, ulcers can be described in many ways; for instance, ulcers have a full-thickness wound, lack a source of re-epithelization in the center, and show poor tendency to heal.

The most common clinical cause of CLUs is venous insufficiency followed by arterial insufficiency, diabetes, or a combination of two or more of these factors [3].

The Wound Healing Society described chronic wounds as "a silent epidemic disorder" correlated to the percentage of the public with this condition. In the United States, approximately 6.5 million patients suffer from chronic nonhealed wounds. Therefore, two million working days are lost annually. In addition, in the United Kingdom, the annual incidence of leg ulcers has been estimated to be 3.5 per 1000 individuals [4].

Venous insufficiency is considered the most common cause of leg ulcers, accounting for 70% of leg ulcers. Inline arterial diseases and mixed venous and arterial disorders account for 10 and 15% of ulcers, respectively. There is a major challenge in the assessment and diagnosis of CLU in regard to miscellaneous disorders such as vasculitis and hematological diseases. These kinds of disorders represent the remaining 5% of the causes of CLUs [5].

Scottish guidelines define a chronic venous leg ulcer as "an open lesion between the knee and the ankle joint that remains unhealed for at least 4 weeks and occurs in the presence of venous disease" [6].

2. Anatomy of venous system in lower limbs

The anatomical variation and nonuniform nomenclature of the lower limb vein system, especially in the literature, supported the constitution of the International Interdisciplinary Committee in 2001 to perform adjustment and uniformity of the anatomical terminology of lower limb veins (**Figure 1**) [8].

The veins of the lower limb can be classified into three systems: superficial, deep, and perforator veins (**Figure 2**). These veins are arranged into two main compartments: superficial and deep compartments. A superficial compartment is present between the skin and muscular fascia, which contain superficial veins. A deep compartment that contains deep veins is present under the deep fascia. The perforator veins are connected to the superficial and deep system [9]. **Figure 3** shows that there is another compartment within the superficial compartment enclosing the saphenous vein, which is called the saphenous compartment.

The principle method for venous return from the lower limb is through the deep vein system, which pairs below the knee and accompanies arteries and then joins to form the popliteal vein that completely ascends as the femoral vein. The main veins in the superficial system that are the target of many venous therapies are the great saphenous vein and small saphenous veins, which are connected with communicator veins [10].

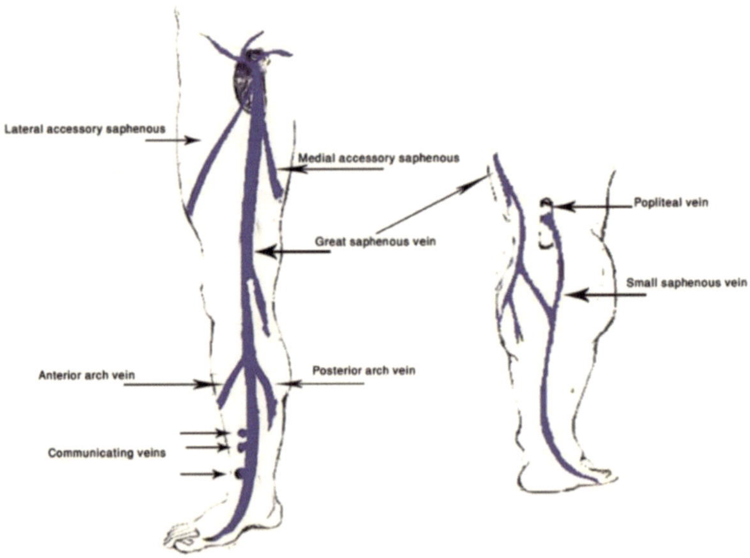

Figure 1.
Diagram of the superficial venous system of lower limbs [7].

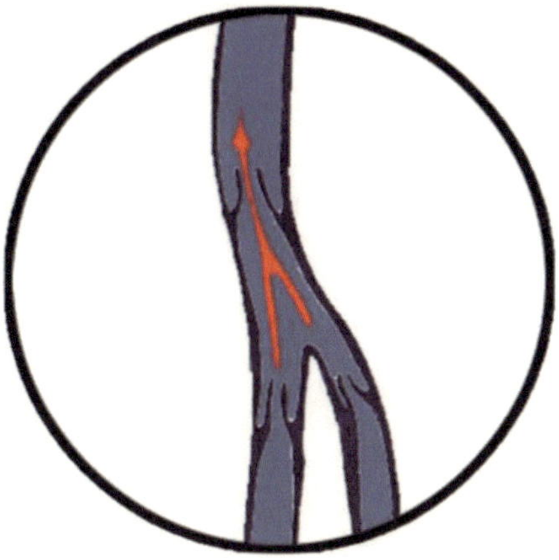

Figure 2.
Normal vein valve.

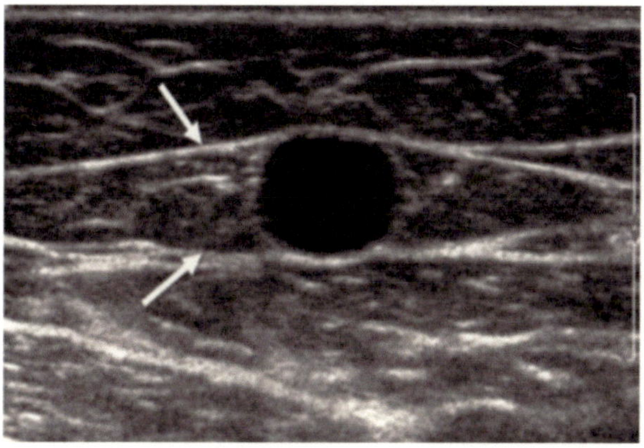

Figure 3.
Ultrasound image of the saphenous compartment.

The perforator veins have normal unidirectional flow from the superficial to deep system, and there are more than 150 perforators in the lower extremities, but most of them are inactive in the normal state. Perforator veins on the medial aspect of the leg represent the most clinically important perforators in chronic vein insufficiency [11].

Valves of lower extremity veins are anatomical features that have clinical importance in cases of incompetence of these valves, transmission of venous pressure to skin venules, and development of skin changes [12].

3. Physiology of lower limb venous system

The venous system functions to support circulation by the venous return mechanism, as 60–80% of blood volume rests in the venous system (25% in the splanchnic network and other residual volumes in postcapillary venules). Therefore, venous return must be equal to cardiac output to maintain homeostasis of tissue perfusion [13]. Many factors have a role in venous return mechanisms, such as central pumps, pressure gradients, venous valves, and muscle pumps (peripheral pumps) [7].

Venous valves are distributed mainly in the distal vein circulation of the lower limb to overcome the effect of gravity and break down the hydrostatic pressure of

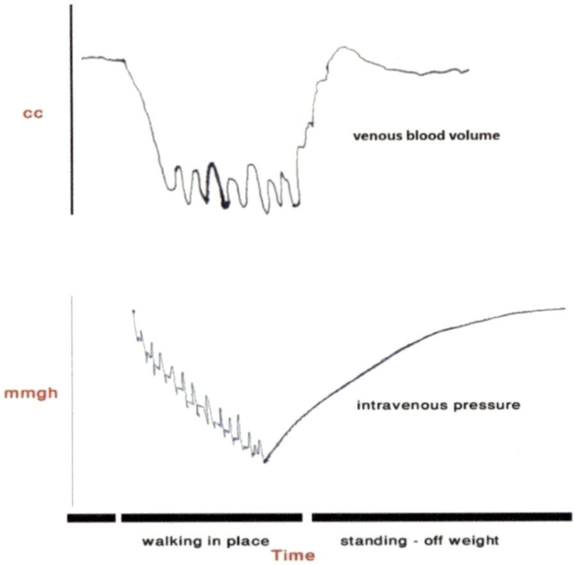

Figure 4.
Schematic summarization of the relationship between pressure and volume in the lower extremities while walking and standing. Note the efficacy of the calf muscle pumping mechanism that leads to a decrease in venous volume and pressure with walking and a slight delay in increasing venous pressure opposite to venous blood volume in the standing position. Alternation in this relationship results in high ambulatory venous pressure.

the blood column into segments. Valve closure is a passive mechanism involving a gradient pressure difference between the supra- and infravalvular segments and normal retrograde flow that lasts for less than 0.5 seconds, which is enough time to close cusps completely [12].

Calf muscle contraction (gastrocnemius and soleus) is an essential part of the mechanism of venous return, and it has been estimated that approximately 60% of venous return from the lower limb depends on the ejection force of the calf muscle. The net result of serial contraction of the calf muscle during exercise produces a streamline and unidirectional blood in the deep venous system toward the heart and improves cardiac output [12].

The efficacy of calf muscle pumps is dependent on the strength of the muscle, range of movement of the ankle joint, and competence of vein valves. We hypothesize that atrophy of the calf muscle decreases the strength of contraction, resulting in a reduction in venous return and chronic vein insufficiency that underlie the pathogenesis of venous ulcers [14].

Accumulation of blood in peripheral venous circulation during rest leads to elevation of venous pressure, especially with the standing position, while contraction of the calf muscle will decrease the venous pressure to a suitable baseline. The measurement of the drop in superficial venous system pressure after exercise is called *ambulatory venous pressure* (AVP), which is an indicator of calf muscle pump function, and an elevation above 30 mm Hg has a linear relationship with leg ulcers (**Figure 4**) [15].

4. Pathophysiology of venous ulcer

The pathophysiology behind chronic leg venous ulcers is still unclear.

Ambulatory venous hypertension (AVH) is the essential pathological factor behind venous ulcers. Venous incompetence can result from immobility, ineffective pumping mechanisms of the calf muscles, and venous valve dysfunction. In addition, venous valve dysfunction that results from venous thrombosis, phlebitis, or trauma leads to alterations in venous hemodynamics and precipitates venous hypertension [16].

Subsequently, chronic blood stasis of the lower limb venous system causes further capillary damage with inflammatory process activation. Leukocyte activation, endothelial damage, platelet aggregation, and intracellular edema are highly related to venous ulcer development and impaired wound healing [17].

4.1 Ambulatory venous hypertension

The calf muscle pump consists of the calf muscle, a superficial venous system, a deep venous system, and perforators that connect both systems. The out-flow vein of this pump is the popliteal vein. Failure of the calf muscle pump to decrease AVP leads to persistent elevation of postexercise pressure or AVH [15].

Therefore, one or more of the following pathological situations can lead to calf muscle pump dysfunction and AVH.

4.1.1 Reflux in superficial veins system

The cause behind the reflux or incompetent valve in superficial veins is still ambiguous. Currently, there is a discussion on congenital and acquired factors that may be behind the structural changes in valve cusps.

The reflux in superficial veins can be compensated with calf muscle contraction if perforator valves are competent. Secondary incompetent valves of deep and perforator veins are likely to occur with large-volume reflux post sapheno-femoral or sapheno-popliteal incompetence [12].

4.1.2 Reflux/obstruction in deep veins system

Post thrombotic damage to deep veins will result in obstruction, reflux, or both and can even lead to reflux in superficial and perforator veins later (*post thrombotic syndrome*) [12].

4.1.3 Incompetent medial calf perforator

An outward flow of incompetent perforators more than 500 milliseconds and equal to or more than 3.5 millimeters in size will have a significant hemodynamic effect with high AVH and skin changes [12].

Muscular dysfunction of the calf muscle, fixed ankle joint, and prolonged immobilization will lead to blood stasis and venous hypertension as a result of pump mechanism failure [18]. In clinical practice, these pathologies present in combination with multilevel involvement in a large group of patients.

4.2 Chronic venous disorder and chronic venous insufficiency

According to updated terminology of chronic venous disorders in the VEIN-TERM transatlantic interdisciplinary consensus document, chronic venous disorder (CVD) is defined as a wide spectrum of functional and morphological abnormalities that involve the vein system from telangiectasia to venous ulcers (C1–C6 clinical classes). The term chronic venous insufficiency (CVI) is reserved for advanced CVD (C3–C6 clinical classes) and includes moderate to severe edema, skin changes, or venous ulcers [19].

CVI is classified into two types. Primary chronic venous insufficiency occurs due to weakness or degenerative changes in wall or venous valves that started as reflux in superficial veins and proceed to perforators and deep veins later due to overload that led to dilatation in the venous wall [20].

Secondary chronic venous insufficiency, known as *post-thrombotic syndrome*, is secondary to acute DVT and later sequelae that can lead to reflux, obstruction, or both in deep veins. Additionally, it could be secondary to superficial thrombophlebitis or arteriovenous fistula [19].

4.3 Revised CEAP classification of chronic venous disorders (CVDs)

The need for clinical assessment, evaluation, and stage identification methods of CVD supported the presentation of the CEAP classification at the American Venous Forum annual meeting in 1994, which was revised in 2004 [21].

CEAP classification is a method for categorizing CVD based on:

Clinical manifestations

Ethological factors

Anatomical distribution of disease

Pathophysiological process behind this disorder (**Table 1**)

Clinical class	
C0	No venous disease
C1	Spider angioma
C2	Varicose veins
C3	Edema of venous etiology
C4	Hyperpigmentation, dermatitis, lipodermatosclerosis
C5	Healed ulceration
C6	Active ulceration
Etiology	
Ec	Congenital
Ep	Primary
Es	Secondary
En	No venous etiology identified
Anatomy	
As	Superficial veins
Ap	Perforating veins
Ad	Deep veins
An	No venous location identified
Pathology	
Pr	Reflux
Po	Obstruction
Pr,o	Reflux and obstruction
Pn	No venous pathology identified

**Each clinical class is further subclassed as "S" if symptomatic and "A" if asymptomatic.*
**The symptoms include aching, pain, tightness, skin irritation, heaviness, muscle cramps, and other symptoms relating to venous disorders.*

Table 1.
Revised CEAP classification.

5. Epidemiology of venous ulcer

According to the Edinburgh study, a cross-sectional study of a random sample, VLUs represent approximately 70% of all leg ulcers and affect 1% of the population; prevalence increases with age [22].

Development in the diagnosis and early management of varicose veins, especially with significant reflux, can decrease the prevalence of venous ulcers by 50%, as superficial vein insufficiency represents 50% of the causes of leg ulcers. The management of risk factors such as obesity has a strong relationship with venous ulcers [23].

Based on estimates of the San Diego epidemiologic study, more than 11 million men and 22 million women between the ages of 40 and 80 years in the United States have varicose veins, and more than two million adults have advanced CVD with skin changes or ulcers [24]. The incidence of postthrombotic venous ulcers has not changed in the past two decades for women and has recently increased in men [25].

6. Clinical presentation and diagnosis of CVI and venous ulcer

There is a wide spectrum of differential diagnoses for ulcers in the lower limbs. Therefore, proper management depends on determining the etiology of ulcers and managing them. Venous ulcers are the most common cause of lower limb ulcers, followed by arterial and diabetic ulcers. There are distinctive clinical presentation and physical examination findings that can help to differentiate venous ulcers from other lower extremity disorders [26].

The diagnosis of venous ulcers is generally clinical; this step in the diagnosis of venous ulcers is often neglected by physicians. Diagnosis is based on radiology reports such as color duplex ultrasonography and venography, which may be helpful in doubtful cases [27].

Inspection and palpation are essential parts of the examination and should be used to search for signs of venous disorder. Auscultation for bruit is particularly helpful in those with vascular malformation and arteriovenous fistula [27]. Examination is always performed with patients in a standing position and should focus on the size and distribution of varicose veins.

Eklof et al. defined signs present in the clinical part of CEAP classification that suggested CVI (**Figures 5–7**) [21]:

Lower limb edema: Venous hypertension edema unilaterally starts at the ankle and pitting pattern and worsens in the evening.

Eczema: Erythematous dermatitis, which is usually distributed on varicose veins because of uncontrolled CVD but can be seen anywhere in response to local management.

Skin pigmentation: Extravasated blood due to venous hypertension in the small vein leads to intradermal accumulation of hemosiderin, which causes brownish darkening of the skin around the ankle region and sometimes the leg.

Lipodermatosclerosis (LDS): This is defined by Eklof et al. as localized chronic inflammation with fibrosis in skin and subcutaneous tissue and may progress to scarring and contracture in the Achilles tendon [21]. Most authors agree that LDS is highly suggestive of severe CVI and provides clues about the poor prognosis of wound healing. LDS frequently leads to the development of venous ulcers in many cases [18].

Atrophic blanche (white atrophy): This is smooth, white atrophic plaque surrounded by dilated capillary and sometimes hyperpigmentation. It is also a sign of severe CVI and should be distinguished from healed ulcers by history, as it develops

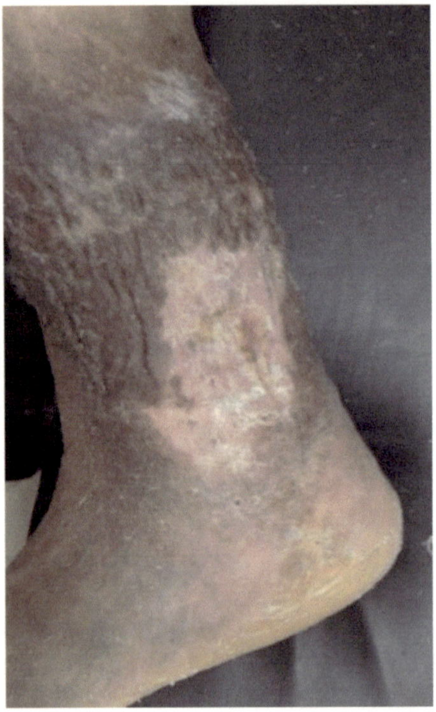

Figure 5.
Atrophie blanche.

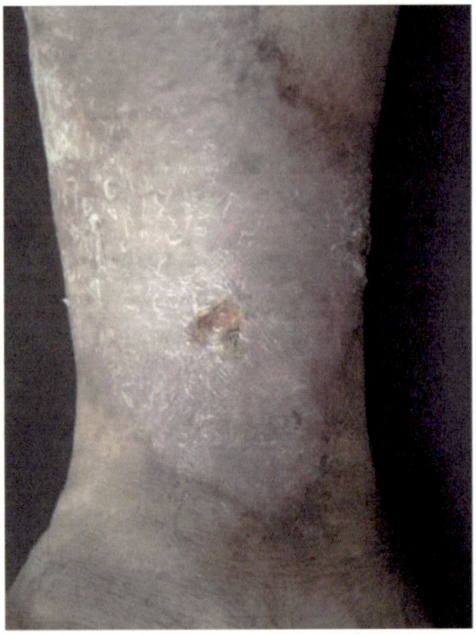

Figure 6.
Lipodermatosclerosis.

independently. Ulcerated atrophie blanche can be extremely painful and has a low tendency for healing [18].

Venous ulcer: Gillespie mentioned the most current updated definition for venous ulcer as *"a full thickness defect of the skin, located in the lower leg, typically with pigmentation and/or skin changes and presence or history of venous disease (documented*

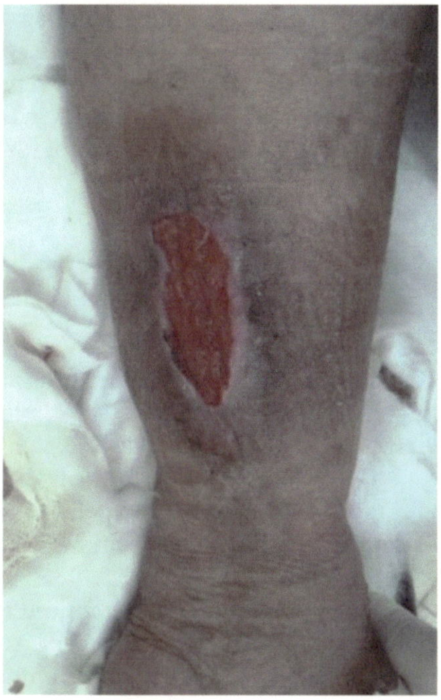

Figure 7.
Eczema.

history of DVT, documented axial venous reflux or deep vein obstruction) in the absence of another condition that could be the essential cause of the ulcer" [28].

A positive history of previous DVT events, family history of varicose veins, or previous intervention to the venous system in line with good clinical examination help to clarify the diagnosis in up to 76% of cases of venous ulcers [18]. The choice of investigation should be based on the severity of the problem and management plan. The noninvasive method is usually used to evaluate patients for venous ablation or preoperative surgery for perforators; invasive diagnostic methods should be used for patients who need complex operations, such as valve reconstruction or venous bypass [12].

The palpable pedal pulse or measurement of ankle-to-brachial blood pressure ratio (ankle/brachial index [ABI]) is one of the critical points in diagnosis of venous ulcer, as it differentiates venous ulcer from arterial ulcer and determines if there is any association of ischemic degree that contraindicated to compression therapy, which is the traditional management approach for venous ulcers. Culture swabs and investigations for vasculitis and connective tissue diseases such as rheumatoid arthritis are helpful in the diagnosis of difficult cases and resistant ulcers [18].

The atypical appearance of ulcers, such as nodular growth, everted edges, deterioration, or delayed healing with appropriate treatment, are indications for biopsy to exclude malignant transformation [29].

Duplex scanning is currently the gold standard for the evaluation of patients with CVIs. It has high sensitivity and specificity in the diagnosis of superficial and deep venous system disorders, and it provides information about the patency of the deep venous system, diameter of the vein, and flow rate. The real-time color duplex scan makes the orientation of venous flow much easier and provides information about reflux in the superficial, deep, or perforator veins. Through interpretation of all previous dates, the differentiation between primary and secondary CVIs is easy. In addition, duplex scans today have an important role in endovenous procedures [23].

Phlebography, such as ascending or descending phlebography, is not a first-line diagnostic tool in cases of venous ulcers and is preserved for evaluation of the venous system before complex procedures such as valve reconstruction or bypass, as it can provide information about the level of obstruction in the deep venous system and the state of valves [23]. CT angiogram is a useful tool for the assessment of the pelvic vein and inferior vena cava (IVC), especially before venous stenting, and MR venogram is preferred for vein malformation cases.

7. Management of venous ulcer

The management of CVUs is a major challenge in terms of healing, preventing recurrence and minimizing social and economic effects. In the Western world, approximately 1% of the annual healthcare balance is expended on venous ulcer care [22]. The future world vision directed more towards the prevention rather than the management of venous ulcers becomes more expensive over time, thus standing in the way of the 2009 Pacific Vascular Symposium's goal to decrease incidence of venous ulcer by 50% in the next 10 years [30].

The key for the management of venous ulcers is reduced AVH, which leads to a decrease in edema and inflammatory reactions in the leg, resulting in stimulated healing of ulcers and preventing recurrence if optimum venous pressure is maintained. The correction of vein disorders that lead to venous hypertension is an important step in addition to ulcer care [31]. The management of venous ulcers includes conservative (lifestyle modification, compression therapy, and ulcer care) and surgical (surgical cover of ulcer and surgical elimination of venous hypertension) procedures.

7.1 Conservative management

7.1.1 Modification of lifestyle

Theoretically, moderate exercise concentrated on mobility of the ankle joint and contraction of the calf muscle (peripheral heart) are beneficial in decreasing venous congestion of the lower limbs and hemodynamics. Although there is not a lot of evidence confirming the effect of exercise on healing venous ulcers, supervised moderate exercise should be considered as adjuvant to main treatment for CVI and venous ulcer.

Another important procedure that is not practical for patients is leg elevation at or above the level of the heart, which can decrease venous pressure around the ankle nearly to zero, resulting in an improvement in lower limb swelling and an increased ulcer healing rate. Leg elevation, if associated with compression therapy, can decrease ulcer recurrence [31].

7.1.2 Compression therapy

Compression therapy is still the cornerstone of CVI and venous ulcer care. It is defined as an applied external pressure on a specific lower limb area to overcome gravity and hydrostatic pressure in veins. The mechanism of action has not been fully understood until now. It depends on preserving interfacing pressure and stiffness (increase of interface pressure with activity as increased limb circumference by muscle contraction).

In applying compression to a patient in a normal standing position, an external pressure of 35–40 mmHg will narrow the vein; however, if pressure exceeds

60 mmHg, it will lead to occluding of the vein. As such, optimum external graduated pressure between 35 and 40 mmHg will improve venous pumping function and microcirculation. In addition, it lowers the level of inflammatory mediators, such as alpha tumor necrosis factor, which causes tissue damage. Therefore, compression promotes ulcer healing [31].

The Unna boot developed in 1885 is the oldest modality of compression therapy. Other more familiar modalities include compressive bandages, compression stockings, and intermittent pneumatic devices. LaPlace's law states that the pressure in the cylinder is inversely related to the radius with uniform tension on the wall, so this modality of compression will provide graduated pressure that is the highest at the ankle, resulting in the cephalic direction of venous flow [32].

A recent Cochrane review found that venous ulcers heal more rapidly with the application of compression therapy than without compression therapy and that high-grade compression with a three- or four-layer bandage or short stretch bandage is better than other systems that deliver low pressure [33].

A meta-analysis out of the United Kingdom found that high-grade compression (sub-bandage pressure 35–40 mmHg at ankle) by standardized four-layer bandage technique shows shorter healing time than short stretch bandages [34]. The average healing rate is approximately 60–70% at 12–24 weeks in various types of compression models [35].

Brien et al. stated that four-layer bandaging is the most effective method for the management of venous ulcers, with a healing rate of 54% at 3 months in a randomized control trial conducted on 200 patients. In addition, they recommend using it routinely in the management of patients with uncomplicated venous ulcers. Additionally, it can decrease the rate of recurrence if maintained lifelong [36].

The following sections discuss the technique and components of these systems, also known as the *Charing Cross Hospital Bandage*, according to recommendations from the Scottish Intercollegiate Guidelines Network (SIGN) guidelines [37] and the International Leg Ulcer Advisory Board (**Figure 8**) [38].

First layer: The padding layer involves application of orthopedic cotton in a spiral fashion with minimal overlap from the base of toes to just under the knee to protect the bony prominence and absorb exudate. In patients with ankle circumference less than 18 cm, an additional layer is needed as an artificial increase in circumference.

Second layer: This is a layer of cotton crepe bandage that oversmooths the first layer and has the last effect in compression. It is applied in a spiral fashion with 50% overlap.

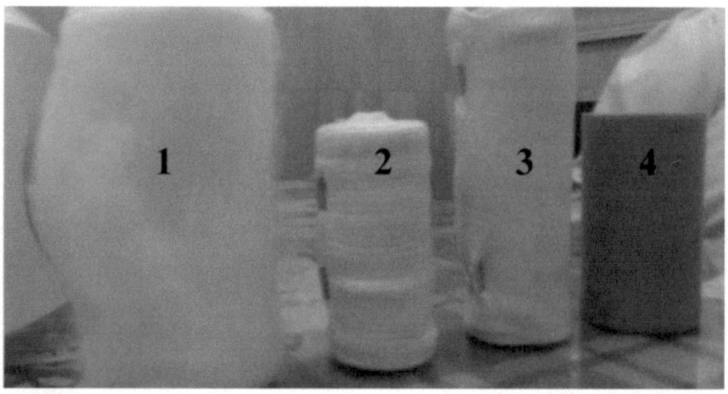

Figure 8.
Component of four-layer bandaging. (1) Orthopedic cotton; (2) cotton crepe bandage; (3) elastic extensible bandage; and (4) elastic cohesive bandage.

Third layer: This is an elastic extensible bandage applied by figure eight winding with 50% extension from base of toes to just under the knee (it provides sub-bandage pressure = 17 mmHg). The ankle joint is kept in dorsiflexion or at a 90-degree angle.

Fourth layer: This layer is an elastic cohesive bandage applied in a spiral fashion with 50% overlap and 50% extension (adds remaining 23 mmHg sub-bandage pressure) (**Figure 9**).

The disadvantage of the four-layer compression bandage is that it needs trained physicians to apply the optimum pressure, whereas compression stockings can be used by the patient and removed at night [39].

Intermittent pneumatic compression is expensive and requires immobilization of the patient. Therefore, it is reserved for bedridden patients who cannot tolerate continuous compression therapy [40].

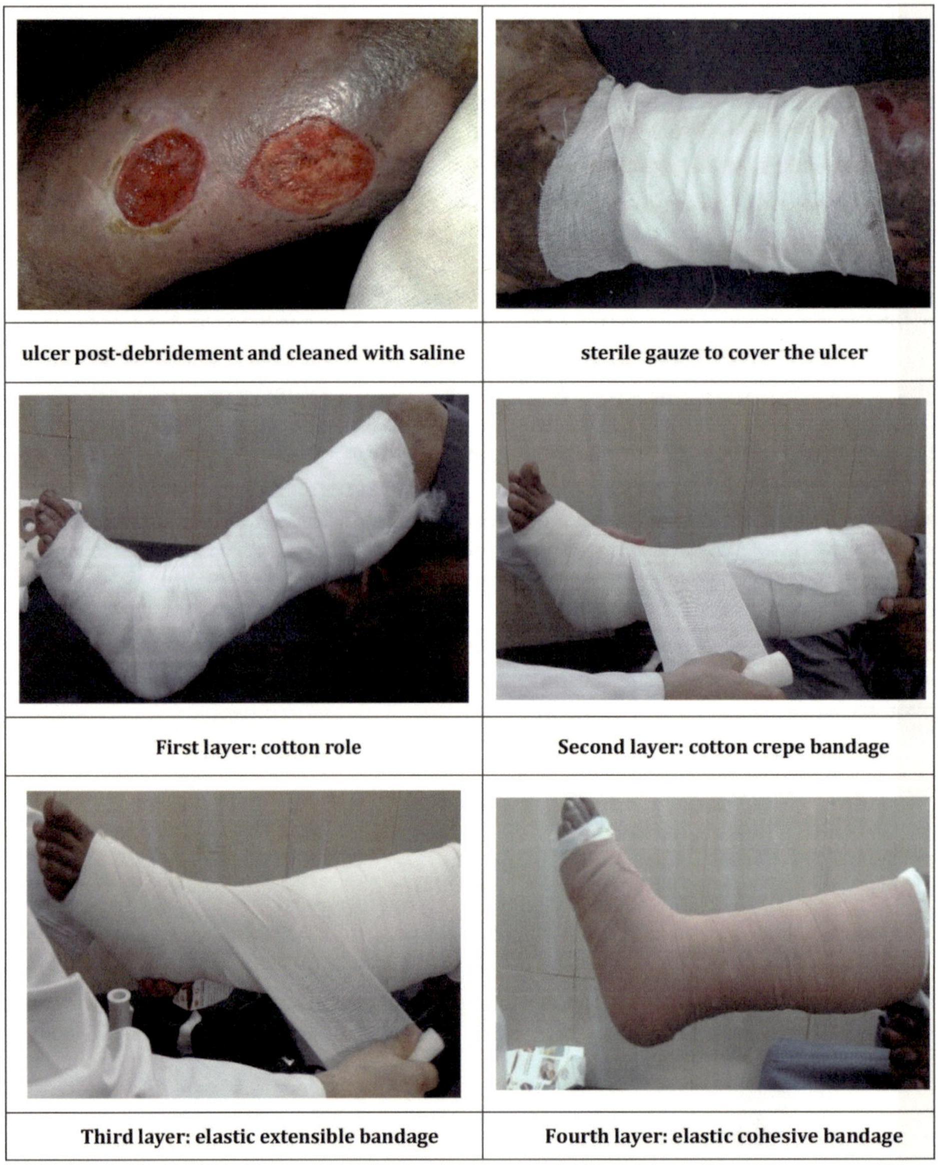

Figure 9.
Four-layer compression bandaging steps.

7.1.3 Ulcer care

Tap water can be used to clean venous ulcers. There is no advantage observed with the use of physiological saline and recommended deep debridement for recalcitrant chronic venous leg ulcers to remove fibrosis that arrests the healing process, but the use of chemical or enzymatic debridement has no special advantage [23].

A meta-analysis of 42 randomized controlled trials showed no major difference between dressing types and expensive hydrocolloid dressings. Medical evidence does not support increased healing with hydrocolloid dressings compared to lower-cost, simple nonadherent dressings. Without clear evidence that supports the use of certain dressings over others, the choice of dressings for venous ulcers can be directed by cost, ease of application, and patient and physician preference [41].

There is no evidence to support that the use of topical antibiotics has a positive effect on the management of infected venous ulcers or promotes healing. A Cochrane review on the use of silver-containing topical material concluded that there is insufficient evidence to support its use in infected venous ulcers. Other articles support avoiding topical application because it sensitizes the skin and recommend managing clinically infected venous ulcers with systemic antibiotics [29].

7.2 Surgical management

7.2.1 Surgical cover of ulcer (skin graft)

Skin grafting may be used for patients with large or refractory venous ulcers that do not show signs of healing within 4–6 weeks with standard care [29]. However, skin grafting is not effective if there is persistent edema, which is common with venous insufficiency, and the underlying venous disease is not addressed. A Cochrane review found few high-quality studies to support the use of skin grafting for the treatment of venous ulcers [42].

7.2.2 Surgery for venous insufficiency

The role of surgery is to reduce venous hypertension, promote healing, and prevent ulcer recurrence. Surgical options for the treatment of venous insufficiency include ablation of the saphenous vein, interruption of the perforating veins with subfascial endoscopic surgery, stenting of iliac vein obstruction, and removal of incompetent superficial veins with phlebectomy, stripping, sclerotherapy, or laser therapy [43].

Scottish guidelines state that there is no evidence to support surgical intervention for venous insufficiency prior to standard management (compression) for healing venous ulcers. One study showed a significant difference in recurrence in favor of surgery [23].

7.3 Platelet concentrates

Platelet concentrates are autologous material prepared from venous blood after various processing of blood samples. Generally, it depends on the centrifugation principle to separate the whole blood sample into red blood cells that heavily precipitate down and concentrate other elements that can be used topically or via infiltration for therapeutic purposes [44].

Platelet concentrates were first presented 20 years ago and were developed with the aim of using blood protein elements as a biological source of growth factors to promote the angiogenesis process and stimulate cells involved in the healing process, such as fibroblasts, neutrophils, and mesenchymal stem cells [45].

Platelet-rich fibrin (PRF) is a natural fibrin matrix developed by Choukroun et al. in France through new technology that is characterized by a simple and open access technique without anticoagulant or bovine thrombin. Just immediate centrifugation of patients' blood samples leads to conversion of fibrinogen to fibrin by physiological thrombin; this slow polymerization of fibrin charges it by platelets, leucocytes, and cytokines to give us autologous biomaterials from platelets and immune cells to support healing [46].

The protocol for preparing PRF is very simple. Blood is extracted from the patient and placed in a glass-coated tube without anticoagulant and immediately centrifuged. Time is an important factor, as the coagulation cascade starts within minutes via activation of platelets through contact with the glass tube in absence of an anticoagulant. Then, physiological thrombin transforms the fibrinogen to a fibrin network charged with active platelets and cytokines that will take the middle portion of the tube between the precipitated red blood cells layer at the bottom and acellular plasma at the top [47].

Any delay in blood handling will lead to the start of coagulation without separation of the blood component, and fibrin will be formed in a diffuse way in all tubes, resulting in a blood clot and not a PRF clot (**Figures 10–12**) [48].

From clinical data, note the ability of PRF to induce healing without any inflammatory excess. Dohan et al. stated that the PRF process not only activates platelets but also activates leucocytes to release important cytokines in response to artificial inflammation induced by these techniques. An initial investigation revealed that PRF also functions as an immune node to increase defense mechanisms and control inflammatory responses, which explains the decrease in surgical site infection treated by PRF because of trapped cytokines in fibrine networks [49].

PRF contains three main components that are important to tissue healing.

The first of these components is the host cells, which constitute the main difference between PRF and previous-generation PRP, as PRF incorporates not only platelets but also incorporates active leucocytes that have a role in anti-infection and regulation of immunity. The natural three-dimensional fibrin network is a

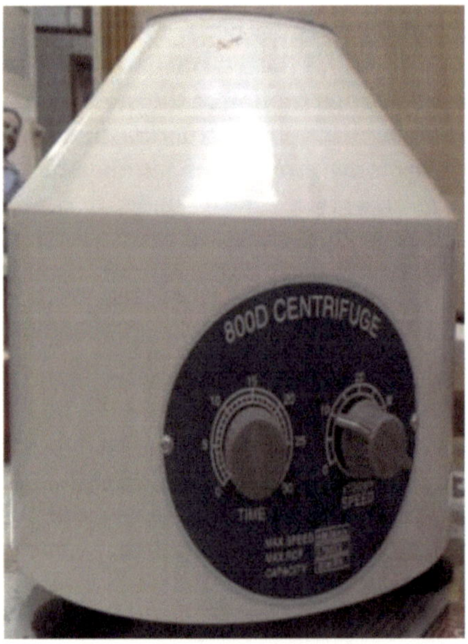

Figure 10.
Centrifuge device used for PRF.

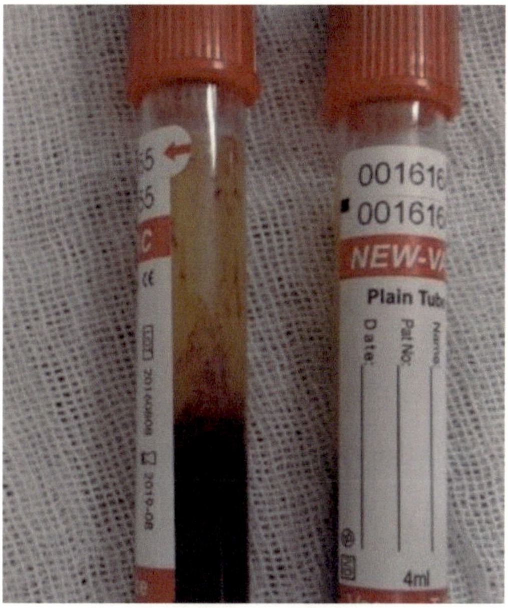

Figure 11.
PRF clot at middle of tube.

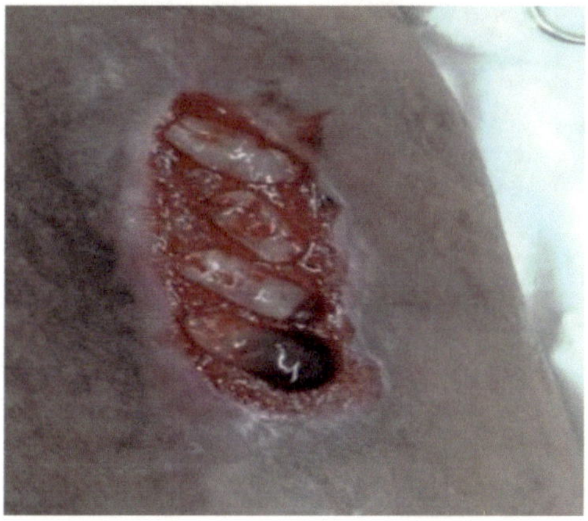

Figure 12.
PRF membranes on the surface of the ulcer.

second component that does not work as a server for host cells only but can also promote cell invasion and help in tissue regeneration. The last items in these structures are the natural growth factors that have an important biological role in the healing process, as platelet-derived growth factor (PDGF) is an essential growth factor for cell migration, differentiation, and proliferation. Vascular endothelial growth factor (VEGF) is also important for the angiogenesis process in granulation tissue, and other growth factors, such as TGF-beta, epidermal growth factor, and insulin-like growth factor, are important for wound healing (**Figures 13** and **14**) [45, 50].

Yazawa et al. stated that the concentration of growth factors in PRF was three times greater than that in PRP due to the use of fibrine as a drug delivery system for growth factors, which helped in the slow release of natural factors over a period of approximately 1 week [51].

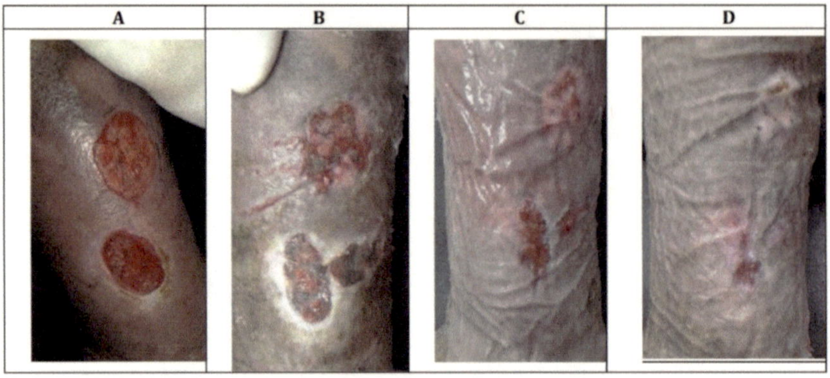

Figure 13.
A male patient, 45 years old, with secondary CVI of the left leg with two ulcers treated with four-layer compression bandages and PRF membrane applied on the proximal ulcer only.

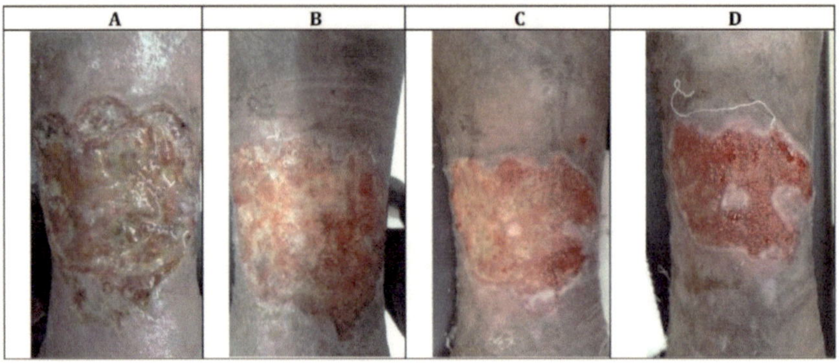

Figure 14.
A 55-year-old female patient with primary CVI of the left leg with ulcers treated with four-layer compression bandages and PRF.

8. Conclusion

- Venous ulcers are the most common cause of CLUs and have a great impact on patient QoL and productive work time.

- Management depends on reversing ambulatory venous hypertension, which is the essential pathological factor behind VLUs, by using compression therapy as the cornerstone of management along with new adjuvant therapies that can provide necessary growth factors to promote the healing process.

- PRF is a promising material for wound healing, as platelets and leukocytes release many growth factors and cytokines that are important for wound healing.

Acknowledgements

Staff of Scientific Board of Vascular Surgery Department, Faculty of Medicine, Zagazig University, Egypt.

Rwida Nori Alati, Zliten Medical College, Asmarya Islamic University.

Conflict of interest

No conflict of interest.

Author details

Walid A.M. Ganod
Vascular Surgery Unit, Zliten Medical Center, Zliten Medical College, Asmarya Islamic University, Zliten, Libya

*Address all correspondence to: walid.ganod@gmail.com

References

[1] Kahle B, Hermanns H-J, Gallenkemper G. Evidence-based treatment of chronic leg ulcers. Deutsches Ärzteblatt International. 2011;**108**:231-237

[2] Mostow EN. Diagnosis and classification of chronic wounds. Clinics in Dermatology. 1994;**12**:3-9

[3] Mekkes JR, Loots MAM, Van Der Wal AC, et al. Causes, investigation and treatment of leg ulceration. The British Journal of Dermatology. 2003;**148**: 388-401

[4] Sen CK, Gordillo GM, Roy S, et al. Human skin wounds: A major and snowballing threat to public health and the economy: Perspective article. Wound Repair and Regeneration. 2009;**17**:763-771

[5] Sarkar PK, Ballantyne S. Management of leg ulcers. Postgraduate Medical Journal. 2000;**76**:674-682

[6] O'donnell TF, Passman MA, Marston WA, et al. Management of venous leg ulcers: Clinical practice guidelines of the Society for Vascular Surgery® and the American Venous Forum. Journal of Vascular Surgery. 2014;**60**:3S-59S

[7] Bergan JJ, Bunke N. The Vein Book. Oxford University Press; 2014

[8] Caggiati A, Bergan JJ, Gloviczki P, et al. Nomenclature of the veins of the lower limb: Extensions, refinements, and clinical application. Journal of Vascular Surgery. 2005;**41**:719-724

[9] Oğuzkurt L. Ultrasonographic anatomy of the lower extremity superficial veins. Diagnostic and Interventional Radiology. 2012;**18**:423-430

[10] Bergan J, Pascarella L. Venous Anatomy, Physiology, and Pathophysiology. 2006. pp. 39-45

[11] May R, Partsch H, Staubesand J. Perforating Veins. 1st ed. München: Urban and Schwarzenberg; 1980

[12] Vaidyanathan S, Menon RR, Jacob P, et al. Chronic Venous Disorders of the Lower Limbs: A Surgical Approach. Springer; 2014

[13] Gloviczki P. Handbook of Venous Disorders: Guidelines of the American Venous Forum. Third ed. CRC Press; 2008

[14] Jane B, Helen E, Kathleen F, et al. Understanding the relationships between the calf muscle pump, ankle range of motion and healing for adults with venous leg ulcers: A review of the literature. Wound Practice and Research. 2012;**20**(2):80-85

[15] Meissner MH, Moneta G, Burnand K, et al. The hemodynamics and diagnosis of venous disease. Journal of Vascular Surgery. 2007;**46S**:4-24

[16] Araujo T, Valencia I, Federman DG, et al. Managing the patient with venous ulcers. Annals of Internal Medicine. 2003;**138**:326-334

[17] Etufugh CN, Phillips TJ. Venous ulcers. Clinics in Dermatology. 2007;**25**:121-130

[18] Valencia IC, Falabella A, Kirsner RS, et al. Chronic venous insufficiency and venous leg ulceration. Journal of the American Academy of Dermatology. 2001;**44**:401-424

[19] Eklof B, Perrin M, Delis KT, et al. Updated terminology of chronic venous disorders: The VEIN-TERM transatlantic interdisciplinary consensus document. Journal of Vascular Surgery. 2009; **49**:498-501

[20] Labropoulos N, Tassiopoulos AK. Vascular diagnosis of venous

thrombosis. In: Vascular Diagnosis. Elsevier; 2005. pp. 429-438

[21] Eklöf B, Rutherford RB, Bergan JJ, et al. Revision of the CEAP classification for chronic venous disorders: Consensus statement. Journal of Vascular Surgery. 2004;**40**:1248-1252

[22] Lal BK. Venous ulcers of the lower extremities: Definition, epidemiology, and economic and social burdens. Seminars in Vascular Surgery. 2015;**28**:35-37

[23] Charit C, Schulze B. Evidence-based S3-guideline on venous leg ulcer developed by the guideline subcommittee 'Diagnostics and Treatment of Venous Leg Ulcers' of the European Dermatology Forum. Journal of the European Academy of Dermatology and Venereology. 2016;**30**:1843-1875

[24] Kaplan RM, Criqui MH, Denenberg JO, et al. Quality of life in patients with chronic venous disease: San Diego population study. Journal of Vascular Surgery. 2003;**37**:1047-1053

[25] Smith JJ, Garratt AM, Guest M, et al. Evaluating and improving health-related quality of life in patients with varicose veins. Journal of Vascular Surgery. 1999;**30**:710-719

[26] McGee S, Boyko E. Physical examination and chronic lower extremity ischemia: A critical review. Archives of Internal Medicine. 1998;**158**:1357-1364

[27] Bradbury A, Ruckley CV. Clinical presentation and assessment of patients. In: Handbook of Venous Disorders: Guidelines of the American Venous Forum. Third ed. CRC Press; 2008. p. 331

[28] Gillespie DL. Venous ulcer diagnosis, treatment, and prevention of recurrences. Journal of Vascular Surgery. 2010;**52**:8S-14S

[29] O'Donnell TF Jr, Passman MA, et al. Management of venous leg ulcers: Clinical practice guidelines of the Society for Vascular Surgery® and the American Venous Forum. Journal of Vascular Surgery. 2014;**60**:3-59

[30] Henke P. The pacific vascular symposium 6: The venous ulcer summit in perspective. Journal of Vascular Surgery. 2010;**52**:1S-2S

[31] Pascarella L, Shortell CK. Medical management of venous ulcers. Seminars in Vascular Surgery. 2015;**28**:21-28

[32] Rudolph D. Standards of care for venous leg ulcers: Compression therapy and moist wound healing. Journal of Vascular Nursing. 2001;**19**:20-27

[33] Cullum N, Nelson E, Fletcher A, et al. Compression for venous leg ulcers. Cochrane Database of Systematic Reviews. 2001;**2**:CD000265

[34] O'Meara S, Tierney J, Cullum N, et al. Four layer bandage compared with short stretch bandage for venous leg ulcers: Systematic review and meta-analysis of randomized controlled trials with data from individual patients. BMJ. 2009;**338**:b1344. DOI: 10.1136/bmj.b1344

[35] Raffetto JD, Marston WA. Venous ulcer: What is new? Plastic and Reconstructive Surgery. 2011;**127**(Suppl):279S-288S

[36] Brien JFO, Grace PA, Perry IJ, et al. Randomized clinical trial and economic analysis of four-layer compression bandaging for venous ulcers. The British Journal of Surgery. 2003;**90**:794-798

[37] British Thoracic Society Scottish Intercollegiate Guidelines Network. British guideline on the management of asthma. Thorax. 2008;**63**(Suppl. 4):iv1-iv121. DOI: 10.1136/thx.2008.097741

[38] Moffat C, Partsch H, Clark M, et al. Understanding Compression Therapy.

Position Document of the EWMA. London, UK: MEP Ltd.; 2003. p. 19

[39] Falanga V, Margolis D, Alvarez O, et al. Rapid healing of venous ulcers and lack of clinical rejection with an allogeneic cultured human skin equivalent. Archives of Dermatology. 1998;**134**:293-300

[40] Nelson E, Mani R, Thomas K, et al. Intermittent pneumatic compression for treating venous leg ulcers. Cochrane Database of Systematic Reviews. 2008;**2**:CD001899

[41] Palfreyman S, Nelson EA, Michaels JA. Dressings for venous leg ulcers: Systematic review and meta-analysis. BMJ. 2007;**335**:244

[42] Jones JE, Nelson EA. Skin grafting for venous leg ulcers. Cochrane Database of Systematic Reviews. 2013, 2013;**1**:CD001737

[43] Robson MC, Cooper DM, Aslam R, et al. Guidelines for the treatment of venous ulcers. Wound Repair and Regeneration. 2006;**14**:649-662

[44] David M, Ehrenfest D, Andia I, et al. Classification of platelet concentrates (Platelet-Rich Plasma-PRP, Platelet-Rich Fibrin-PRF) for topical and infiltrative use in orthopedic and sports medicine: Current consensus, clinical implications and perspectives. Muscles, Ligaments and Tendons Journal. 2014;**4**:3-9

[45] Miron RJ, Choukroun J. Platelet Rich Fibrin in Regenerative Dentistry: Biological Background and Clinical Indications. John Wiley & Sons; 2017

[46] Saluja H, Dehane V, Mahindra U. Platelet-rich fibrin: A second generation platelet concentrate and a new friend of oral and maxillofacial surgeons. Annals of Maxillofacial Surgery. 2011;**1**:53

[47] Toffler M, Toscano N, Holtzclaw D, et al. Introducing Choukroun's platelet rich fibrin (PRF) to the reconstructive surgery milieu. Journal of Implant and Advanced Clinical Dentistry. 2009;**1**:21-30

[48] Dohan DM, Choukroun J, Diss A, et al. Platelet-rich fibrin (PRF): A second generation platelet concentrate. Part I: Technological concepts and evolution. Oral Surgery, Oral Medicine, Oral Pathology, and Oral Radiology. 2006;**101**:39-44

[49] Dohan DM, Choukroun J, Diss A, et al. Platelet-rich fibrin (PRF): A second generation platelet concentrate. Part III: Leucocyte activation: A new feature for platelet concentrates? Oral Surgery, Oral Medicine, Oral Pathology, and Oral Radiology. 2006;**101**:51-55

[50] Ehrenfest DMD, Corso MD, Diss A, et al. Three-dimensional architecture and cell composition of a Choukroun's platelet-rich fibrin clot and membrane. Journal of Periodontology. 2010;**81**(4): 546-555. DOI: 10.1902/jop.2009.090531

[51] Yazawa M, Ogata H, Nakajima T, et al. Basic studies on the clinical applications of platelet-rich plasma. Cell Transplantation. 2003;**12**:509-518

Section 3

Biomaterials for Wound Healing

Chapter 6

Polymeric Biomaterials for Wound Healing Incorporating Plant Extracts and Extracellular Matrix Components

Margaret O. Ilomuanya, Ibilola M. Cardoso-Daodu, Uloma N. Ubani-Ukoma and Adannaya C. Adebona

Abstract

Biomaterials are constructed to promote or stimulate the processes of wound healing. Polymeric biomaterials can be used to hydrate the wound and serve as barrier to pathogens with plant extracts, antimicrobial agents and extracellular components incorporated to stimulate the healing process. The biological and physical augmentation provided by extracellular matrix derived implants continues facilitate innovation in biomaterials utilized in management of nonhealing wounds. Tissue-processing methodologies can birth extracellular matrix-based devices with characteristic post-implantation responses ranging from the classic foreign body encapsulation of a permanent implant, to one where the implant is degraded and resorbed, to one where the processed extracellular matrix implant is populated by local fibroblasts and supporting vasculature to produce, a viable and metabolically active tissue. Extracellular matrix components and plant extracts have been shown to possesses pharmacological properties with potential for use in the treatment of skin diseases and wound healing. Antioxidant, anti-inflammatory assays, and wound healing assays have been shown to support the dermatological and wound healing usage of these medicinal plants extracts.

Keywords: Wound healing, Biomaterials, extracellular matrix, chronic wounds, plant extracts, Electrospun fibers

1. Introduction

Biomaterials are polymers that are compatible with the body system introduced into the body to correct an anomaly or used for therapeutic purposes. These materials are broadly divided into three classes – synthetic polymers (usually hydrophobic), natural polymers and inorganic polymers [1]. These polymeric materials have found usefulness in various aspects of medicine such as tissue engineering [1], drug delivery [2], gene therapies [3], wound healing etc. Wounds occur when an intact body organ or tissue is compromised. The body immediately sets off several processes to ensure healing. The successful completion of this healing process is dependent on several factors such as immune cells, infection at the wound site, external factors such as drugs and underlying conditions like diabetes, and hypoxia. Wounds can either be classed as acute where the healing period is

IntechOpen

between 8 to 12 weeks and chronic where healing is delayed beyond 12 weeks [4] as in vascular ulcers, diabetic foot ulcers and pressure ulcers [5].

Wound healing involves four sequential but partially overlapping processes of hemostasis, inflammation, proliferation, and remodeling [3, 5]. Ideally, with proper wound care such as regular cleaning, debridement and change of dressing, the healing process should proceed uninterrupted to completion. However, due to underlying conditions, poor nutrition, possible contamination of wound site and sometimes overactive immune responses, conventional therapy is introduced to control and ensure complete healing. Wound management also involve primary close by suturing, plastering or use of adhesives at first presentation to ensure proper healing [6]. The major objectives of wound care are to prevent infection, ensure proper wound closure and reduce scar formation [7].

1.1 Biomaterials and wound healing

Conventional treatment of wounds some of which have been alluded to above include drug therapies for pain, prevention or treatment of infections and wound cleaning. Bandages and closure systems are commonly used to create an enabling environment for healing. Polymeric biomaterials, synthetic or natural are an improvement on conventional wound therapy. These polymeric materials are constructed to ensure moisture and warmth is retained at the wound site while also sealing the wound from infectious agents [4]. Some of the materials are naturally occurring such as hyaluronan, chitosan, alginates. Others include hydrocolloids, polycaprolactone (PCL), polylactide-co-glycolide (PLGA), polyethylene glycol (PEG), polyurethane (PU) etc. A major advantage of biomaterials in wound care is their biocompatibility at the site of application [1]. These materials are also biodegradable; a quality that is particularly needed when the aim is to deliver medication to a wound site. This ensures that the biomaterial will degrade after drug delivery and so does not require surgical removal. Biomaterials are constructed to promote or stimulate the processes of wound healing. For instance, hydrogels can be used to hydrate the wound and serve as barrier to pathogens; curcumin, zinc nanoparticles and antibacterial can also be incorporated to stimulate the healing process [7, 8]. Polyethylene glycol when combined with polymyxin B or alginate has antibacterial activity and promotes wound regeneration respectively [9]. Biomaterials also act as scaffolds for incorporation of growth factors and as skin substitutes using hyaluronan and collagen to mimic the extracellular matrix (ECM) [9].

Injuries or wounds are currently treated via autografting or allografting. However, due to organ rejection by the immune system in some cases and lack of donors, the use of scaffolds has become increasingly popular. These scaffolds used in tissue repair are expected to be biocompatible, biodegradable, easily sterilizable and structurally desirable [10]. They can be cell or drug loaded to enhance healing; however, the constituent materials of the scaffolds can also have innate tissue repair properties. Depending on the desired properties, scaffolds are fabricated using synthetic or natural polymers which come with their unique characteristics.

Some synthetic polymers like polyurethane are used in the fabrication of semi-permeable dressings because of its permeability to moisture and vapor while acting as barrier to bacteria [4]. Fibrous scaffolds made with Poly(lactide-co-glycolide) polymers have been employed in the regeneration of bone tissues, they are also formulated as injectable in situ scaffolds [10]. Polyethylene glycol (PEG) polymers are used as carriers for growth factors i.e., EGF for targeted delivery to the wound site [11] and electrospun scaffolds of polycaprolactone (PCL), a biocompatible and bioresorbable polymer mimics the extracellular matrix (ECM) and therefore suitable for the treatment of acute and chronic wounds [4]. Polyvinyl alcohol and eudragit polymers are also useful additions in tissue engineering.

Natural polymers employed in wound healing include collagen, gelatin, chitosan, and hyaluronic acid. Chitosan is used in burns and wound healing because of its biocompatibility, tissue repair ability and lack of side effects [12, 13]. It serves as a carrier for heavy molecules such as proteins, antigens, and peptides. Ahmad et al. [14] investigated the wound healing properties of mupirocin-loaded chitosan-based hydrogel membrane. The study showed promising reports of good wound healing potentials with controlled release and no skin irritation. Conventional treatment with topical mupirocin ointment requires multiple applications and is less acceptable because of complaints associated with soiling of patient wears. Similarly, an investigative study of high molecular weight chitosan in wound healing showed exceptionally good re-epithelialization and fast wound closure compared to fucidin-ointment treated wounds [13]. Collagen and gelatin nanofibrous scaffolds are fabricated for wound healing and cartilaginous tissue regeneration respectively [15, 16] and nanofibrous scaffolds of hyaluronic acid mimics the ECM essential in controlling cellular function [2, 17].

2. Extracellular matrix targeted for chronic wound

Extracellular Matrix (ECM) is a structural scaffold that organizes cell adhesion and migration it also controls cellular growth, metabolism, and differentiation signals. It is composed of a wide variety of dynamic macromolecules and their regulatory factors which provide structural aid and physical protection [18]. Novel research has dynamically changed our understanding of the role of the extracellular matrix in tissue regeneration. The extracellular matrix is thought to provide passive structural support for cells however it has now been discovered that the individual or fragmented Extracellular matrix can send signals vital for cell processes during wound healing through integrin reactions coupled with growth factor activation [19]. Studies have shown that the Extracellular Matrix plays an active role in chronic wound healing. In a study by Baek et al. [20], the extracellular matrix was fabricated as a porous sheet matrix derived from human adipose tissue. Its aim was to act not just as a scaffold but a tool to enhance the overall process of wound healing through its components. Application of the extra cellular matrix sheet dressing showed enhanced wound healing rate compared to the control which was foam wound dressing [20]. The extracellular matrix is a broad molecule network made up of protein glycosaminoglycan and glycoconjugate, elastin and collagen. The extracellular matrix is a nonvascular structure that controls a vast number of cellular functions. The extracellular matrix is a complex structural network and undergoes constant restructuring of its network through matrix degrading enzymes [21]. The extra cellular matrix is composed of multiple matrix proteins that make up its main part. Proteins provide structural support to cells and tissues. The proteins that make up the extracellular matrix can be structural or non-structural depending on their roles and responsibilities [22]. In a study by Hui et al. [23], growth factor re-enforced extracellular matrix was prepared, and the wound healing properties were evaluated using a mouse model. It reflected that the extra cellular matrix promotes wound healing in the early stage of adipocyte recruitment. Rapid re-epithelization, enhanced granulation, tissue growth and supported angiogenesis were also observed. Growth factor re-enforced extracellular matrix was used to treat the wounds and total wound healing was observed on day seven of wound healing [23]. To accelerate healing processes and decrease the complication occurrence various agents, growth factors, natural and synthetic antioxidants (coenzyme Q10-CoQ10), are applied. Amajuoyi et al. incorporated natural ECM matrix co-enzyme Q10 and keratin in electrospun keratin/Co Enzyme Q10/Poly vinyl alcohol nanofibrous scaffold [24]. This potential dressing for infected wounds was effective in preventing the proliferation of microorganism. Encapsulation of

CoQ10 in nanoliposomes has also been shown to enhance CoQ10 activity by accelerating wound healing process after tooth extraction [24, 25]. A reduction in inflammatory reaction and increase in collagen deposition following surgical procedure, were previously obtained in animals when CoQ10 was applied in a form of ointment resulting. The expression of IL-1β, TNF-α, NF-κB and HO-1, cytokines involved in inflammation and oxidative tissue damage, were significantly suppressed by CoQ10 application for 3 days following surgical procedure [25]. The ECM was shown to be more stimulated to facilitate wound healing when formulated with biomaterials. **Table 1** show in details the Drug delivery technologies incorporating Extracellular matrix and Plant extract targeted for management of chronic wounds.

Drug delivery Technology incorporating biomaterials	Plant extract(s)	Extracellular matrix component	Pharmacological action	Ref.
1. Hydrogels				
a. Alkyl acrylate polymer	*Aspalathus linearis*	.	Therapeutic properties of green and fermented rooibos extract loaded hydrogels have been established in vivo, with the best wound healing indices shown by the hydrogels containing fermented rooibos extract. This is possibly a result of a shorter inflammatory phase resulting in quicker wound closure and reduced fibrosis.	[26]
b. Hyaluronic acid and chitosan		Angiogenic promoting growth factor vascular endothelial growth factor	The hydrogels possessed both antibacterial and angiogenic, suggesting it might have potential as a wound healing therapeutic. The hydrogels that have incorporated hyaluronan have been shown to promote blood clotting and possess antibacterial properties	[27]
2. Electrospun scaffolds				
a. Polycaprolactone (PCL) for skin tissue engineering	*Memecylon edule*	—	PCL/ *Memecylon edule* show minimal cytotoxicity and the epidermal differentiation of adipose derived stem cells on PCL/ *Memecylon edule* scaffolds demonstrated the potential of electrospun PCL/ ME nanofibers as substrates for skin tissue engineering in chronic wound healing.	[28]
b. Chitosan nanoparticles and electrospun scaffolds	—	Novel chondrogenic growth factors (Nell-1)	Nell-1 specifically promotes inducing human bone mesemchymal cells *in vitro*, and chondrogenic differentiation by increasing expression of chondrogenic related genes and proteins. Thus enhancing its potential utility for cartilage tissue engineering	[29]

Drug delivery Technology incorporating biomaterials	Plant extract(s)	Extracellular matrix component	Pharmacological action	Ref.
3. Skin substitutes				
a. Epidermal/dermal substitute		Fibroblast	Apligraf® neonatal dermal fibroblasts grown in a matrix that consists of bovine-derived type I collagen with layers of human neonatal epidermal keratinocytes on top that have been exposed to air to promote stratification in order to mimic the stratum corneum hence facilitating chronic wound healing.	[30]
b. Allogenic dermal substitutes		Neonatal fibroblasts	TransCyte™ a collagen-coated nylon matrix with an outer silicon film seeded with human neonatal fibroblasts, has been used for both partial and full-thickness burn wounds. Dermagraft™, used both for burns and chronic wounds, consists of a bioresorbable polyglactin scaffold containing human neonatal fibroblasts	[31]
4. Nanomedicines				
a. Silver Nanoparticles	*Cassia auriculata*	—	Cassia auriculata L.-mediated silver nanoparticles were effective on both incision and excision wound models in Wistar albino rats exhibiting better performance in wound healing process rather than the extract and Povidone Iodine ointment.	[32]
b. Dual growth factor-releasing nanoparticle-in-nanofiber system		Vascular endothelial growth factor	Normal full thickness rat skin wound models demonstrated that nanofiber/nanoparticle scaffolds significantly accelerated the wound healing process by promoting angiogenesis, increasing re-epithelialization and controlling granulation tissue formation.	[33]
c. Liposomal nanocarriers	Curcumin	—	The antibacterial activity of the Curcumin-liposomal formulation was found to be like silver sulfadiazine cream 1% regarding the inhibition of the bacterial growth. At low dose of curcumin nano-liposomal formulation efficiently improved injuries and infections of burn wounds	[34]

Table 1.
Drug delivery technologies incorporating extracellular matrix and plant extract targeted for management of chronic wounds.

2.1 GAG (Glycosaminoglycans)

GAG is a lengthy linear polysaccharide chain. It is a sulphated di-saccharide formed by uronic acid and N-acetyl- glucosamine or N-acetyl -galactosamine. GAG in partnership with proteoglycans control the wound healing process, GAG is involved in the remodeling phase as it supports capillary growth, fibronectin, and collagen formation at the site of the injury so that vascular density of the wound can be restored. GAG also participates in cell to cell and cell to matrix interactions cell proliferation migration and cytokine and growth factor signaling associated with wound healing. GAG chain reflects an impressive structural diversity because of the dynamic biosynthesis that is tightly controlled in biological systems allowing modified GAG to particularly interact with various ligands in a controlled and timely manner [35]. In a study by Amaral et al. [35], Collagen-GAG scaffolds were fabricated with platelet rich protein infused in the pores of its scaffold. The composite scaffold containing collagen, GAG and platelet rich protein was observed to release key growth factors such as, TGFβ, FGF, VEGF and PDGF for vascular regeneration for 14 days. Growth factors released were enough to enhance the proliferation of major cells involved in wound healing. It also increased the angiogenic and vascularization abilities which are key indices for progress in wound healing, conclusively indicating promising results as therapy for wound healing [36].

2.2 Collagen

Collagen is the most common protein in the body. It is highly populated in the extracellular matrix of the connective tissue like the tendon, cartilage, and skin. It is the most abundant structured protein found in the extra cellular matrix. It gives tensile strength and takes part in adhesion and migration. In the extra cellular matrix collagen is aligned as fibrils to allow for support of the structural framework of the tissues. Collagen type I is in all tissues, tendon, and skin. Collagen type II is found in the cartilage and cornea. Collagen type III is found in the walls of blood vessels [18, 19]. In a study by Lei et al. [37], Collagen hydrogel was fabricated for wound dressing. It was shown to enhance the rate and quality of wound healing. It also improved the tensile strength of regenerated tissue and skin at the wound site. In the study the effect of collagen hydrogel dressing on chronic wound healing and capillary regeneration was explored in diabetic Sprague Dawley rat models. Rats treated at the wound site with collagen hydrogel showed faster healing with smaller wound areas by days seven and fourteen compared to the untreated rats [37]. In another study by Morteza et al. [38] bacterial cellulose/collagen hydrogel as wound dressing was compared to collagenase ointment and the control was an untreated wound. Bacterial Cellulose Collagen hydrogel showed better regeneration and tissue repair when applied at the wound site than the collagenase ointment or control. The study concluded that Bacterial Cellulose/Collagen hydrogel serves as a promising biologically active hydrogel dressing for skin regeneration [38, 39].

2.3 Elastin and fibronectin

It is found in the extra cellular matrix spaces of tissues and is responsible for the flexibility and distensibility of tissues. Elastin is responsible for the dermis stretching ability along with fibrillin and fibulin. The study by Kawabata et al. [40], highlighted cutaneous ulcers treated with silk elastin-based hydrogels. It was shown that silks elastin enhanced rapid wound healing in chronic ulcers of diabetic mice. Silk elastin hydrogels showed enhanced epithelialization rate compared to conventional hydrogels in chronic ulcer models. Indicating that elastin hydrogel is a promising material for accelerating the healing of chronic ulcers [40].

Fibronectins exist in two different forms, firstly as plasma that migrates the blood, secondly as cellular protein created by fibroblast. Fibronectin is aligned into a network of fibrils. It is created in the form of a disulphide-bonded dimer that can be broken down. Fibronectin is involved in the development and response to injury. It plays an important role in enhancing and modulating cell functions in the extracellular matrix [18, 19, 40]. In a study by Norris et al. [41] an Acoustic fabrication of Collagen -Fibronectin composite gels were carried out to accelerate microtissue regeneration. The ultrasound-based fabrication altered the collagen fiber structure and arrangement this led to improvement in its bioactivity. The study investigated how the synergistic effect of collagen and fibronectin coupled with the ultrasound effect altered the protein alignment and bioactivity of composite hydrogels. Results from the investigation showed that the fibronectin can be redistributed within three-dimensional hydrogels under the influence of ultrasound to produce composite hydrogels which lead to the improvement of microtissue regeneration. Conclusively ultrasound waves can lead to protein realignment and fibronectin rearrangement which can enhance wound healing. This is a promising and novel tool and provides a less invasive treatment for chronic wounds [12].

Extra cellular matrix also plays an indirect role in the modulation of extra cellular protease production and activation it also modifies growth factor availability and activity for wound healing [42]. In a study by Riis et al. 2020, adipose derived stem cells which have the ability to deposit extracellular matrix are being investigated for novel treatment of chronic wound and enhancement of wound healing. The extracellular matrix eventually forms a scaffold which is composed of collagen I and III and fibronectin, all of which are essential for progress in wound healing processes [13]. PLA-based electrospun fibers loaded with hyaluronic acid-valsartan hydrogels have been shown to be stable and possess proven diabetic wound healing property. This was as a result of the known biomimetic effect of the fibers and increased re-epithelization facilitated by the hydrogels containing angiotensin inhibitors which is facilitated by the presence of hyaluronic acid as the ECM components [43].

3. Biomaterials and drug delivery incorporating plant extracts targeted for management of chronic wounds

Biomaterials such as biomimetic polymers have been utilized as carrier systems for plant extracts utilized in management of chronic wounds. The problems of resistance and environmental degradation associated with irrational use of orthodox medicines have increased interests in natural and safer alternatives when managing chronic of wounds. Chah et al. [44] evaluated the antibacterial and wound healing activities of methanolic extracts of *Ageratum conyzoides* L (Asteraceae), *Anthocleista djalonen*, A. Chev (Loganiaceae), *Napoleonaea imperialis*, P. *Beauv (Lecythidaceae)*, *Ocimum gratissimum*, *Briq (Lamiaceae)* and *Psidium guajava*. The antibacterial and wound healing properties of *Napoleona imperialis*, *Ocimum gratissimum* and *Ageratum conyzoides* were established however utilization of these extracts as crude portends a setback for quality control and wide utilization of these herbal products. Incorporation of herbal extracts into biomaterials have been shown to increase the stability of the herbal extracts within the biomaterial whilst ensuring that plant extract elicits its desired effect. The polyherbal antioxidant preparation containing extracts of *T. conophorum* and *O. gratissimum* was shown to exhibit excellent antioxidant and wound healing properties. The formulation served to protect the skin from reactive oxygen species created by UV radiation and environmental toxin, thus protecting the skin from photo aging. This hence showed a migration from the work of Shah et al., where the extracts elicit wound healing activities to the instance where extracts incorporated into biomaterials could effectively be utilized as a dosage form in management of chronic wounds [44, 45]. Elegbede et al. [26] studied the therapeutic properties of green and fermented *Aspalanthus linearis* extract loaded hydrogels in surgical wound healing. The best wound healing indices shown by the hydrogels containing fermented rooibos extract due to shortening the inflammatory phase which resulted in quicker wound closure and reduced fibrosis (**Table 1**). Biomaterials have also incorporated both plant extracts and conventional medicine in management of chronic wounds.

Panax ginseng, extracted by soxhlation from the clean and dried root and incorporated into PCL (polycaprolactone nanofibers) by electrospinning for bone tissue regeneration was demonstrated to induce the expression of osteogenic genes like osteocalcin and collagen type 1 [46]. The mineralization and phosphatase activity of the ginseng extract was shown to be significantly higher due to the presence of *Panax ginseng* hence its usefulness in bone engineered scaffold development in management of surgical wounds [3, 45, 46]. Nanoscaffolds of polycaprolactone have been incorporated and electrospun with the medicinal extracts of *Tecomella undulata*, *Asparagus racemosus*, *Glycyrrhiza glabra*, and *Linum usitatissimum* to impart their wound healing properties and antimicrobial activity. Morphological examination shows that the supplement of these plant extracts did not alter the final morphology of the nanofibers, but the average diameter was increased in all the extract loaded nanofibers. The release studies using acetate buffer with a pH of 5.5 shows that the nanoscaffolds released the antibacterial extracts in a sustained manner up to a 24-hour period and also shows zones of inhibition when cultured on agar plates with growth of *S. aureus* and *K. pneumoniae* [9, 47]. The fabricated wound dressings exhibited significant moisture vapor transmission rate, which is a suitable criterion for gases permeability in facilitating wound healing. When correlated and compared with commercially accessible dressing materials, it was established that nanofiber incorporated with herbal drug was 50% more efficient [46, 47]. The plant extract from *Garcinia manostana* have been found to have usefulness as wound dressing material. Charernsriwilaiwat et al. [46–48], *in vitro* analysis using Franz's diffusion cells method and an *in vivo* analysis using Male Wistar rats shows that the plant extract fabricated with chitosan-ethylenediaminetetraacetic acid/polyvinyl alcohol composite reduces inflammation and also leads to increase in antioxidant activity. It also demonstrated antimicrobial activity against *Staphylococcus aureus* and *Escherichia coli* [48].

Curcumin is a known natural polyphenolic compound which is gotten from the rhizome of the natural plant *Curcuma longa*. It is a novel, proven treatment that facilitates faster wound healing due to its possessing antioxidant and anti-inflammatory properties. It helps in accelerating healing of wounds by contributing to the three phases of wound healing such as the inflammatory, proliferatory and the remodeling phases [49]. Curcumin has been reported to have a wide range of pharmacologic actions ranging from anti-inflammatory, anti-HIV, an antibacterial, anti-oxidant activity, anti-parasitic, anti-mutagenic and anti-cancer, with very low or no intrinsic toxicity [49, 50]. Curcumin has significant effect on the inflammatory phase during wound healing. The Inflammatory phase is one of the most important phases during wound healing, and it is often counted as the first step in optimal wound healing. Since tissue damage causes early acute inflammation, the control of inflammation can help optimize the wound healing process [49–52].

The *in vitro* analysis using myoblast cells and an *in vivo* analysis using Female mice when curcumin was electrospun with polylactic acid demonstrated greater cell mobility, early remodeling and inhibition of nitric oxide which usually impede wound healing [49, 53].

Momordica charantia is a traditional herbal commonly used for its antidiabetic, antioxidant, contraceptive, and antibacterial properties [54]. When formulated as a powder ointment, *Momordica charantia* showed a stastically significant response ($P < 0.01$), in terms of wound-contracting ability, wound closure time and period of epithelization, with increased tissue regeneration at wound bed when compared with povidone iodine which served as control [54, 55]. Hussan et al. developed biomaterial based *Momordica charantia* ointment which was evaluated as an alternative topical medication for diabetic wounds. The ointment showed intense TGF-β expression and a high level of total protein content, showing that it accelerated wound healing in diabetic rats, via enhancing TGF-β expression [55].

Utilization of medicinal plants with known wound healing activities such as *Tetracarpidium conophorum* in collaboration with known conventional medicine have been shown to increase their activity as well as shorten wound healing times. Ezealisiji *et al.* [56] reported that the n-hexane and methanol extracts of the *Tetracarpidium conophorum* seed nut established accelerated dose-dependent wound healing activity of the extracts. This was attributed to the presence of some secondary metabolites like flavonoids with repeated antioxidant and immune stimulating activities. However, Ilomuanya et al. [45, 57] utilized response surface methodology coupled with statistically designed experiments to optimize the multivariable processes in developing *Tetracarpidium conophorum* hydrogel containing gentamicin. The extract synergistically facilitated a potential wound healing activity that either active ingredient wound not have been able to achieve.

4. Conclusion and future trends

Wound healing is a complex and dynamic process of restoring cellular structures and tissue layers in damaged tissues as closely as possible to its normal state. Plant extracts and human extra cellular matrices that have been seen to possess wound healing activities have the capability of facilitating re-epithelization and tissue regeneration which accelerates the wound healing process. Utilization of appropriate biomaterials as carrier systems can enhance the activity of the plant extracts in hastening the inflammatory, proliferative and the remodeling phases of chronic wounds without the inherent problem of antibiotic resistance and hypersensitivity to the very few medications available. Increased utilization of folkloric plant extracts with proven wound healing activities will ensure an increased option and platform for management of Chronic wounds. There still exits inherent challenges in the use of extracellular matrix loaded biomaterials, cellular and extra cellular treatments options which can enable delivery of multiple molecules at the wound site without degradation is required. The cost of these technologies should also be affordable to encourage scale up.

Conflict of interest

The authors have no conflict of interest.

Author details

Margaret O. Ilomuanya[1*], Ibilola M. Cardoso-Daodu[1], Uloma N. Ubani-Ukoma[1] and Adannaya C. Adebona[2]

1 Department of Pharmaceutics and Pharmaceutical Technology, Faculty of Pharmacy, University of Lagos, Lagos, Nigeria

2 Department of Pharmaceutics and Pharmaceutical Technology, Faculty of Pharmacy, Federal University Oye Ekiti, Ekiti, Nigeria

*Address all correspondence to: milomuanya@unilag.edu.ng

References

[1] Kohane DS, Langer R. Polymeric Biomaterials in Tissue Engineering. Paed. Research. 2008: 67, 487 – 491

[2] Samson AO, Ilomuanya MO, Gbenebor OP, Dada MO, Odili CC. Biomaterials for Drug Delivery: Sources, Classification, Synthesis, Processing and Applications. In Advanced Functional Materials. IntechOpen. 2020: 1-25 Http://dx.doi.org/10.5772/intechopen.93368

[3] Piraino F. and Selimovic S.: A Current view of Functional Biomaterials for Wound Care, Molecular and Cellular Therapies. Biomed Research International 2015: 1-11 http://dx.doi.org/10.1155/2015/403801

[4] Mir M, Ali MN, Barakullah A, Gulzar A, Arshad M, Fatima S, Asad M. Synthetic Polymeric Biomaterials for Wound Healing: A Review. Progress in Biomaterials. 2018: 7, 1-21. Https://doi.org/10.1007/s40204-018-0083-4

[5] Frykberg RG, Banks J. Challenges in the Treatment of Chronic Wounds. Advances in Wound Care. 2015: 4 (9): 560 – 582. Http://dx.doi.org/10.1089/wound.2015.0635

[6] Percival JN: Classification of Wounds and their Management. Surgery. 2002: 20(5) 114 – 117. https://doi.org/10.1383/surg.20.5.114.14626

[7] He F, Jiao H, Zhao L, Liao X, Fan Z. Facile and Large-scale Synthesis of Curcumin/PVA hydrogel: effectively kill bacteria and accelerate cutaneous wound healing in the rat. J. Biomater Sci Polym Ed. 2018; 29: 325 – 343. https://doi.org/10.1080/09205063.2017.1417002

[8] Khorasani MT, Joorabloo A, Moghaddam A, Shamsi H, MansooriMoghadam Z. Incorporation of ZnO nanoparticles into haparinised polyvinyl alcohol/chitosan hydrogels for wound dressing application. Int J Biol Macromol. 2018; 114: 1203 – 1215. https://doi.org/10.1016/j.ijbiomac.2018.04.010

[9] Murray RZ, West ZE, Cowin AJ, Farrugia BL. Development and use of biomaterials as wound healing therapies. Burns and Trauma. 2019; 1-9. https://doi.org/10.1186/s41038-018-0139-7

[10] Elkasabgy NA, Mahmoud AA. Fabrication Strategies of Scaffolds for Delivering Active Ingredients for Tissue Engineering. AAPS PharmSciTech (2019) 20: 256 https://doi.org/10.1208/s12249-019-1470-4

[11] Shahverdi S, Hajimiri M, Esfandiari MA, Larijan B, Atyabi F, Rajabiani A, Dehpour AR, Gharehaghaji AA, Dinarvand R. Fabrication and structure analysis of poly(lactide-co-glycolic acid)/silk fibroin hybrid scaffold for wound dressing applications. Int J Pharm (2014) 473:345-355. 10.1016/j.ijpharm.2014.07.021

[12] Deng C-M, He LZ, Zhao M, Yang D, Liu Y. Biological properties of the chitosan-gelatin sponge wound dressing. Carbohydrate Polym. 2007;69(3):583-589

[13] Alsarra IA. Chitosan topical gel formulation in the management of burn wounds. Int J Biol Macromol. 2009;45(1):16-21.

[14] Ahmad S, Minhas MU, Ahmad M, Sohail M, Abdullah O, Badshah SF. Preparation and Evaluation of Skin Wound Healing Chitosan-Based Hydrogel Membranes. AAPS PharmSciTech. 2018: 19(7) 3199 – 3209. Http://doi.org/10.1208/s12249-018-1131-z

[15] Yeo IS, Oh JE, Jeong L, Lee TS, Lee SJ, Park WH, et al. Collagen-based biomimetic nanofibrous scaffolds: preparation and characterization of collagen/silk fibroin bicomponent nanofibrous structures. Biomacro molecules. 2008;9(4):1106-16. 65.

[16] Aliakbarshirazi S, Talebian A. Electrospun gelatin nanofibrous scaffolds for cartilage tissue engineering. Mater Today Proc. 2017;4(7):7059-64. 66

[17] Lian Y, Yuan L, Ji L, Zhang K. Gelatin/hyaluronic acid nanofibrous scaffolds: biomimetics of extracellular matrix. Acta Biochim Biophys Sin. 2013;45(8):700-703. https://doi.org/10.1093/abbs/gmt032

[18] Jaspreet K, Shouvik B, Ram S. The extracellular matrix: Structure, composition, age-related differences, tools for analysis and applications for tissue engineering. Journal of Tissue Engineering. 2014;20(5):2041731414557112. PMID: 25610589; PMCID: PMC4883592. https://doi.org/10.1177/2041731414557112

[19] Agren S, Werthen M. The Extracellular Matrix in Wound Healing: A Closer Look at Therapeutics for Chronic Wounds. The International Journal of Lower Extremity Wounds. 2007;6(2):82-97. doi:10.1177/1534734607301394

[20] Baek S, Lee S, Jeong Y, Kim Young K, Rhie J. Wound-healing effect of adipose stem cell-derived extracellular matrix sheet on full-thickness skin defect rat model: Histological and immunohistochemical study. Int. Wound Journal. 2019; 16: 286–296. https://doi.org/10.1111/iwj.13030

[21] Godfrey M. Extracellular Matrix. Asthma and COPD (Second Edition), Basic Mechanisms and Clinical Management. Academic Press. 2009 274p. ISBN 9780123740014, https://doi.org/10.1016/B978-0-12-374001-4.00022-5

[22] González-Díaz, E.C.; Varghese, S. "Hydrogels as Extracellular Matrix Analogs." Gels. 2016 2(3):20. doi:10.3390/gels2030020

[23] Hui-Cong D, Jiang L, Wen-Xin G, Li J, Zhang R, Dang J, Shu M, Li L. "Growth Factor- Reinforced ECM Fabricated from Chemically Hypoxic MSC Sheet with Improved In Vivo Wound Repair Activity". BioMed Research International. 2017 11p. https://doi.org/10.1155/2017/2578017 ID 2578017

[24] Amajuoyi, J.N., Ilomuanya, M.O., Asantewaa-Osei, Y. et al. Development of electrospun keratin/coenzyme Q10/poly vinyl alcohol nanofibrous scaffold containing mupirocin as potential dressing for infected wounds. Futur J Pharm Sci 6, 25 (2020). https://doi.org/10.1186/s43094-020-00043-z

[25] Todorovic K, Jovanovic G, Todorovic A, et al. Effects of coenzyme Q10 encapsulated in nanoliposomes on wound healing processes after tooth extraction. J Dent Sci. 2018;13(2):103-108. doi:10.1016/j.jds.2017.10.004

[26] Elegbede, R.D., Ilomuanya, M. O., Sowemimo, A.A., Nneji, A., Joubert, E., De Beer, D., Koekemoer, T., van de Venter, M. (2020) Effect of fermented and green Aspalathus linearis extract loaded hydrogel on surgical wound healing in Sprague Dawley rats. Wound Medicine, 29, 100186, ISSN 2213-9095, https://doi.org/10.1016/j.wndm.2020.100186

[27] Huang J, Ren J, Chen G, Li Z, Liu Y, Wang G, et al. Tunable sequential drug delivery system based on chitosan/hyaluronic acid hydrogels and PLGA microspheres for management of non-healing infected wounds. Mater Sci Eng C. 2018;89:213-222

[28] Jin G, Prabhakaran M P, Kai D, Annamalai S K, Arunachalam K D, Ramakrishna S, Tissue engineered plant extracts as nanofibrous wound dressing, Biomaterials, 34 (3): 724-734. 2013, https://doi.org/10.1016/j.biomaterials.2012.10.026

[29] Wang C, Hou W, Guo X, Li J, Hu T, Qiu M, Liu S, Mo X, Liu X. Two-phase electrospinning to incorporate growth factors loaded chitosan nanoparticles into electrospun fibrous scaffolds for bioactivity retention and cartilage regeneration. Mater Sci Eng C Mater Biol Appl. 2017 Oct 1;79:507-515. doi: 10.1016/j.msec.2017.05.075

[30] Vig K, Chaudhari A, Tripathi S, Dixit S, Sahu R, Pillai S, et al. Advances in skin regeneration using tissue engineering. Int J Mol Sci. 2017;18:789.

[31] Shevchenko RV, James SL, James SE. A review of tissue-engineered skin bioconstructs available for skin reconstruction. J R Soc Interface. 2010;7:229-258.

[32] Kumarasamyraja D, Swamivelmanickam M. Evaluation of wound healing activity of biosynthesized silver nanoparticles from aqueous extract of Cassia Auriculata L. Int J Phytopharm. 2014;5:201-209

[33] Xie Z, Paras C B, Weng H, Punnakitikashem P, Su L-C, Vu K, Tang L, Yang J, Nguyen K T, Dual growth factor releasing multi-functional nanofibers for wound healing, Acta Biomaterialia 2013,9 (12) 9351-9359, https://doi.org/10.1016/j.actbio.2013.07.030

[34] Kianvash, N., Bahador, A., Pourhajibagher, M. et al. Evaluation of propylene glycol nanoliposomes containing curcumin on burn wound model in rat: biocompatibility, wound healing, and anti-bacterial effects. Drug Deliv. and Transl. Res. 7, 654-663 (2017). https://doi.org/10.1007/s13346-017-0405-4

[35] Amaral R, Zayed N, Pascu E, Cavanagh B, Hobbs C, Santarella F, Simpson C, Murphy C, Sridharan R, Gonzalez- Vazquez A, O Sullivan B, O Brein F, Kearney C. Functionalising Collagen-Based Scaffolds with platelet-rich plasma for enhanced skin wound healing potential. Frontiers in Bioengineering and Biotechnology. 2019; 7:371 DOI: 10.3389/fbioe.2019.00371

[36] Ghatak S, Maytin E, Vincent J, Ilia H, Ricardo A, Rodriguez M, Markwalt R, Misra S. Roles of Proteoglycans and Glycosaminoglycans in wound healing and fibrosis. International Journal of Cell Biology. 2015; 2015:834893. doi: 10.1155/2015/834893

[37] Lei J, Chen P, Li Y, Wang X, Tang S. Collagen hydrogel dressing for wound healing and angiogenesis in diabetic rat models. International Journal Clinical Experimental Medicine. 2017;10(12): 16319-16327

[38] Morteza B, Naimeh M, Moghtader M. An Introduction to Hydrogels and Some Recent Applications, Emerging Concepts in Analysis and Applications of Hydrogels. Sutapa B Majee.editor. Intech Open, DOI: 10.5772/64301

[39] Rodrigues P, Fontes de Sousa M, Saskac S, Barud H, Roncalho de Limac L, Virgínia da Conceição Amaro M, de Guzzi Plepisa A, José Lima Ribeiroc S, Minarelli Gaspara A. Bacterial Cellulose/Collagen Hydrogel for Wound Healing. Materials Research, 2016 19(1): 106-116.https://doi.org/10.1590/1980-5373-MR-2015-0249

[40] Kawabata S, Kanda N, Hirasawa Y, Noda K, Matsuura Y, Suzuki S, Kawai K. The Utility of Silk-elastin Hydrogel as a New Material for Wound Healing.

Plastic Reconstruction Surgery Global Open 2018;6: e1778 doi: 10.1097/GOX.0000000000001778

[41] Norris E, Dalecki D, Hocking D. Article Acoustic Fabrication of Collagen–Fibronectin Composite Gels Accelerates Microtissue Formation. Applied Science 2020; 10: 2907. doi:10.3390/app10082907

[42] Nicks BA, Ayello E, Woo K, Nitzki-George D, Sibbald G. Acute wound management: revisiting the approach to assessment, irrigation and closure considerations. Int J Emerg Med. 2010:3. 399 – 407. Http://dx.doi.org/10.1007/s12245-010-0217-5

[43] Ilomuanya M.O, Okafor P.S., Amajuoyi J.N., Onyejekwe J., Okubanjo O.O., Adeosun S.O., Silva B.O. (2020) Polylactic acid-based electrospun fiber and Hyaluronic acid- valsartan hydrogel scaffold for chronic wound healing. Beni Suef University J. Basic and Applied Sci. 9:31 https://doi.org/10.1186/s43088-020-00057-9

[44] Chah KF, Eze CA, Emuelosi CE, Esimone CO. Antibacterial and wound healing properties of methanolic extracts of some Nigerian medicinal plants. J Ethnopharmacol. 2006 Mar 8;104(1-2):164-167. doi: 10.1016/j.jep.2005.08.070. Epub 2005 Oct 13. PMID: 16226414

[45] Ilomuanya M.O., Akhimien T., Aghaizu C., Adeyinka O., Ajayi T. (2018) Polyherbal Antioxidant Topical Preparation Comprising Ethanol Extract of Tetracarpidium conophorum and Ocimum gratissimum: Formulation and Evaluation. Dhaka Univ. J. Pharm. Sci. 17(2): 213-219, DOI: http://dx.doi.org/10.3329/dujps.v17i2.39178

[46] Pajoumshariati S, Yavari S.K, Shokrgozar M.A, Physical and biological modification of polycaprolactone electrospun nanofiber by panax ginseng extract for bone tissue engineering application, Ann. Biomed. Eng. 44 (2016) 1808-1820

[47] Chellamani K, Vignesh Balaji R, Veerasubramanian D, Sudharsan J, Wound healing ability of herbal drug incorporated PCL (Poly (ε-caprolactone)) wound dressing, Journal of Academia and Industrial Research, April 2 (2014) 622-626

[48] Charernsriwilaiwat N, Rojanarata T, Ngawhirunpat T, Sukma M, Opanasopit P, Electrospun chitosan-based nanofiber mats loaded with Garcinia mangostana extracts, Int. J. Pharm. 452 (2013) 333-343

[49] Javadi, B., & Sahebkar, A. (2017). Natural products with anti-inflammatory and immunomodulatory activities against autoimmune myocarditis. Pharmacological Research, 124, 34-42

[50] Asefi S, Seifi M, Fard GH, Lotfi A. Innovative evaluation of local injective gel of curcumin on the orthodontic tooth movement in rats. Dent Res J (Isfahan). 2018 Jan-Feb;15(1):40-49. doi: 10.4103/1735-3327.223618

[51] Haagsma JA, Graetz N, Bolliger I et al. The global burden of injury: incidence, mortality, disability-adjusted life years and time trends from the Global Burden of Disease study 2013. Inj. Prev. 22(1), 3-18 (2015).

[52] Abdollahi, E., Momtazi, A. A., Johnston, T. P., & Sahebkar, A. (2018). Therapeutic effects of curcumin in inflammatory and immune mediated diseases: A nature made jack of all trades? J. Cellular Physiology, 233(2), 830-848

[53] Nguyen T.T.T, Ghosh C, Hwang S-G, Dai Tran L, Park J.S, Characteristics of curcumin-loaded poly (lactic acid) nanofibers for wound healing, J. Mater. Sci. 48 (2013) 7125-7133.

[54] Pişkin A, Altunkaynak BZ, Tümentemur G, Kaplan S, Yazıcı OB, Hökelek M. The beneficial effects of Momordica charantia (bitter gourd) on wound healing of rabbit skin. J Dermatolog Treat. 2014 Aug;25(4):350-357. doi: 10.3109/09546634.2012.713459.

[55] Hussan F, Teoh SL, Muhamad N, Mazlan M, Latiff AA. *Momordica charantia* ointment accelerates diabetic wound healing and enhances transforming growth factor-β expression. J Wound Care. 2014 Aug;23(8):400, 402, 404-7. doi: 10.12968/jowc.2014.23.8.400

[56] Ezealisiji, K.M., Stanley, C.N. & Ekanem, E.S., 2016, 'Evaluation of anti-cholesterol activity of ethyl acetate and n-hexane extracts of Tetracarpidium conophorum (Mull. Arg.) Hutch and Dalziel (African walnut) towards hypercholesterolemic rats', Intl. J. Pharmacog. Phytochem. Res. 8(8), 1372-1376.

[57] Ilomuanya M.O., Amenaghawon N.A., Odimegwu J., Okubanjo O.O., Aghaizu C., Adeyinka O., Akhimien T., Ajayi T. (2018) Formulation and optimization of gentamicin hydrogel infused with *tetracarpidium conophorum* extract via Central composite design for topical delivery. Turkish J. Pharm. Sci. 15(3):319-327 https://doi.org/10.4274/tjps.33042

Chapter 7

Bionanomaterials: Advancements in Wound Healing and Tissue Regeneration

Priyanka Chhabra and Kajol Bhati

Abstract

Abnormal wound healing represents a major healthcare issue owing to upsurge number of trauma and morbid physiology which ultimately posed a healthcare burden on patient, society and health care organization. A wound healing is a complex process so effective management of chronic wounds is often hard. Recently in addition to many conventional wound treatment's advances in bionanomaterial are attaining much attention in wound care and skin tissue engineering. Bionanomaterials are biomolecule-based nanocomposite synthesized by plants, microbes and animals which possess high degree of biocompatibility, biodegradability, non-toxicity and bioactive assets. Bioactive assets like antimicrobial, immune modulatory, cell proliferation and angiogenesis of biomolecules forms fortunate microenvironment for the wound healing process. Nature has provided us with a significant set of biomolecules like chitosan, hyaluronic acid, collagen, cellulose, silk fucoidan etc. have been exploited to construct engineered bionanomaterials. These biopolymeric nanomaterials are currently researched comprehensively as they have higher surface to volume ratio and high chemical affinity showing a promising augmentation of deadly wounds. In this chapter we aimed to highlight the biological sources and bioengineering approaches adapted for biopolymers so they facilitate wound healing process.

Keywords: Biopolymers, Bionanomaterials, wound healing, nanocomposites, tissue engineering

1. Introduction

Wound healing process involves a series of intricate cellular events involving organized and regulated events such as hemostasis, inflammation, cell migration, proliferation, and remodeling [1]. Upon the onset of the inflammatory response, fibroblasts begin to proliferate and migrate into the wound area which involve the interaction and participation of different types of growth factors, cells and supporting cell-ECM interaction and ultimately reconstitute the wounded skin after injury [2]. Sometimes the normal wound healing process gets altered due to morbid physiology for example, in case of burns, accidents, diabetic foot ulcers, wound healing is delayed. This leads to the compromised mobility, amputation of limbs, even death, which cause the foremost social, and financial burden for decades [3]. Nowaday's nanotechnology and nanomedicine has created a new way to treat acute and chronic wound which ultimately encourage tissue regeneration and remolding. Indeed, many research studies and clinical trials data have already been published [4]. This chapter summarized the systematic evaluation of different types of bionanomaterials which promote wound healing process and introduce their future scope [5].

2. Physiology of normal wound healing

The normal wound healing cascade involves a complex series of cellular and biochemical events which begin with hemostasis and inflammation, proliferation, maturation, remodeling, and wound contraction. These phases are not exactly distinguishable from each other, because occasionally they overlap or proceed concurrently [6].

2.1 Hemostasis

It is the first stage of wound healing which start immediately after the injury and cause the stoppage of bleeding. In hemostasis various platelets factors are released by the degranulation thrombocytes cells like insulin-like growth factor (IGF-I), Platelet-derived growth factor (PDGF), Transforming growth factor beta (TGF-β) and Epidermal growth factor (EGF) followed by coagulation cascade. Coagulation cascade is the multifaceted chain reaction which begin at the site of injury in which the conversion of prothrombin to enzyme thrombin takes place. Thrombin converts the fibrinogen in to fibrin monomers at the site of the wound surface. Fibrinogen polymerizes the fibrin monomers to form a fibrin chain which are interlinked by coagulation factor XIII and form a stable fibrin network.

2.2 Inflammatory phase

After the hemostasis is achieved inflammation is initiated at the site of injury. Immediately after the rupturing of blood vessel mast cells releases various inflammatory factors like thromboxanes, histamins and prostaglandins which causes the vasoconstriction to prevent blood loss.

Initially, Polymorphonuclear neutrophils (PMNs) are arrived at the wounded area within an hour of injury. PMNs cells are the predominant cells for the first two days at the site of injury, which are attracted to the site by growth factors and fibronectins. Neutrophils release free radicals which phagocyte the debris and kill bacteria at the site of injury. This process is known as respiratory burst. Other leukocytes like helper T cells also present in the wounded area helps in the secretion of cytokine which divide T cells and increases inflammation, vasodilatation, vessel permeability and activity of macrophage. Macrophages are essential for the tissue regeneration and wound healing. Macrophages are stimulated by the low oxygen content to produce various factors which enhance the angiogenesis, stimulate the cells to re-epithelialise the wound, form granulation tissue, built a new ECM ultimately pushing the wound healing process into next phase. Macrophages become prominent by replacing the PAMs cells at the wound site. As inflammation decreases, few inflammatory factors are secreted and numbers of neutrophils and macrophages are decreased at the wound site create a clean wound bed which indicate that inflammatory phase is ending and enters in to the proliferative phase [7].

2.3 Migration and proliferation phase

After few days of injury migration and proliferation phase starts and last up to 21 days from the day of the wound takes place. This phase is characterized by angiogenesis, epithelisation and fibroplasias. In proliferation phase wound start to rebuilt with healthy granulation tissue. To form the granulation tissue sufficient supply of oxygen and nutrient is required by the blood vessels. A new network of blood vessels is replaced by the damaged one by the process of angiogenesis, formation of extra cellular matrix (ECM) and collagen takes place. With the formation of the granulation tissue damaged mesenchymal cells are converted into the fibroblast cells which act as a bridge for the movement of the cells around the affected area. In healthy wound these fibroblasts start to appear within three days of the injury and liberate liquids and collagen which help to strengthen the wound site. The wound continues to grow stronger in the proliferation phase with the reorganization of the fibroblast cells and help in the formation of new tissue and speed up the wound healing process [7].

2.4 Remodeling phase

Remodeling or maturation phase is the last phase of healing process which finalizes the wound healing process. Remodeling phase start approximately 21 days after the injury and can go up to 2 years with the change in the matrix composition over the time. During this phase, the collagen formation and organization takes place with the help of collagenases and matrix metalloproteinases. The tensile strength of the dermal tissue increases and nonfunctional fibroblasts are recouped by the functional ones. With the passage of the time cellular activity decreases and the blood vessels in the affected area reduced. Wound contraction takes place and type III collagen is remodeled in type I collagen which increase the tensile strength of the wound and wound is fully closed [8, 9].

3. Pathophysiology of chronic wounds

A chronic wound is defined as one in which the normal process of healing is disrupted at one or more points in the phases of hemostasis, inflammation, proliferation and remodeling and do not heal completely within 90 days after the onset of any injury [10]. Chronic wounds, unlike acute wounds, do not undergo the ordered molecular and cellular processes of physiological tissue repair previously discussed. However, the healing process of chronic wounds is thought to be stuck in inflammation [11]. Chronic wounds can also be considered to be an imbalance between tissue deposition stimulated by growth factors, and tissue destruction mediated by proteases. Hereby, the imbalance favors the destructive process [10]. Thus, the molecular and cellular processes are disrupted leading to significant differences in the microenvironment of the wound, both in terms of the constituents of the exudates and the cellular components of the wound area. In addition, oxidative damage by free radicals, condition specific factors of underlying diseases, and accumulated necrotic tissue as well contributes to the chronic state. The further healing of those wounds results in skin defects of excessive fibrous appearance, for instance keloids and scar contractures, or alternatively in insufficient tissue replacement, i.e., a non-healing wound [12].

4. Challenges in tissue regeneration

The role of ECM in wound healing has been traditionally thought of as a passive structural support for cells. It is now clear that cell-ECM interactions, in concert with growth factors, are necessary for rapid wound healing. Hence, the main challenge in wound therapeutics is to provide an ideal microenvironment for optimal cell migration and proliferation [13]. Many strategies have been adopted for accelerating tissue repair. Exogenous growth factors, ECM molecules, and short peptide sequences targeting specific integrin receptors have been shown to accelerate wound healing both *in vitro* and *in vivo*. However, native ECM molecules or growth factors lack structural properties, and are expensive to produce in large quantities [14]. On the other hand, polymeric materials offer excellent physical support, and enhance biological activity. To circumvent these disadvantages, polymeric materials have also been functionalized with bioactive peptide sequences, nanoparticles and growth factors in to bionanomaterial [4].

5. Biomaterials for wound healing

Recent years have witnessed extraordinary growth of research and applications in the field of nanoscience and nanotechnology. The field of nanoscience is one of the most dynamic research areas in modern material science and combination of physics, chemistry, biology, material science & medicine has materialized as nanotechnology. Nanoparticles and nanostructure are rapidly increasing for new application in the field of biomedicine and wound healing.

Nanomaterials are the materials which are having a maximum diameter of 100 nm and nanoproducts which lies in nanoscale are known as nanomaterial. Nanomaterial possesses large surface to volume ration due to which they offer wide-ranging application in the field of science and technology. There are variety of biomaterials which acquire excellent candidature for numerous biomedical applications. When these biomaterials are used in nanoforms like nanotubes, nanocomposite, nano pockets and nanoparticles they are known as bionanomaterial [15, 16].

The size of the bionanomaterial hold an important parameter in terms of biological application because of its similarity in size as compared to genetic material i.e., around 2.5 nm in width and to building block of cell i.e., protein which is around 1-20 nm. So, for biological application the size and surface properties of the bionanomaterial can be personalized as per the prerequisite.

The nature has provided us with a significant set of biomaterials like chitosan, cellulose, silk, hyaluronic acid, alginate, fucoidan, pectin, gelatin, keratin, carboxymethyl cellulose, Bovine serum albumin. These proteins and polysaccharides-based biomaterials possess a physiochemical property like biocompatibility, biodegradability and non-toxicity which makes them apposite for inclusion in living systems thereby accelerate or replace the function of bodily tissues, organs or damaged tissue & augment wound healing process. Polymeric biomaterials can be fabricated in to variety of nanostructures like nanotubes, nanoparticles, nano- capsules, nanopockets, nanocrystals, nanowhiskers which ultimately possess the potential to encourage self-healing mechanisms that can mimic tissue regeneration [17, 18]. The summery of all the biomaterials in provided in the **Table 1**.

5.1 Nano-biomaterials in wound healing

As we know wound healing is well orchestrated process involving a significant number of physiochemical events in different phases of healing process involving hemostasis, inflammation, proliferation and remolding. There are variety of factors which significantly influence the wound healing course and slow down their activities, completely disturb the wound healing process. It is difficult to visualize the necessity of altered tissue and ample the requirements for tissue regeneration. Nature has provided with us a significant set of biomaterials which possess fundamental properties like non-toxicity, biocompatibility, biodegradability and

DOI: http://dx.doi.org/10.5772/intechopen.97298

Biomaterial	Monomer units and linkage	Biological Role in wound healing	Characteristics	Nano-biomaterial	Reference
Chitosan	*N*-acetyl glucosamine linked by β-1, 4 glycosidic linkages	It act as a hemostat during early blood clotting cascade It activates neutrophils infiltration & migration It also stimulates PMN leucocytes, macrophages & fibroblast for phagocytosis and cell proliferation. It provides non-protein matrix for 3D growth of tissue.	It is bio- degradable, biocompatible, antimicrobial, antifungal and non-toxic in nature	Chitosan can be engineered in to nanoparticles, nano- fibrils, nanotubes and nanorods	[18, 19]
Cellulose	β-d-Glucose linked by β-1,4-glycosidic linkage	It aids in the absorption of exudates resulting in the intake of cell debris (such as necrotic tissue and fibrinous coating) and the porous cellulose structure mimics ECM of skin thus helping in tissue regeneration	It is non-toxic, non-allergic and biocompatible, unique rheological properties, crystalline behaviors, sustainability and biodegradability	Nanocrystals, nanofibers, nano whiskers, nanorods, nanofibrils, and nanocellulose.	[20–22]
Silk fibroin	Disulphide bonds	Silk arouse cell migration and proliferation It trigger collagen formation & encourage epithelization by enhancing fibroblast and keratinocytes proliferation	It is bio- degradable, biocompatible, easily factionalized and its many physical properties can be modified non-immunogenic and bioresorbable material	Silk can transformed in to silk nanoparticles, nanofilms, nanocomposites	[23, 24]
Hyaluronic acid	β-d -glucuronic acid and *N*-acetyl-d-glucosamine linked by β-1,4 and β-1,3 glycosidic linkages	Hyaluronic acid attunes vital phases of wound healing like inflammation, cellular migration, and angiogenesis, It also stimulates TGFβ-1, b-FGF, PDGF, and EGF growth factors production and enhance keratinocytes proliferation in wound bed	Highly biocompatible, Biodegradable, Bacteriostatic, non-immunogenic and possess high water retention capacity	It can be architectures in to nanoparticles and nanotubes	[25]

Biomaterial	Monomer units and linkage	Biological Role in wound healing	Characteristics	Nano-biomaterial	Reference
Alginate	β-d-Mannuronic acid and α-l-guluronic acid linked by α-1, 4 glycosidic linkages	Calcium alginates assist in hemostasis by releasing calcium ions at the wound site. Provide moist wound environment and confines pathogenic and bacterial access into the wound. It also augments proliferation and cell adhesion	Alginates and alginic acids are antibacterial, Biocompatible, Biodegradable moisture absorbent in nature	They can be transformed in to nanogels nanoparticles and nanofibers	[26]
Fucoidan	α-l-Fucose linked by α-1, 3 glycosidic linkages	It can bind and activate growth factors production at the wound site It also enhance the formation of neovascularization & collagen matrix and augment the wound healing process	Anti-inflammatory, antioxidant Anticoagulant, antiviral and immunomodulatory	It can be molded in to nanoflakes, nanospikes,nanofilms, nanoparticles	[27, 28]
Pectin	D-galacturonic acid linked by α-(1 → 4)-glycosidic bond...	pectin is hydrophilic in nature. It allows removal of wound exudates from wound bed. It also allows maintenance of acid environment which is impermeable to microbes.	Due to the presence of large number sof esters and galacturonic acid it possess anti-inflammatory properties It is also Antithrombogenic, biodegradable and biocompatible in nature	Nanocomposites, Nanofilms	[29, 30]
Gelatin	Sugar and amino acids	Gelatin stimulates signal transduction and cell adhesion in well-coordinated progression of wound healing process.	It is highly absorbent, biodegradable, Biocompatible, and non immunogenic in nature	Nanocomposites, nanofilms	[31]
Collagen	Amino acids linked by amide linkage	It fascinates fibroblast and boost collagen deposition. It inactivates matrix metalloproteinases (MMPs), also stimulates tissue growth, angiogenesis,autolytic debridement &reepithelization	Collagen is biodegradable, anti-inflammatory and non-toxic	Nanofibers, nanoparticles	[4, 32]

Table 1.
Biomaterials and their wound healing properties.

also mimic with the host extra cellular environment. Moreover, several of them are non-immunogenic and fulfill the demands of suitable wound healing dressing material. Biomaterials and their composites are comprehensively investigated by the researchers which can be tailored in nanostructure like nanoparticles, nanofilms, nanoflakes, nanocomposites, nano capsules, nanotubes, nanogels, nanofibrils, nanospikes and nanowhikers. These nanostructures encourage the potential to endorse self-healing mechanism that can mimic tissue regeneration. With the extended knowledge of nanotechnology and nanomedicine they represent a great prospect to improve currently available medical treatments and prognosis impaired wound healing [33].

5.1.1 Nanoparticles

As a functioning field of nano-research, the molecular designing of different self-assembling biocompatible nanoparticles has been created in recent years. Nanoparticle, exhibit unique physiochemical properties and maximized its use for biomedical and therapeutic application, including for wound healing. Using the nanoparticles, delayed wound healing and burn care has been enhanced. Polymeric nanoparticles are manufactured from biodegradable polymers or copolymers to remove, capture, encapsulate or bind the drug. They can be made up of natural ones, Synthetic and semi-synthetic polymers and their copolymers, such as alginate, chitosan, gelatin, poly (glycolic acid), albumin, poly-alkyl cyanoacrylate, PLGA, etc. They have the benefits of controlled and sustained discharge, enhanced bioavailability, elevate level of exemplification, and biocompatibility with tissues and cells. Chitosan nanoparticles have traditionally been among the most commonly researched groups of natural biopolymer products for biomaterials. Using either "bottom-up" or "top-down" methods or a mixture of both techniques, Chitosan nanoparticles can be synthesized. Chitosan can be used as a wound-healing agent due to its antimicrobial, haemostatic, film-forming, anti-inflammatory, and anticoagulant activities. Curcumin loaded chitosan nanoparticles accelerate the wound healing by regulating inflammation and neovascularisations. As chitosan is remarkable antimicrobial agent which modulate the production of reactive oxygen species, IL-6 secretion and augment proinflammatory activation and ultimately augment healing in chronic wound [34].

Hyaluronic acid (HA-NPs) nanoparticles also showed good stability and had a potential to be applied as blood contact material. Studies showed that HA-NPs showed excellent comprehensive biocompatibility, strongly promoting adhesion and proliferation of extra cellular while still exerting inhibitory effects on platelets, and macrophages [35].

Gelatin is a naturally produced collagen-derived polymer utilized specifically in the manufacture of biodegradable materials, and biocompatible fabrics for wound dressing. Fibrin is also a natural polymer which, in the presence of the enzyme thrombin, is made from fibrinogen polymerized into fibrin. Fibrin has distinctive properties, including inflammation reduction and enhanced immunological response and cell permeability, and has been broadly included in wound healing and tissue engineering [36]. Under acidic conditions, pectin has the ideal consistency also at higher temperatures, making it the perfect choice for use in the drug delivery system. In the presence of divalent cations, pectin has a peculiar gel forming capacity that makes it an excellent carrier for supplying bioactive agents. At low pH, pectin forms an accumulation of macromolecules, but the pectin aggregates appear to dissociate at neutral pH and form an extended network. Thiolated pectin-based nanoparticles have recently been explored and their potential for delivery of ocular drugs has been studied. The thiolated pectin nanoparticles have been prepared using magnesium chloride as an ionic crosslinker by ionotropic gelation and timolol maleate as the model drug. They indicated that the addition of crosslinker imparts a more pronounced effect on the nanoparticles' particle size, whereas the drug trap is influenced by polymer concentration. Mucoadhesive nanoparticles have been shown to extract the substance from the particles trapped in the cul-de-sac for a long period of time. Developed pectin nanoparticles through mechanical homogenization and showed enhanced drug dissolution [7].

Silk fibers are used by the textile industries and as suture material. Silk fibers are generated by the silkworm cocoons named *Bombyx mori*. Nowadays, silk is valuable in the biomedical sector because of its mechanical and biological properties like biodegradability, stiffness, biocompatibility, water vapor permeability, and antibacterial properties. Due to its different properties, silk can be used as a material for wound dressing. Hydrocolloid dressings loaded with silk fibroin nanoparticles showed enhanced effectiveness of medical dressing due to the hydrophobic nature of silk fibroin polymers, result in enhanced physical properties. It also maintains the environment of extra cellular matrix, furthermore cell viability is also increased in burn wound animals models [7].

5.1.2 Nanofilms

In current scenario of nanotechnology research, nanostructure of polymeric biomaterial has been attracted a great attention of researchers. Nanofilms are among them one type of nanomaterials which is widely used for wound healing applications. Nanofilms are the thin single or multilayer biomaterials structure which vary from few nanometers to several micrometers in thickness. They are flexible sheets and generally used in wound dressing. The nanofilms synthesized for wound healing applications are transparent in nature, also allow exchange of gases like oxygen and carbon dioxide and but impermeable to water, bacteria and other pathogens. The variety of biomaterials can easily be tailored in to nanofilms. Carboxymethylcellulose nano films own high absorption capacity of exude and also triggers the formation of new blood vessels and remove necrotic debris and devitalized tissues from a wound bed.

Chitosan and alginates based nanofilms augment the wound healing process in both excision and incision animal wound model studies and also facilitated cell viability, collagen deposition, tissue regeneration and remolding [37]. Nanofilms based on hyaluronic acid effectively accelerate wound healing process and cause less trauma while removing these nanofilms based wound dressing. Studies showed that low proportion of hyaluronic acid in chitosan-hyaluronic acid composite nanofilms will decrease the water vapor permeability and fibroblast adhesion which is beneficial to accelerate wound healing process. Collagen based nanofilms demonstrated in study enhance fibroblast migration which markedly improved wound healing process.

Fucoidan- is an emerging biomaterial from a family of sulfated polyfucose polysaccharides extracted from brown marine algae. Fucoidan comes under spotlight due to its significant properties like antioxidant, antivirus, anticoagulant and anti-inflammatory and non-toxicity. It was studied that fucoidan based nanofilms increase the potential wound healing in burns wounds by significantly induce wound contraction. It reacts with the basic fibroblast growth factor and transforming growth factor and mediate the wound healing process [38].

5.1.3 Nanofibers

Nanofibers display two main characteristics: a pore size and high surface/volume ratio which placed it under spot light in variety of biomedical application like drugs delivery and wound healing. High surface area and different fabrication process used for adjusting the composition of nanofibrils make it responsible to speed the wound healing process. It augments cell adhesion, proliferation and differentiation at the wound bed. The traditional method of processing these biomaterials is through the technique of electrospinning, which provides the possibility of operating with a high yield at a nano-scale. Low spinnability can be manage by adding synthetic polymers into the natural polymers. As we known natural polymers offers extensive variety of bioactive properties which makes then suitable for biomedical and wound healing applications. Many studies showed that nano porosity and large surface to volume ratio makes the nanofibers competent to smooth the wound healing process. Mesh like structure of nanofibers promote high absorption of wound exudate. It also promotes cell respiration and exchange of gases. Biopolymeric nanofibers boom the ability of fibrous mesh to react with biological components of wound healing process [39].

Gelatin is a natural polymer derived from collagen that is biocompatible and biodegradable. It enhanced the regeneration of tissue and helps in healing of wound. When used as a wound dressing material, gelatin nanofibers comply with all required specifications like haemostatic, low cytotoxicity, reduced antigenicity [40]. Their scarcity of antimicrobial properties, restricts the use of gelatin. The antimicrobial properties of gelatin have been enhanced by adding other substances into it like poly([2-(methacryloyloxy)ethyl] trimethylammonium chloride) (PMETAC) and showed good bacterial activity against *Staphylococcus aureus*, *Escherichia coli*, methicillin-resistant, and Acinetobacter baumannii. Further study on cell adhesion revealed that cells attached and proliferate on the nanofiber surface, resulted in the safe use of gelatin nanofibers as material for wound dressing [41].

Collagen type I nanofibers were also favored to enhance cell proliferation. 3D nanofibrous scaffolds as dressings of collagen accelerate the wound closure in 14 days [42].

Chitosan nanofibers are also emerging candidate in the area of biomaterials. Studies showed that many different types of drugs like chemotherapeutics agents, antibiotics and proteins can be successfully loaded in electrospun nanofibers. Chitosan nanofibers possess several bioactive properties and can be utilized for wound dressing, tissue engineering and drug delivery system [43].

Due the small pore size of chitosan nanofibers they reduce the bacterial infection at wound bed and also decrease dehydration during wound healing process [44].

As Ideal wound dressing should maintain the water loss at a range of 2000 and 2500 g^{-2} day^{-1} at the wound site indicates that the higher values dry the wound rapidly and cause hindrance in smooth wound healing progression. Studies showed that chitosan-based nanofibers has water vapor transmission rate of 1950 to 2050 g^{-2} day^{-1} makes it ideal candidate for wound healing dressing [45].

In addition to that nanofibers of hyaluronic acid [HA] also hold a potent position in the field of biomedical application due to their unique properties as an extracellular-matrix and accelerating wound healing. Hyaluronic acid nanofibers have very mechanical properties due to which they cannot be used alone as a wound healing dressing material. Thus, reinforcement agent is required to incorporate into nanofibers. Hyaluronic acid has carboxygroup, which is capable of forming hydrogen bond with the protonates amines. Chitosan possesses an amine group that helps in the formation of hydrogen bonds with hyaluronic acid. In turn, it increases the mechanical strength of hyaluronic acid nanofibers dressing [46].

5.1.4 Nanocomposites

Currently, due to the rapid development in the field of nanotechnology and nanomedicine formation of nanocomposites for biomedical and wound healing is more facile and development of biopolymer nanocomposites has bloomed due to its outstanding endorsements in structural, electrical, mechanical applications. They are enlightened materials to transport nanoparticles [47]. The distinct features of nanocomposite may reflect the mutual properties of their components; they can serve for different biomedical purpose. In wound dressing, nanocomposites aims to reinforce structural stability and increase antimicrobial activity [48].

Biopolymer nanocomposite loaded with nanoparticles of antimicrobial agent play a vital role in the tissue repair and regeneration. Due to high surface to volume ratio of nanoparticles, they significantly increase the efficacy of the wound dressing against different microorganisms by reducing the risk of developing bacterial resistance. Chitosan own functional amino group that can be further engineered for a wide range of applications. Studies showed that chitosan-based nanocomposites loaded with antimicrobial agent are attractive not only in food preservation but also in biomedical field. Antimicrobial nanoparticle loaded chitosan nanocomposites encourage controlled release of drug through the matrix at wound site which prevent the unwanted bacterial infection. Montmorillonite–chitosan–silver sulfadiazine nano composites were evaluated on skin lesions which showed increased efficacy of prepared nanocomposites and can be used as potent wound dressing material [49].

Silk nanocomposites also investigated for wound healing applications as silk own good permeability to oxygen and water vapors, also possess high thermal resistance, good tensile strength and antimicrobial properties [50].

Hyaluronic acid-based nanocomposite showed satisfied properties of an ideal wound dressing in terms of porosity, swelling, biocompatibility, biodegradation. They also showed haemostatic potential and antibacterial properties. Hyaluronic acid nanocomposite incorporated with silver nanoparticles own effective response against *S. aureus*, *E. coli*, *P. aeruginosa* and *K. pneumoniae* microbes. So they can be used as potential bio nanocomposite for wound dressing of chronic wound loaded with bacterial infections [51].

Guar gum loaded Carboxymethyl nanocomposites showed enhanced re- epithelial growth and very less inflammatory cells which confirm that they reduce microbial infections. Therefore, Guar gum loaded Carboxymethyl nanocomposites has the potential of effectively accelerate wound healing process and are a suitable candidate for wound dressing material [52].

6. Conclusions

The nanotechnology and nanomedicine-based therapies are an emerging trend in the field of biomedical and wound healing application. Plentiful researchers have designed and innovate nanoplatforms to enhance wound healing process which demonstrate promising results in the field of wound healing. Recently biopolymeric nano systems have attracted much attention which showed a great response and benefits in treating acute and chronic wounds. The potential of bionanomaterials for biomedical and wound healing application is enormous due to their bioactive physiological properties like biocompatibility, biodegradability, non-toxicity, non-immunogenic which synthetic polymers do not possess. These nanomaterials play a significant role in cell attachment, differentiation and proliferation as well as delivery of target protein, drugs, stem cells and growth factors. Various types of nanomaterial can be engineered using these biomaterials like nanoparticles, nanofilms, nanocomposites, nanofibers which enhance the administration of different drugs and reduce the cytotoxicity. Topical application of bionanomaterials not only improve controlled drug delivery but also favors cell fibroblast proliferation, and reduced tissue inflammation. Furthermore, the detailed insight of molecular mechanism in wound healing and the role of bionanomaterial in this process is needed attention to translate basic research into clinical application.

Conflict of interest

There are no conflicts of interest.

Author details

Priyanka Chhabra* and Kajol Bhati
Department of Forensic Science, School of Basic and Applied Sciences, Galgotias University, Greater Noida, Uttar Pradesh, India

*Address all correspondence to: pchhabra188@gmail.com

References

[1] Hou B, Qi M, Sun J, Ai M, Ma X, Cai W, et al. Preparation, characterization and wound healing effect of vaccarin-chitosan nanoparticles. Int J Biol Macromol [Internet]. 2020 Dec;165:3169-79. Available from: https://linkinghub.elsevier.com/retrieve/pii/S0141813020348340

[2] Rajoo A, Ramanathan S, Mansor SM, Sasidharan S. Formulation and evaluation of wound healing activity of *Elaeis guineensis* Jacq leaves in a *Staphylococcus aureus* infected Sprague Dawley rat model. J Ethnopharmacol [Internet]. 2021 Feb;266:113414. Available from: https://linkinghub.elsevier.com/retrieve/pii/S0378874120332992

[3] Rodrigues M, Kosaric N, Bonham CA, Gurtner GC. Wound healing: A cellular perspective. Physiol Rev. 2019;99(1):665-706.

[4] Barroso A, Mestre H, Ascenso A, Simões S, Reis C. Nanomaterials in wound healing: From material sciences to wound healing applications. Nano Sel. 2020;1(5):443-60.

[5] Chhabra P, Tyagi P, Bhatnagar A, Mittal G, Kumar A. Optimization, characterization, and efficacy evaluation of 2% chitosan scaffold for tissue engineering and wound healing. J Pharm Bioallied Sci [Internet]. 2016;8(4):300. Available from: http://www.jpbsonline.org/text.asp?2016/8/4/300/199346

[6] Steenfos HH. Growth Factors and Wound Healing. Scand J Plast Reconstr Surg Hand Surg [Internet]. 1994 Jan 8;28(2):95-105. Available from: http://www.tandfonline.com/doi/full/10.3109/02844319409071186

[7] Sharma R, Ahuja M, Kaur H. Thiolated pectin nanoparticles: Preparation, characterization and ex vivo corneal permeation study. Carbohydr Polym [Internet]. 2012 Jan;87(2):1606-10. Available from: https://linkinghub.elsevier.com/retrieve/pii/S0144861711008642

[8] Janis JE, Harrison B. Wound Healing. Plast Reconstr Surg [Internet]. 2016 Sep;138:9S–17S. Available from: http://journals.lww.com/00006534-201609001-00004

[9] Broughton G, Janis JE, Attinger CE. The Basic Science of Wound Healing. Plast Reconstr Surg [Internet]. 2006 Jun;117(SUPPLEMENT):12S–34S. Available from: http://journals.lww.com/00006534-200606001-00005

[10] Han G, Ceilley R. Chronic Wound Healing: A Review of Current Management and Treatments. Adv Ther [Internet]. 2017;34(3):599-610. Available from: http://www.ncbi.nlm.nih.gov/pubmed/28108895

[11] Bucalo B, Eaglstein WH, Falanga V. Inhibition of cell proliferation by chronic wound fluid. Wound Repair Regen [Internet]. 1993 Jul;1(3):181-6. Available from: http://www.ncbi.nlm.nih.gov/pubmed/28108895

[12] Dhall S, Do DC, Garcia M, Kim J, Mirebrahim SH, Lyubovitsky J, et al. Generating and reversing chronic wounds in diabetic mice by manipulating wound redox parameters. J Diabetes Res [Internet]. 2014;2014:562625. Available from: http://www.ncbi.nlm.nih.gov/pubmed/25587545

[13] Eriksson J, D'Angelo W, Badylak SF. Common Challenges in Tissue Regeneration. In: Epigenetics and Regeneration [Internet]. Elsevier; 2019. p. 217-29. Available from: https://linkinghub.elsevier.com/retrieve/pii/B9780128148792000091

[14] Peng J, Zhao H, Tu C, Xu Z, Ye L, Zhao L, et al. In situ hydrogel dressing loaded with heparin and basic fibroblast growth factor for accelerating wound healing in rat. Mater Sci Eng C [Internet]. 2020 Nov;116:111169. Available from: https://linkinghub.elsevier.com/retrieve/pii/S0928493120305221

[15] Rivero PJ, Urrutia A, Goicoechea J, Arregui FJ. Nanomaterials for Functional Textiles and Fibers. Nanoscale Res Lett [Internet]. 2015 Dec 29;10(1):501. Available from: http://www.nanoscalereslett.com/content/10/1/501

[16] Gao L, Gan H, Meng Z, Gu R, Wu Z, Zhu X, et al. Evaluation of genipin-crosslinked chitosan hydrogels as a potential carrier for silver sulfadiazine nanocrystals. Colloids Surfaces B Biointerfaces [Internet]. 2016 Dec;148:343-53. Available from: https://linkinghub.elsevier.com/retrieve/pii/S0927776516304465

[17] Liu X, Wong KKY. Application of Nanomedicine in Wound Healing. In: Nanotechnology in Dermatology [Internet]. New York, NY: Springer New York; 2013. p. 221-9. Available from: http://link.springer.com/10.1007/978-1-4614-5034-4_21

[18] Wong K, Lee, Zhang, Liu, Sun, Che. Enhancement of anticancer efficacy using modified lipophilic nanoparticle drug encapsulation. Int J Nanomedicine [Internet]. 2012 Feb;731. Available from: http://www.dovepress.com/enhancement-of-anticancer-efficacy-using-modified-lipophilic-nanoparti-peer-reviewed-article-IJN

[19] Shukla SK, Mishra AK, Arotiba OA, Mamba BB. Chitosan-based nanomaterials: A state-of-the-art review. Int J Biol Macromol [Internet]. 2013 Aug;59:46-58. Available from: https://linkinghub.elsevier.com/retrieve/pii/S0141813013002262

[20] Pei Y, Ye D, Zhao Q, Wang X, Zhang C, Huang W, et al. Effectively promoting wound healing with cellulose/gelatin sponges constructed directly from a cellulose solution. J Mater Chem B. 2015;3(38):7518-28.

[21] Portela R, Leal CR, Almeida PL, Sobral RG. Bacterial cellulose: a versatile biopolymer for wound dressing applications. Microb Biotechnol [Internet]. 2019 Jul 5;12(4):586-610. Available from: https://onlinelibrary.wiley.com/doi/10.1111/1751-7915.13392

[22] Moon RJ, Schueneman GT, Simonsen J. Overview of Cellulose Nanomaterials, Their Capabilities and Applications. Jom. 2016;68(9):2383-94.

[23] Patil PP, Reagan MR, Bohara RA. Silk fibroin and silk-based biomaterial derivatives for ideal wound dressings. Int J Biol Macromol [Internet]. 2020;164:4613-27. Available from: https://doi.org/10.1016/j.ijbiomac.2020.08.041

[24] Shen G, Hu X, Guan G, Wang L. Surface Modification and Characterisation of Silk Fibroin Fabric Produced by the Layer-by-Layer Self-Assembly of Multilayer Alginate/Regenerated Silk Fibroin. Matsusaki M, editor. PLoS One [Internet]. 2015 Apr 28;10(4):e0124811. Available from: https://dx.plos.org/10.1371/journal.pone.0124811

[25] Snetkov P, Morozkina S, Uspenskaya M, Olekhnovich R. Hyaluronan-Based Nanofibers: Fabrication, Characterization and Application. Polymers (Basel) [Internet]. 2019 Dec 9;11(12):2036. Available from: https://www.mdpi.com/2073-4360/11/12/2036

[26] Najafiasl M, Osfouri S, Azin R, Zaeri S. Alginate-based electrospun core/shell nanofibers containing dexpanthenol: A good candidate for wound dressing. J Drug Deliv Sci Technol. 2020;57(March).

[27] Hao Y, Zhao W, Zhang L, Zeng X, Sun Z, Zhang D, et al. Bio-multifunctional alginate/chitosan/fucoidan sponges with enhanced angiogenesis and hair follicle regeneration for promoting full-thickness wound healing. Mater Des [Internet]. 2020;193:108863. Available from: https://doi.org/10.1016/j.matdes.2020.108863

[28] Lim SJ, Wan Aida WM. Extraction of Sulfated Polysaccharides (Fucoidan) From Brown Seaweed [Internet]. Seaweed Polysaccharides: Isolation, Biological and Biomedical Applications. Elsevier Inc.; 2017. 27-46 p. Available from: http://dx.doi.org/10.1016/B978-0-12-809816-5/00003-7

[29] Munarin F, Tanzi MC, Petrini P. Advances in biomedical applications of pectin gels. Int J Biol Macromol [Internet]. 2012;51(4):681-9. Available from: http://dx.doi.org/10.1016/j.ijbiomac.2012.07.002

[30] Kodoth AK, Ghate VM, Lewis SA, Prakash B, Badalamoole V. Pectin-based silver nanocomposite film for transdermal delivery of Donepezil. Int J Biol Macromol [Internet]. 2019 Aug;134:269-79. Available from: https://linkinghub.elsevier.com/retrieve/pii/S0141813019317039

[31] Galdopórpora JM, Morcillo MF, Ibar A, Perez CJ, Tuttolomondo M V., Desimone MF. Development of Silver Nanoparticles/Gelatin Thermoresponsive Nanocomposites: Characterization and Antimicrobial Activity. Curr Pharm Des [Internet]. 2019 Dec 17;25(38):4121-9. Available from: http://www.eurekaselect.com/175414/article

[32] Deng A, Yang Y, Du S, Yang S. Electrospinning of in situ crosslinked recombinant human collagen peptide/chitosan nanofibers for wound healing. Biomater Sci [Internet]. 2018;6(8):2197-208. Available from: http://xlink.rsc.org/?DOI=C8BM00492G

[33] Mogoşanu GD, Grumezescu AM. Natural and synthetic polymers for wounds and burns dressing. Int J Pharm [Internet]. 2014 Mar;463(2):127-36. Available from: https://linkinghub.elsevier.com/retrieve/pii/S0378517313010831

[34] Wang T, Zheng Y, Shen Y, Shi Y, Li F, Su C, et al. Chitosan nanoparticles loaded hydrogels promote skin wound healing through the modulation of reactive oxygen species. Artif Cells, Nanomedicine, Biotechnol [Internet]. 2018 Oct 31;46(sup1):138-49. Available from: https://www.tandfonline.com/doi/full/10.1080/21691401.2017.1415212

[35] Jiang T, Xie Z, Wu F, Chen J, Liao Y, Liu L, et al. Hyaluronic Acid Nanoparticle Composite Films Confer Favorable Time-Dependent Biofunctions for Vascular Wound Healing. ACS Biomater Sci Eng [Internet]. 2019 Apr 8;5(4):1833-48. Available from: https://pubs.acs.org/doi/10.1021/acsbiomaterials.9b00295

[36] İnal M, Mülazımoğlu G. Production and characterization of bactericidal wound dressing material based on gelatin nanofiber. Int J Biol Macromol. 2019;137:392-404.

[37] Sarhan WA, Azzazy HME, El-Sherbiny IM. Honey/Chitosan Nanofiber Wound Dressing Enriched with *Allium sativum* and Cleome droserifolia : Enhanced Antimicrobial and Wound Healing Activity. ACS Appl Mater Interfaces [Internet]. 2016 Mar 16;8(10):6379-90. Available from: https://pubs.acs.org/doi/10.1021/acsami.6b00739

[38] Sezer AD, Hatipoğlu F, Cevher E, Oğurtan Z, Baş AL, Akbuğa J. Chitosan film containing fucoidan as a wound dressing for dermal burn healing: Preparation and in vitro/in vivo evaluation. AAPS PharmSciTech. 2007;8(2):1-8.

[39] Iacob AT, Drăgan M, Ionescu OM, Profire L, Ficai A, Andronescu E, et al. An overview of biopolymeric electrospun nanofibers based on polysaccharides for wound healing management. Pharmaceutics. 2020;12(10):1-49.

[40] Gaspar-Pintiliescu A, Stanciuc AM, Craciunescu O. Natural composite dressings based on collagen, gelatin and plant bioactive compounds for wound healing: A review. Int J Biol Macromol [Internet]. 2019;138:854-65. Available from: https://doi.org/10.1016/j.ijbiomac.2019.07.155

[41] İnal M, Mülazımoğlu G. Production and characterization of bactericidal wound dressing material based on gelatin nanofiber. Int J Biol Macromol [Internet]. 2019 Sep;137:392-404. Available from: https://linkinghub.elsevier.com/retrieve/pii/S0141813019322202

[42] Mihai MM, Dima MB, Dima B, Holban AM. Nanomaterials for Wound Healing and Infection Control. Materials (Basel) [Internet]. 2019 Jul 6;12(13):2176. Available from: https://www.mdpi.com/1996-1944/12/13/2176

[43] AL-Jbour ND, Beg MD, Gimbun J, Alam AKMM. An Overview of Chitosan Nanofibers and their Applications in the Drug Delivery Process. Curr Drug Deliv. 2019 Apr 10;16(4).

[44] Kai D, Liow SS, Loh XJ. Biodegradable polymers for electrospinning: Towards biomedical applications. Mater Sci Eng C. 2014 Dec;45.

[45] Archana D, Dutta J, Dutta PK. Evaluation of chitosan nano dressing for wound healing: Characterization, in vitro and in vivo studies. Int J Biol Macromol. 2013 Jun;57.

[46] Hussein Y, El-Fakharany EM, Kamoun EA, Loutfy SA, Amin R, Taha TH, et al. Electrospun PVA/hyaluronic acid/L-arginine nanofibers for wound healing applications: Nanofibers optimization and in vitro bioevaluation. Int J Biol Macromol [Internet]. 2020;164:667-76. Available from: https://doi.org/10.1016/j.ijbiomac.2020.07.126

[47] Wang M. Developing bioactive composite materials for tissue replacement. Biomaterials. 2003 Jun;24(13).

[48] Zafar R, Zia KM, Tabasum S, Jabeen F, Noreen A, Zuber M. Polysaccharide based bionanocomposites, properties and applications: A review. Int J Biol Macromol. 2016 Nov;92.

[49] Mala R, Rani MJ, Prasath NH, Celsia ASR. Nano composite material of chitosan for wound healing: A review. In 2019. p. 020013. Available from: http://aip.scitation.org/doi/abs/10.1063/1.5100698

[50] Chouhan D, Mandal BB. Silk biomaterials in wound healing and skin regeneration therapeutics: From bench to bedside. Acta Biomater [Internet]. 2020;103:24-51. Available from: https://doi.org/10.1016/j.actbio.2019.11.050

[51] Anisha BS, Biswas R, Chennazhi KP, Jayakumar R. Chitosan–hyaluronic acid/nano silver composite sponges for drug resistant bacteria infected diabetic wounds. Int J Biol Macromol [Internet]. 2013 Nov;62:310-20. Available from: https://linkinghub.elsevier.com/retrieve/pii/S0141813013004844

[52] Orsu P, Matta S. Fabrication and characterization of carboxymethyl guar gum nanocomposite for application of wound healing. Int J Biol Macromol [Internet]. 2020 Dec;164:2267-76. Available from: https://linkinghub.elsevier.com/retrieve/pii/S0141813020340824

Chapter 8

Current Understanding to Accelerate Wound Healing: Mechanism and Clinical Importance

Sunil Kumar, Shravan Kumar Paswan, Pritt Verma, Akanksha, RamKishor Sah, Sajal Srivastava and Chandana Venketeswara Rao

Abstract

Wound mending is a complex organic cycle that brings about the reclamation of tissue honesty. Physiologically, it very well may be separated into four particular periods of hemostasis, inflammation, proliferation, and tissue remodeling (redesigning). This chapter portrays the cellular premise of wound mending and extracellular flagging cycles, which is responsible to control them. The capacity of fibroblasts, neutrophils, platelets, and macrophages is contemplated exhaustively. The idea of mending by essential and optional expectation is talked about. Numerous components are known to unfavorably influence mending including undernourishment, hypoxia, immunosuppression, ongoing sickness, and medical procedure. It is fundamental that specialists comprehend the key physiological cycles associated with mending to limit patient illness from postponed recuperating.

Keywords: hemostasis, inflammation, proliferation, remodeling, physiology of wound, wound healing

1. Introduction

An injury is characterized as harm or disturbance to the typical anatomical construction and function [1]. This can go from a straightforward break in the epithelial veracity of the skin, or it tends to be more profound, stretching out into subcutaneous tissue with harm to different constructions such as ligaments, muscles, vessels, nerves, parenchymal organs, and even bone [2].

In ordinary pathology, wounds stay a difficult clinical issue, with ahead of schedule and late inconveniences introducing a regular reason for dismalness and mortality [2, 3]. Trying to decrease the injury trouble, much exertion has alerted on comprehension of the physiology of recuperating and twisted consideration with an accentuation on new helpful methodologies and the proceeding with improvement of innovations for intense and long tenure of wound management [1, 4]. The massive social and monetary effect of wounds overall is an outcome of their high pace of event as a rule and their expanding recurrence in the maturing populace.

Notwithstanding a high number of intense injuries, there is likewise countless persistent, difficult-to-mend wounds related with sicknesses and irregularities that straightforwardly or by implication finish in harm of the cutaneous inclusion, including arterial, venous, diabetic, and pressure ulcers. The commonness of these ongoing injuries augmented with age [5–7].

2. Types of wounds: acute and chronic wounds

Despite the etiology of the injury, the maintenance measures are comparative. Intense injuries are regularly because of some type of injury that could be direct or entering (surgical cuts, discharges, creature chomps, and so forth). An injury harms the tissue that arouses a designed physiological reaction to provide hemostasis and initiate the cycles of tenderness, development, and remodeling [8]. Intense injuries, with careful entry points, ordinarily follow these steps somewhat rapid.

Wounds showing postponed recuperating 84 days after primary injury are called as constant injuries, regularly because of delayed neurotic tenderness. Surgical cuts are classically spotless and lead to nonsignificant tissue disturbance and thrashing. Injuries that occur on surgery are controlled type of injury, which can be grouped based on level of pollution (for example, spotless, clean infected, infection, and grimy) to foresee the danger of wound disease following a medical procedure. These injuries can be shut quickly with stitches and will in general mend quickly. This is named as conclusion by essential expectation. At the point when injury is tainted and left open to forestall disease and lesion (wound), conclusion is performed following a couple of days, it is named as deferred essential recuperating. At point where tissue thrashing has been broader, the boundaries cannot be estimated, or injury should be left open due to sepsis, reparative cycle is delayed, as deformity should fill up with extensive tissue of granulation type. This cycle is named as conclusion by auxiliary goal. Marvelous deformities can recuperate thusly, yet end corrective outcome is regularly subpar in comparison to those closed up basically [9–11].

3. Arrangement of occasions in injury recuperating

Following tissue injury by means of an entry point, the underlying reaction is typically blood loss. The course of coagulation and vasoconstriction begins with thickened blood promptly impregnating injury, prompting hemostasis, with parchedness, a scab structures. A convergence of provocative cells follows, with the arrival of cell substances and arbiters. Re-epithelialization and angiogenesis happen

Healing phases	Post-injury time	Concerned cells	Activities/functions
Hemostasis	Immediate	Platelets	Clotting
Inflammation	1–4 days	Macrophages, neutrophils,	Phagocytosis
Proliferation (granulation and contraction)	4–21 days	Lymphocytes, macrophages, neurocytes, angiocytes, keratinocytes, fibroblasts	Re-establish and fill defect, skin function closure
Remodeling (maturation)	21 days to 2 years	Fibrocytes	Tensile strength development

Table 1.
Phases of wound therapeutic.

and statement of new cell and extracellular segments follows. **Table 1** represents the phases of wound healing [12, 13].

3.1 Beginning stage—hemostasis

The underlying injury causes blood and lymph fluid to shed. It is also the interaction during which the underlying repairing coagulum formed. Both exterior and natural thickening components are implemented. The distinguishing tool is extracted from the thrombocytes and the foreign component from the injured tissues. After vasoconstriction, the platelets adhere to the damaged endothelium and release adenosine diphosphate (ADP), which advances the clustering of thrombocytes, which stops the injury. After the ephemeral vasoconstriction ends, the vessels dilate, allowing more thrombocytes and other platelets to be flooded [14, 15].

At this point, one can consider the initiation of incendiary phase. While some argue for a different provocative phase, it starts during the hemostasis stage, which again proves the mending abstract cover idea. These thrombocytes, just as the selected white platelets, release various elements to augment recovery cycle. α-Granules free platelet factor IV, transforming growth factor-β (TGF-β), and PDGF (platelet-determined growth factor). The initiation of aggravation cycles, collagen genesis and collagen corruption, myoblastic formation from altered fibroblasts, fresh blood vessels developments, and epithelialization occur [14, 15].

These cycles are mediated by numerous cytokines and developmental factors. Interleukins emphatically have a strong influence on fiery interaction. VEGF (vascular endothelial growth factor) and various variables improve venous arrangement, and some have numerous uses, such as FGF-2 (fibroblast growth factor), which affects interaction of epithelialization and angiogenesis. Vasoactive amines (serotonin and histamine) are delivered from thick bodies present in thrombocytes. PDGF acts as chemotactic for fibroblasts, whereas TGF-β acts as powerful modulator for mitosis in fibroblastic, causing productive development of collagen fibrils in later phases. Fibrinogen is separated into fibrin, and the structure for finishing of the coagulation interaction is shaped. Fibrin offers primary aid for cell components responsible for irritation. This cycle begins following the injury and can last for a few days [14, 15].

3.2 Inflammation

The core point of this wound recuperating phase is to forestall disease. Notwithstanding the etiology of wound, the mechanical hindrance, which was the forefront against attacking microorganisms, is not at this stage flawless. Neutrophils, the "initial responders," are exceptionally mobile cells that penetrate the wound within an hour of insult and move at sustained levels for the initial 48 h. This took place through various multiple indicators, including the supplement course; TGF-β indication and interleukin enactment, which prompt neutrophils to descend a substance angle toward the injury, a cycle called chemotaxis [8]. Neutrophils have three fundamental components for annihilating garbage and microbes. First and foremost, they can straightforwardly ingest and obliterate unfamiliar particles, a cycle called phagocytosis. Additionally, neutrophils can degranulate and deliver an assortment of harmful substances (cathepsin, neutrophil elastase, proteases, and lactoferrin) that will obliterate microorganisms just as host's dead tissue. Late proof has shown that neutrophils can also create chromatin and protease "traps" that capture and abolish microbes in extracellular space. Oxygen-free extremists are a side effect of neutrophil movement, which is recognized to have bactericidal features, but also can join with chlorine to cleanse the wound. By the time neutrophils have completed their mission, they go through apoptosis, break away from the surface of lesion, or are phagocytosed by macrophages. Macrophages are much larger phagocytic cells that arrive at top fixation in an injury at 2–3 days after injury. They are drawn to wound by the synthetic couriers delivered from platelets and harmed cells and can cope in the more acidic climate of injury present at this phase [16].

Macrophages harbor a huge repository of growth factors, for example, epidermal growth factor (EGF) and TGF-β, which are significant for improving the arrangement of granulation tissue, directing the fiery reaction and animating angiogenesis. Lymphocytes appear in wound after 72 h and are considered important in management of twisted recuperating, *via* the creation of an extracellular lattice scaffold and regeneration of collagen. Investigative examinations have shown that hindrance of T-lymphocytes leads to reduced wound strength and impeded collagen deposition [17]. The incendiary wound repair period will continue as long as necessary ensuring that all bacteria, flotsam, and jetsam from injury are removed. Extended irritation can, however, result in extensive tissue damage, delayed expansion and lead to the development of a continuous injury. Numerous variables, such as lipoxins and outcomes of arachidonic corrosive digestion, are believed to have calming features, which mitigate reaction harmlessly and allow the next twisted recovery period to occur [18].

3.3 Proliferation (multiplication)

When the harming boost has stopped, hemostasis has been achieved, the provocative reaction is attuned, and wound is waste-free, the proliferative stage of mending course can begin to fix imperfection. This unpredictable cycle fuses angiogenesis, arrangement of granulation tissue, collagen affidavit, epithelialization as well as wound withdrawal that occur all time [16].

3.3.1 Angiogenesis

Angiogenesis is set off from the second the hemostatic plug takes the shape as platelets discharge FGF, PDGF, and TGF-β. In reaction to hypoxia, VEGF is delivered that is mixed with different cytokines, initiate endothelial cells to activate neovascularization and the maintenance of harmed veins. A group of catalysts such as blended metalloproteinase (MMP) are enacted by attacking neutrophils in hypoxic tissue. They advance angiogenesis *via* freedom of VEGF and redesigning of extracellular framework (ECM) [19, 20]. At first, the focal point of injury is generally avascular, since it depends exclusively on dispersion from unharmed vessels at the edge of injury. While the cycle of angiogenesis continues, a rich vascular organization of vessels is framed all through injury from branches of sound vessels. At first, the vessels are delicate as well as porous, further providing tissue edema and the presence of mending granulation tissue [19].

3.3.2 Fibroblast movement

After the injury affront, fibroblasts are invigorated to multiply by development factors delivered by hemostatic coagulation and afterward move to injury (overwhelmingly by PDGF and TGF-β). On third day, the injury gets wealthy with fibroblasts that deposit extracellular framework proteins (proteoglycans, fibronectins, and hyaluronan) and accordingly produce fibronectin and collagen. The subsequent pink, tough, vascular tissue that replaces the coagulation at injury site is named granulation tissue. This is made out of an alternate span of collagens (a greater extent of type 3 collagen) than that seen in uninjured tissue. When adequate grid has been put in place, the fibroblasts transform into myofibroblasts aggregate and build up pseudopodia. This empowers them to associate with the encompassing proteins collagen and fibronectin and aid to compress the wound. Myofibroblasts likewise advance angiogenesis *via* intercession MMP action [21]. Collagens incorporated by fibroblasts are the critical segment to give tissue solidarity. In injuries shut by essential expectation, concentration of collagen is the highest on fifth day, and this can frequently be touched underneath the skin as a "wound edge." At the point when an injury edge is not obvious, it means that injury is in danger of dehiscence. Overproduction of collagen can lead to the improvement of a hypertrophic scar. Hypertrophic scars remain augmented and erythematous while remaining within limits of the first twist. Dangers for their advancement include injury-related illnesses and those where there is unreasonable pressure [21, 22].

3.3.3 Epithelialization

Epithelial cells move from the edges of wound shortly after the underlying slash until a complete sheet of cells covers wound and connects with network beneath. An embryological cycle, called epithelial-mesenchymal transform (EMT), permits epithelial cells to acquire motility and travel across the lesion surface [23]. In injuries that are basically closed, this step can be completed in 1 day. Alterations in cytokine bindings cause epithelial cells to shift from a mobile aggregate to a proliferative aggregate for repopulating epithelial cell levels and complete injury repair [24]. In injuries that recuperate *via* auxiliary goal, the area devoid of epithelial cells can be huge, and injury should fundamentally contract before epithelialization can be completed. At times this may never occur, and the unification of skin can be used to cover up the imperfection [24].

3.3.4 Wound withdrawal

Wounds start to contract around 7 days after the injury, interceded primarily by myofibroblasts. Associations among myosin and actin bring the cell bodies nearer together to diminish the space of tissues that expect to repair themselves. Constriction can happen at a pace of 0.75 mm per 24 h prompting abbreviated scaring. This is affected by various elements such as twisted shape, with roundabout injuries the slowest and direct injuries contracting quickest. Issues in this recovery period can prompt deformation and arrangement of contractures [25].

3.4 Maturation (remodeling)

The last phase of wound recovery is development stage and incorporates the cross-connection of collagen, redesign, and constriction of wound. At first, fibroblasts incorporate collagen (type 3) that is thinner than it develops. Collagen (type 1) presents abundantly in solid skin. During development stage, collagen (type 1) replaces collagen (type 3) present in scar structures and granulation tissue. This expansion in collagen (type 1) relates with expanded potency of wounds seen 28–35 days subsequent to mending. The 80% of recapturing of injury will occur in 3 months after the injury. Sadly, accomplishing the original capacity of the skin before injury is inconceivable [26].

Wound constriction happens in injuries (open type) to diminish the measure of connective tissue needed to recover injury bed. A planned hypothesis recommends that compression be done using myofibroblasts and their combination of α-smooth muscle actin. Both portability and area of tissue encompassing the injury bed play a role in how well the injury contracts. In zones with low portability, withdrawal might be inconvenient and can be avoided by using different flaps or skin seal [27].

Arrangement of another defensive epithelial layer is combined by epithelial cells moving internal from the edges of injury. Shifting movement rates consider both the definition of the epithelial layer and expansion of tissue depth to restore the typical thickness of epithelium [28].

When mended, an injury leaves a scar. The scar tissue will be somewhat raised, firm, expanded vascularity, and reddish from abundance of collagen. Regularly, it would stay that way for initial 6–9 months, and afterward starts to mellow, straighten up, and turn paler [29].

4. Pathophysiology

Wounds periodically bring about a misrepresented recuperating reaction and show the way for formation of hypertrophic scars and keloids. By meaning, hypertrophic scars are maintained at the edges of the first injury bed though keloids exceed these limits. It is believed that the pressure of overabundance due to the development of abundance on a joint, a hidden hard conception, or loss of tissue may play a role in the advancement of these specific scars. Keloids likewise happens all the more regularly in patients having more obscure skin [30].

The specific component of the structure of these scars is obscure; however, overactive or strange fibroblasts have been observed in keloids. These fibroblasts make plentiful measures of proteoglycan, fibronectin, elastin, and collagen and react unnecessarily to incitement. This reaction is probably identified with the upward directive of insulin-like development factor receptors on keloid fibroblasts. Insulin-like development factor excites creation of collagen. In contrast to ordinary scars, the collagen stored in keloids is organized heedlessly and assumes a part in their development after injury [30, 31].

Collagen present in hypertrophic scars is packaged and organized in curly examples corresponding to surface of epithelia. This fairly coordinated example separates hypertrophic scars from the tumultuous direction found in keloids. In contrast to keloidal fibrablasts, fibroblasts present in hypertrophic scars typically react to development factors and thereby generate just a little overabundance of collagen. Hypertrophic scars likewise have novel nodular designs of α-smooth muscle actin myofibroblasts, like those associated with compression of scar. It is believed that after some time period, hypertrophic scars can relapse, while keloids will not [30, 31].

5. Clinical importance

The numerous cycles engaged with wound recuperating encourage an enormous metabolic interest, which is met with glucose and oxygen conveyed to the site of injury by recently framed endothelial vessels. This blood supply is restricted by elements prompting vasoconstriction and consequently forestalls legitimate injury mending. Medical services suppliers taking care of patients with recuperating wounds ought to know about these components and control for them whenever the situation allows. Reasons for vasoconstriction incorporate agony, cold, dread, nicotine, hypovolemia, beta antagonists, and alpha-1 agonists. Patients should be assessed for substance and drug use and referred for their potential to interfere with or delay wound healing [26, 32].

Smoking is especially unfavorable to wound recuperating as well as influences different phases of the mending interaction. Smoking has vasoconstrictive impacts and diminishes the supply of oxygen supply. Nicotine likewise builds danger of blood clot development because of expanded platelet actuation and diminishes macrophage, fibroblast, and erythrocyte multiplication. Weakness of macrophage and fibroblast relocation affects formation of collagen and subsequently twisted to fix.

This postpone also puts the patient who smokes at an expanded danger for contamination. For patients going through elective methods, conversation about quitting the smoking is significant with respect to legitimate injury recuperating [33–35].

Diabetes, a developing worry for every doctor, can adversely affect twisted fix too. Diabetic patients have expanded prone to microvascular sickness that may debilitate blood stream to site of injury. Hyperglycemia influences storm cellar film porousness and hinders blood stream also. Raised blood sugars alongside diminished invulnerability place this populace in danger for contamination [26].

It is hence fundamental to oversee blood glucose cautiously in patients with mending wounds [36, 37].

Effective injury mending depends on a few factors and includes different high energy measures. Information on the essential physiology of wound mending is indispensable for anticipating potential inconveniences and limiting helpless results. Constant injuries, hypertrophic scars, and keloids can be hard to oversee once these happen. Hence, it is ideal to keep away from the mentioned issues completely. Attention to and evaluating for regular danger factors identified with such complexities can prompt better understanding consideration.

Acknowledgements

The author, Mr. Sunil Kumar, is thankful to Indian Council of Medical Research, New Delhi, for providing Senior Research Fellowship [Letter No: 45/44/2018-Nan/BMS].

Conflict of interest

The authors have no conflict of interest to declare and are responsible for the content and writing of the manuscript.

Author details

Sunil Kumar[1†], Shravan Kumar Paswan[2†*], Pritt Verma[3†], Akanksha[4], RamKishor Sah[4], Sajal Srivastava[5] and Chandana Venketeswara Rao[6]

1 Department of Pharmaceutical Sciences, Guru Jambheshwar University of Science and Technology, Hisar, Haryana, India

2 Pharma Talk Research Foundation, Lucknow, India

3 Goel Institute of Pharmacy and Sciences, Lucknow, India

4 Dr. R.P. Centre for Ophthalmic Sciences, AIIMS, New Delhi, India

5 Pharmacology Division, CSIR-National Botanical Research Institute, Lucknow, Uttar Pradesh, India

6 Amity Institute of Pharmacy, Amity University, Lucknow, Uttar Pradesh, India

*Address all correspondence to: paswanshravan@gmail.com

† Equally contributed authors.

References

[1] Robson MC, Steed DL, Franz MG. Wound healing: Biologic features and approaches to maximize healing trajectories. Current Problems in Surgery. 2001;**38**(2):72-140

[2] Alonso JE et al. The management of complex orthopedic injuries. Surgical Clinics of North America. 1996;**76**(4): 879-903

[3] Natarajan S et al. Advances in wound care and healing technology. American Journal of Clinical Dermatology. 2000;**1**(5):269-275

[4] Szycher M, Lee SJ. Modern wound dressings: A systematic approach to wound healing. Journal of Biomaterials Applications. 1992;**7**(2):142-213

[5] Pragnell J, Neilson J. The social and psychological impact of hard-to-heal wounds. British Journal of Nursing. 2010;**19**(19):1248-1252

[6] Ren H, Ding Y, Hu H, Gao T, Qin Z, Hu Y, et al. Relationships among economic stress, social support, age and quality of life in patients with chronic wounds: A moderated mediation model. Journal of Advanced Nursing. 2020;**76**(8):2125-2136

[7] Keeling D, Price P, Jones E, Harding KG. Social support for elderly patients with chronic wounds. Journal of Wound Care. 1997;**6**(8):389-391

[8] George Broughton I, Janis JE, Attinger CE. The basic science of wound healing. Plastic and Reconstructive Surgery. 2006;**117**(7S):12S-34S

[9] Bryant R, Nix D, editors. Acute and Chronic Wounds: Current Management Concepts. 5th ed. St. Louis: Elsevier Health Sciences; 2015

[10] Monaco JL, Lawrence WT. Acute wound healing: An overview. Clinics in Plastic Surgery. 2003;**30**(1):1-12

[11] Dai C, Shih S, Khachemoune A. Skin substitutes for acute and chronic wound healing: An updated review. Journal of Dermatological Treatment. 2020;**31**(6): 639-648

[12] Gilmore MA. Phases of wound healing. Dimensions in Oncology Nursing: Journal of the Division of Nursing. 1991;**5**(3):32-34

[13] Kirsner RS, Eaglstein WH. The wound healing process. Dermatologic Clinics. 1993;**11**(4):629-640

[14] Laurens N, Koolwijk PD, De Maat MPM. Fibrin structure and wound healing. Journal of Thrombosis and Haemostasis. 2006;**4**(5):932-939

[15] Mercandetti M, Cohen A. Wound healing and repair. eMedicine. 2017; **14**(1):12-20

[16] Velnar T, Bailey T, Smrkolj V. The wound healing process: An overview of the cellular and molecular mechanisms. Journal of International Medical Research. 2009;**37**(5):1528-1542

[17] Peterson JM et al. Significance of T-lymphocytes in wound healing. Surgery. 1987;**102**(2):300-305

[18] Nathan C. Points of control in inflammation. Nature. 2002;**420**(6917): 846-852

[19] Siefert SA, Sarkar R. Matrix metalloproteinases in vascular physiology and disease. Vascular. 2012;**20**(4):210-216

[20] Landén NX, Li D, Ståhle M. Transition from inflammation to proliferation: A critical step during wound healing. Cellular and Molecular Life Sciences. 2016;**73**(20):3861-3885

[21] Mayrand D et al. Angiogenic properties of myofibroblasts isolated from normal human skin wounds. Angiogenesis. 2012;**15**(2):199-212

[22] Desjardins-Park HE, Foster DS, Longaker MT. Fibroblasts and wound healing: An update. Regenerative Medicine. 2018;**13**(5):491-495

[23] Yang J, Weinberg RA. Epithelial-mesenchymal transition: At the crossroads of development and tumor metastasis. Developmental Cell. 2008;**14**(6):818-829

[24] De Donatis A, Ranaldi F, Cirri P. Reciprocal control of cell proliferation and migration. Cell Communication and Signaling. 2010;**8**(1):1-4

[25] Hinz B. Masters and servants of the force: The role of matrix adhesions in myofibroblast force perception and transmission. European Journal of Cell Biology. 2006;**85**(3-4):175-181

[26] Janis JE, Harrison B. Wound healing: Part I. Basic science. Plastic and Reconstructive Surgery. 2014;**133**(2): 199e-207e

[27] Berry DP et al. Human wound contraction: Collagen organization, fibroblasts, and myofibroblasts. Plastic and Reconstructive Surgery. 1998; **102**(1):124-131, discussion 132

[28] Park S et al. Tissue-scale coordination of cellular behaviour promotes epidermal wound repair in live mice. Nature Cell Biology. 2017;**19**(3):155-163

[29] Burd A, Huang L. Hypertrophic response and keloid diathesis: Two very different forms of scar. Plastic and Reconstructive Surgery. 2005;**116**(7): 150e-157e

[30] Alster TS, Tanzi EL. Hypertrophic scars and keloids. American Journal of Clinical Dermatology. 2003;**4**(4): 235-243

[31] Li J, Chen J, Kirsner R. Pathophysiology of acute wound healing. Clinics in Dermatology. 2007;**25**(1):9-18

[32] Rodriguez PG, Felix FN, Woodley DT, Shim EK. The role of oxygen in wound healing: A review of the literature. Dermatologic Surgery. 2008;**34**(9):1159-1169

[33] McDaniel JC, Browning KK. Smoking, chronic wound healing, and implications for evidence-based practice. Journal of Wound, Ostomy, and Continence Nursing: Official Publication of the Wound, Ostomy and Continence Nurses Society/WOCN. 2014;**41**(5):415

[34] Frick WG, Seals RR Jr. Smoking and wound healing: A review. Texas Dental Journal. 1994;**111**(6):21-23

[35] Kean J. The effects of smoking on the wound healing process. Journal of Wound Care. 2010;**19**(1):5-8

[36] Okonkwo UA, DiPietro LA. Diabetes and wound angiogenesis. International Journal of Molecular Sciences. 2017;**18**(7):1419

[37] Brem H, Tomic-Canic M. Cellular and molecular basis of wound healing in diabetes. The Journal of Clinical Investigation. 2007;**117**(5):1219-1222

Section 4

Wound Healing and Treatments

Chapter 9

Copper, an Abandoned Player Returning to the Wound Healing Battle

Gadi Borkow and Eyal Melamed

Abstract

Copper has two key properties that endow it as an excellent active ingredient to be used in the "wound healing battle". First, copper plays a key role in angiogenesis, dermal fibroblasts proliferation, upregulation of collagen and elastin fibers production by dermal fibroblasts, and it serves as a cofactor of Lysyl oxidase needed for efficient dermal extracellular matrix (ECM) protein cross-linking. Secondly, copper has potent wide-spectrum biocidal properties. Both gram-positive and gram-negative bacteria, including antibiotic resistant bacteria and hard to kill bacterial spores, fungi and viruses, when exposed to high copper concentrations, are killed. Copper has been used as a biocide for centuries by many different civilizations. Impregnation of copper oxide microparticles in wound dressings allows continuous release of copper ions. This results not only in the protection of the wounds and wound dressings from pathogens, but more importantly, enhances wound healing. The article discusses the molecular mechanisms of enhanced wound healing by the copper oxide impregnated dressings, which include in situ upregulation of pro-angiogenic factors and increased blood vessel formation. It also includes clinical cases showing clearance of infection, induction of granulation and epithelialization of necrotic wounds, reduction of post-operative swelling inflammation and reduction of scar formation, in wounds when they were treated with copper oxide impregnated dressings. We show the positive outcome at all wound healing stages of using the copper impregnated wound dressings, indicating the neglected critical role copper plays in wound healing.

Keywords: copper oxide, wound dressings, wound healing, angiogenesis, extracellular matrix, chronic wounds

1. Introduction

Wounds normally heal in finely balanced, efficient, and ordered sequence of repair events distinguished by four distinct, but overlapping, phases: Hemostasis, Inflammation, Proliferation and Remodeling [1, 2]. These coordinated cellular and molecular events involve numerous processes such as cell proliferation, migration and differentiation. All of these processes demand a continued and efficient supply of oxygen and nutrients, due to the increased cellular biosynthetic activities. Following wounding, the altered microenvironment, such as the reduced oxygen supply, initiates the release of factors by epidermal cells, fibroblasts, macrophages and vascular endothelial cells, all of which stimulate neo-vascularization. The secreted factors include vascular endothelial cell growth factor (VEGF), fibroblast growth factor (FGF) and transforming growth factor (TGF)-β. VEGF is believed to be the most prevalent, efficacious, and long-term signal that is known to stimulate angiogenesis in wounds. TGF-β, especially TGF-β1, is also a key cytokine that regulates the production and secretion of elastin and collagen [3]. Fibroblasts, which attach to fibrin and integrin cables, produce and secrete collagen and elastin that become cross-linked, forming the dermal extracellular matrix (ECM). This allows the restoration of the structure and function to the injured tissue [4, 5].

1.1 Chronic wounds

Chronic wounds or "hard to heal wounds" are characterized by extensive loss of the integument, clear necrosis, or signs of circulation impairment either localized or more extensive, usually in the limbs, or in pressure areas, leading to extensive loss of substance. Chronic wounds seem to be detained in one or more of the phases of wound healing, and some chronic wounds may never heal or may take years to do so. These wounds have lost the fine balance needed for wound repair, leading to chronic non-healing ulcers, associated with morbidity and mortality due to tissue inflammation and infection [6]. Chronic wounds are usually associated with systemic pathologies [7] that cause ischemia, a restriction in blood supply to tissues. Ischemia occurs in diabetic patients due to atherosclerosis as well as microangiopathic disease [8], in chronic venous ulcers due to chronic venous insufficiency [9], in patients with autoimmune disease or under immunosuppressive drug therapy due to vasculitis [10] and in pressure sores due to necrosis of the integument [11]. Chronic wounds cause patients severe emotional and physical stress and create a significant financial burden on patients and the whole healthcare system. Chronic wounds require special attention and wound care.

1.2 Involvement of systemic copper in wound healing

Copper is an essential mineral involved in many of the physiological processes in all body tissues [12, 13], including the skin and integumentary system [14]. Many of the finely balanced wound healing repair mechanisms are dependent on their interaction with copper (thoroughly reviewed in [6]). This includes, Platelet-derived growth factor (PDGF), involved in the hemostasis phase of wound healing, [15, 16]; VEGF and angiogenin, key growth factors that stimulate angiogenesis, an essential process during the Proliferation Phase [17–23]; secretion of collagens (types I, II, and V), HSP-47 and elastin fiber components (elastin, fibrillins) by dermal fibroblasts during the Proliferation and Remodeling Phases [16, 24, 25]; activity of Lysyl oxidase (LOX) needed for efficient extracellular matrix (ECM) protein cross-linking between elastin and collagen [26]; stabilization of the skin ECM once formed [27, 28]; modulation of integrins by differentiated keratinocytes during the Remodeling phase [29], and Matrix metalloproteinases (MMPs, mainly MMP-1, MMP-2, MMP-8, MMP-9) and the serine proteases (human neutrophil elastase, HNE) are the major groups of proteases involved in the wound healing process. It is thus not surprising that copper chelation delays wound closure [30]. Copper is also a cofactor of superoxide dismutase, an antioxidant enzyme found in the skin that inhibits cellular oxidative effects, such as membrane damage and lipid peroxidation and protects against free radicals [19]. Copper is also a cofactor of tyrosinase, a melanin biosynthesis essential enzyme, responsible for skin and hair pigmentation.

1.3 Copper and wound infections

Infections of the wound may delay wound healing, cause wound deterioration and even cause failure of healing [31]. This may occur through several different mechanisms: consistent and high production of inflammatory mediators, metabolic wastes and toxins; tissue hypoxia; causing hemorrhagic and fragile granulation tissue; reducing fibroblast number and total collagen production; and interfering with reepithelization [32, 33]; reducing the available nutrients and oxygen needed by the host cells and causing neutrophils to be in an activated state producing cytolytic enzymes and free oxygen radicals [34]. In chronic wounds bacteria may be covered by biofilm and be protected from the host defenses and develop antibiotic resistance [31]. Thus, reducing the microbial contamination of wounds increases the capacity of the wound to heal.

Copper is also a needed mineral for the normal function of microorganisms [35]. However, the microorganisms need to carefully control the intracellular copper levels. This is since copper under anaerobic condition is found in the highly reactive cuprous form (Cu^{1+}), and as such it can readily react with the microbial proteins, causing disruption of the protein structures by forming thiolate bonds with iron–sulphur clusters [36]. Thus, above an exposure to a certain concentration of copper, microorganisms cannot cope with the excess copper and are killed [37, 38]. Several mechanisms for the potent biocidal activity of copper have been proposed, which include alteration of proteins and inhibition of their biological assembly and activity; plasma membrane permeabilization; and membrane lipid peroxidation [37]. In contrast to the resistant microbes that have evolved to antibiotics in less than 50 years of use, tolerant microbes to copper are extremely rare even though copper has been a part of the earth for millions of years. This lack of resistance to copper may be explained by the capacity of copper to damage in parallel many key factors in micro-organisms [37].

2. Cuprous oxide impregnated wound dressing

2.1 General description

Copper oxide impregnated wound dressings, hereafter called COD, have been cleared for treatment of acute and chronic wounds, including diabetic ulcers, pressure sores, and venous ulcers, by the USA FDA, EU and other regulatory bodies worldwide. The COD are soft, single use wound dressings composed of an absorbent highly absorbent needle punch layer and one or two external non-binding nonwoven orange polypropylene layers. All layers are impregnated with copper oxide microparticles. The orange external layer(s) is intended to be in contact with the wound bed. The wound dressings are provided with or without an adhesive contour, sterile, in a sterilization pouch (**Figure 1**). The non-adhesive wound dressings can be cut, trimmed or fold over according to the size and shape of the wound. The dressings can be used up to 7 days or until they are completely soaked with wound exudate.

2.2 Antimicrobial efficacy

The COD exert potent wide spectrum antimicrobial efficacy (>4 log reductions), including when the dressings are completely soaked with wound exudate surrogate for 7 days, as demonstrated by us and by independent laboratories using the AATCC Test Method 100. Furthermore, the potent antimicrobial efficacy is maintained even after 7 consecutive microbial inoculations for 7 consecutive days (**Figure 2**).

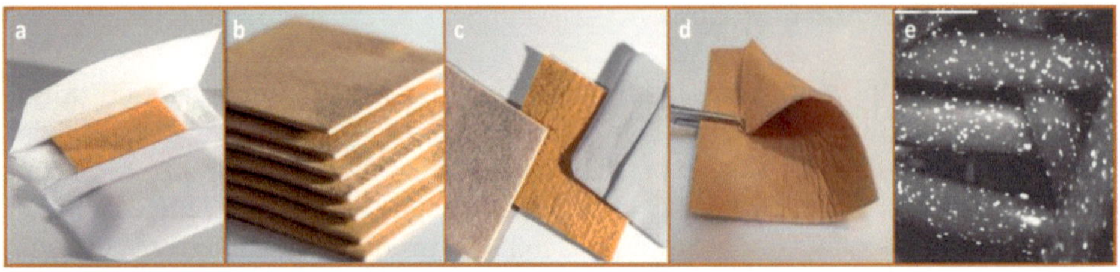

Figure 1.
Copper oxide impregnated wound dressings. The COD are composed of an absorbent layer and one or two external layers. The dressings are provided (a) with or (b) without an adhesive contour. The external layer (c, orange layer) is a non-adherent polypropylene layer placed in contact with the wound bed, which allows the passage of the wound exudates into the internal layer (c, beige layer) that absorbs the wound exudates. COD with two external layers (d) are more appropriate for application in wound cavities and deep wounds. All layers are impregnated with copper oxide microparticles (e, white dots) that endow them with potent biocidal properties.

The antimicrobial efficacy was demonstrated against the following microorganisms: *Escherichia coli, Enterococcus faecalis, Enterobacter aerogenes, Klebsiella pneumoniae, Staphylococcus epidermis,* Methicillin-resistant *Staphylococcus aureus* (MRSA) and *Candida albicans.* When compared with commercially available silver wound dressings, the antimicrobial efficacy was significantly higher than 9 out of the 12 silver dressings studied, and as good as 3 silver dressings (**Figure 3**, unpublished data).

2.3 Molecular mechanisms of enhanced wound healing

The capacity of copper to enhance faster closure of full-thickness wounds was demonstrated in several wound animal models, [30, 39, 40], including in diabetic mice [41].

The capacity of the COD to directly enhance repair of chronic wounds by supplying *in situ* essential copper lacking due to poor systemic blood supply (such as in diabetic ulcers), was demonstrated in a murine diabetic model considered to be the

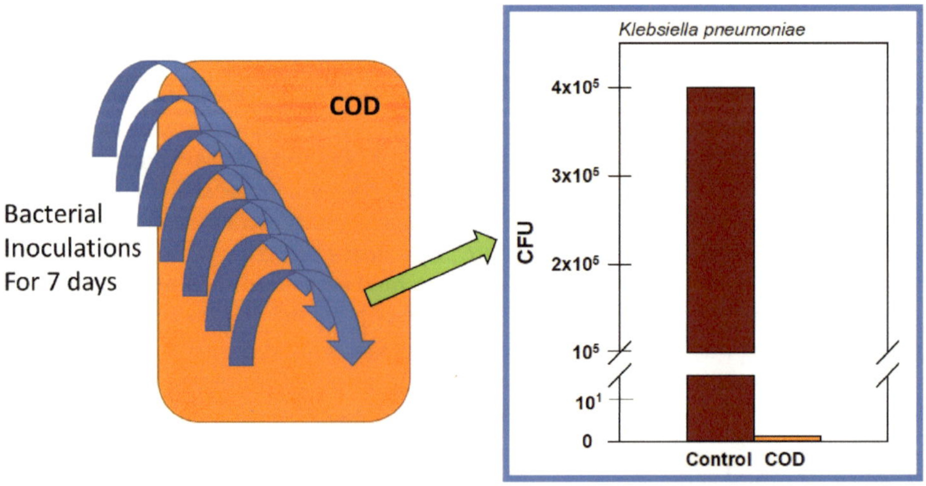

Figure 2.
Continuous antimicrobial efficacy of COD even after 7 consecutive bacterial inoculations. Duplicate COD were inoculated with ~1 x 10^5 Klebsiella pneumonae CFU for 6 consecutive days and incubated at 37 °C. On the seven days the CODs and a Control wound dressings without copper were inoculated with ~4x10^5 CFU. After additional 24 hours of incubation at 37 °C, the bacteria were recovered and their viability determined. While no bacteria survived on the CODs, 4x10^5 viable bacteria were recovered from the control dressings.

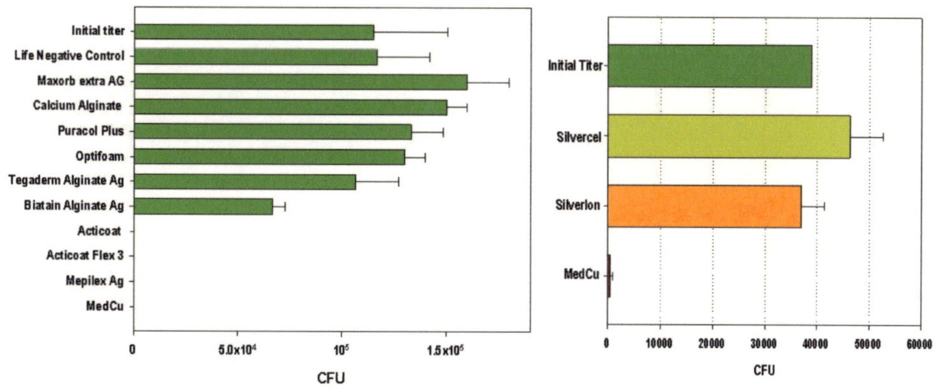

Figure 3.
Antimicrobial efficacy comparison between the COD and commercially available silver dressings. The wound dressings were inoculated with ~10^6 (left panel) and $4x10^4$ (right panel) MRSA CFU. After 1 hour of incubation at 37 °C the bacteria were recovered from the dressings and their viability was determined.

most suitable in diabetic wound healing studies [42]. Wounding and subsequent treatments were performed under aseptic conditions, so that the possible effects of the copper dressings would not be related to their biocidal properties.

A phenotype similar to diabetes type 2 in mice is achieved via a homozygous point mutation on the leptin receptor gene (LEPR) in the hypothalamus. Genetically engineered diabetic mice (db/db) show significant wound-healing impairment compared to wild-type mice [42]. Full-thickness single skin wounds were inflicted under sterile conditions on the dorsum of each animal followed by continuous dermal application of either COD or identical dressings without copper on the entire wound test site. Histological analysis of skin specimens taken from the diabetic mice treated with the COD 6, 12 and 17 days after wounding demonstrated a normal wound-healing process, including epidermal regeneration and granulation tissue formation, with numerous new blood vessels, chronic inflammatory infiltrate, generation of new hair follicles and sebaceous glands, and fibroplasia [41].

The very clear increase in angiogenesis in the copper treated mice was confirmed by immunohistochemistry staining using the Von Willebrand Factor that stains capillaries. Analysis of mRNA expression levels in the wound sites of 84 genes using real-time PCR gene-array analysis together with immunohistochemistry staining revealed the upregulation of several angiogenic factors, such as Vascular endothelial growth factor (VEGF). Based on the analysis performed a molecular mechanism was suggested in which a redox between cuprous oxide and cupric oxide generates hypoxia that induces the upregulation of Hypoxia-inducible factor-1alpha (Hif-1α) in the dermal layer, apparently in macrophages [41]. The upregulation of Hif-1α then induces a chain of events, depicted in **Figure 4**, which lead to endothelial cell migration and proliferation, production of new blood capillaries (angiogenesis), immune cell recruitment, fibroblast migration, intense metabolism, increased secretion of extracellular matrix proteins, and increased epithelialization.

2.4 Clinical cases showing the enhancement of the COD at all stages of wound healing

The following cases illustrates the ability of COD to affect infection reduction, angiogenesis and granulation tissue formation, as well as epithelial tissue formation, in hard to heal wounds. In addition, we describe cases of reduction

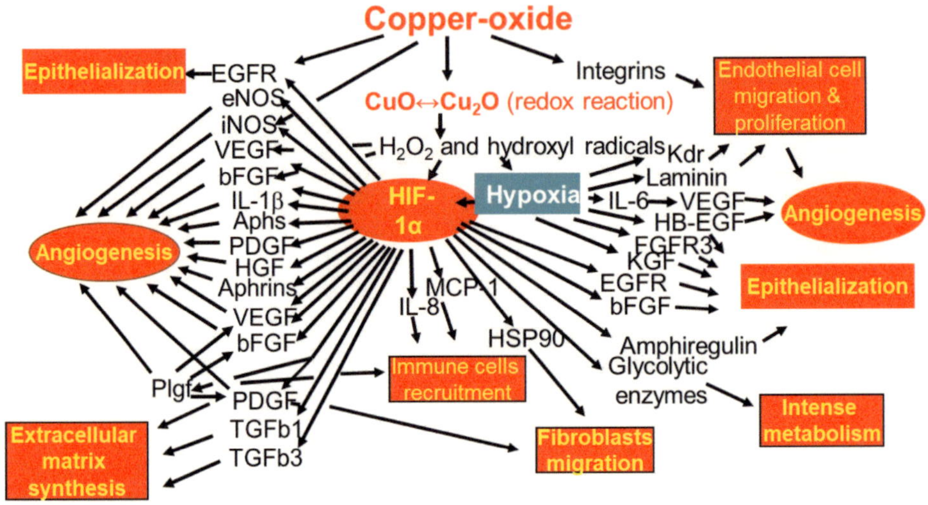

Figure 4.
Molecular mechanisms of enhanced wound healing by COD. (based on the model published in ref. [41]).

of post-operative swelling and better post-surgery scar formation. All photos are published in the book with the patients' consent.

2.4.1 Clearance of infection, induction of granulation and epithelialization

Fifty-seven years old male, with history of non-insulin-dependent diabetes mellitus (NIDDM), suffering from ulcers in both feet, mainly on the right side (**Figure 5a**). The etiology was mainly due to vasculitis type reaction (acute leukocytoclastic vasculitis), with minor large arteries involvement (for which angiographic intervention with percutaneous opening of the superficial femoral artery was carried out). The patient was treated with high dose steroids, immunosuppressive medication (Azathioprine, Imuran) and broad-spectrum antibiotic treatment. The patient right foot worsened with development of necrosis mainly in the medial toes, with the infection spreading to involve the tendons and the plantar fascia. Deep ulcers were present over the medial aspect of the heel and the lateral aspects of the foot (**Figures 5a** and **b**).

The patient underwent surgery to debride the wound including 1st and 2nd ray amputation. Cultures taken at surgery yielded *Pseudomonas aeruginosa* resistant to quinolones and the patient was treated with Imipenem. Five days later the patient underwent trans-metatarsal amputation. The wound was partially closed to prevent a loose flap. Nevertheless, necrosis of the edges of the flap was seen few days following surgery (**Figure 5c**). Bedside debridement was carried out. At that time, culture taken from the second surgery revealed that the pseudomonas has now developed resistance to carbapenems and it was decided to stop the antibiotic treatment. The medial heel wound had at least 30% necrotic tissue. The lateral anterior wound had 80–90% necrosis (**Figure 5c** and **d**).

Trans-tibial amputation deemed to be the next step. WBC count was 18,000, which was an improvement from previous higher levels, and the CRP was 3.0 (normal <0.5). However, since the patient's overall condition was stable, it was decided to continue only with local wound care with COD. The dressings were placed deep in the plantar-fascial part of the amputation wound, on the edges of it and on the ulcers (**Figure 5d** and **e**). The dressings were replaced twice a week. Prontosan® irrigation was recommended during dressing change. No supplemental antibiotic was given.

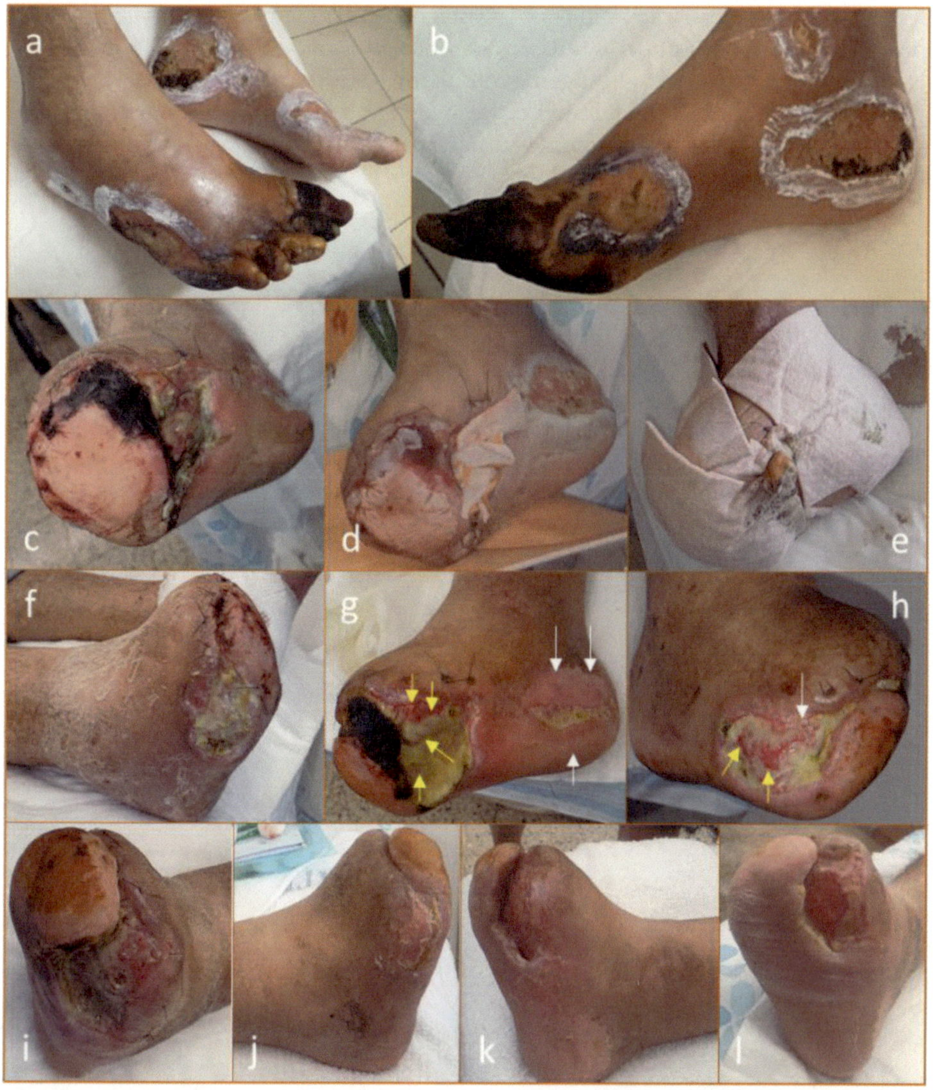

Figure 5.
Clearance of infection, induction of granulation and epithelialization of necrotic wounds. a. Ulcers colonized with Pseudomonas aeruginosa were present on both feet, mainly on the right foot. b. The ulcers were present over the medial aspects of the heel and the lateral aspect of the foot. c. Two weeks following trans metatarsal amputation necrotic tissue was present on the edges of the partially closed flap. d. The COD dressings started to be used (Day 0) by placing them deep in the plantar-fascial part of the amputation wound and e. by covering the medial and latera ulcers. f. One week later, a reduction in the necrotic tissue and beginning of granulation tissue was observed in all wounds. g and h. After 2 months of COD treatment there was clear epithelialization (white arrows) in the lateral and medial ulcers and granulation tissue formation (yellow arrows) in the lateral and medial ulcers and in the main bulk of the amputation wound that can be seen through the remaining thin necrotic tissue. Cultures from the necrotic tissue were negative for pseudomonas (the resistant original pathogen). i. The granulation tissue seemed to affect the necrotic tissue with autolysis (self-debridement). j and k. After 5 months of COD treatment, the medial and lateral wounds were closed. l. The main wound was partially closed and the rest of the wound was with pink to red granulation tissue.

The foot condition improved gradually. The superficial semi-necrotic ulcer at the heel and lateral aspect of the foot showed gradual absorption of the necrotic tissue, granulation and epithelization (**Figures 5f–i**). The main amputation wound, with large area and volume and inner cavity of 6–7 cm, gradually filled with granulation tissue (**Figure 5g**). The granulation tissue seemed to affect the necrotic tissue with autolysis (self-debridement, **Figure 5i**). New epithelium gradually covered the healing wounds (**Figure 5g** and **h**). Microbial culture, taken from the necrotic tissue three months after cessation of antibiotic administration, did not yield pseudomonas, although normal non-pathogenic colonizing bacteria were identified.

After 5 months of COD treatment, the medial and lateral wounds were closed (**Figure 5j** and **k**). The main wound was partially closed and the rest of the wound was with pink to red granulation tissue (**Figure 5l**).

2.4.2 Increased epithelization

The powerful ability of COD to promote epithelization is illustrated in the following case of a 71 years old man with NIDDM and diabetic neuropathy. The patient had osteomyelitis of the calcaneus, which necessitated extensive debridement of the heel and the infected calcaneus bone. The wound did not heal and the calcaneus broke through area of weakness due to the missing bone, thus creating a rocker deformity. Repeated surgery with debridement of the soft tissue, correction of the foot alignment and fixation with Steinman pins was carried out (**Figure 6a** and **b**, 1-week

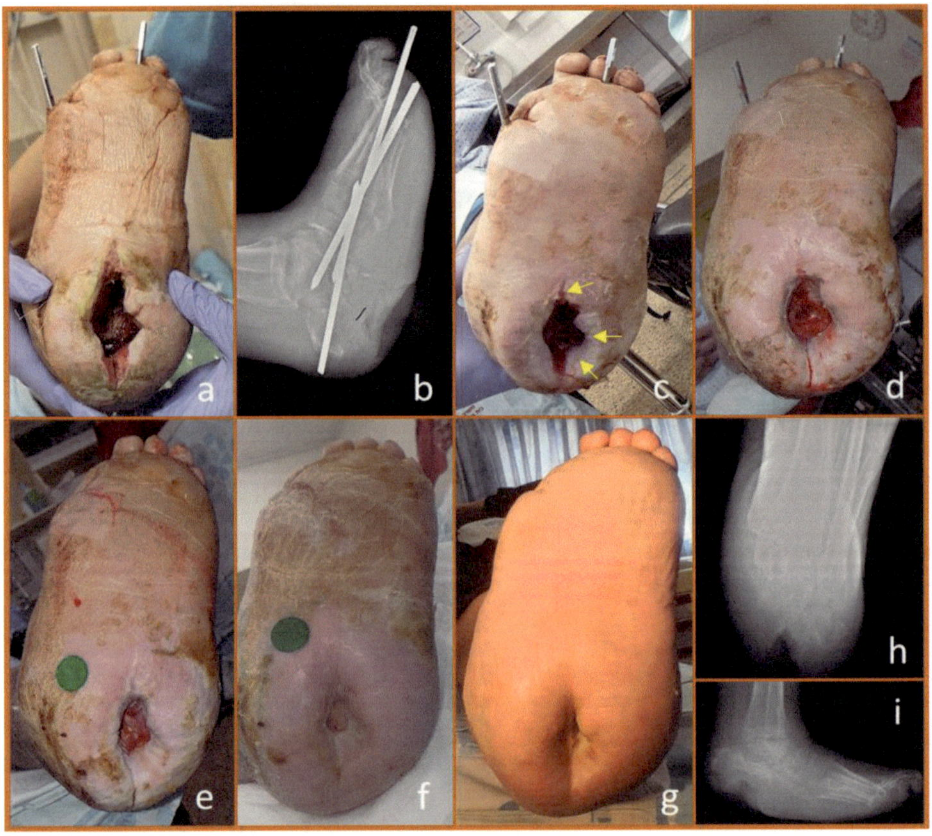

Figure 6.
Epithelization of a rocker deformity related plantar deep wound. The patient had resection of infected calcaneal bone with correction and stabilization of ensuing rocker deformity with Steinman pins. COD was applied at surgery. a. one week following surgery the deep calcaneal wound is evident' without signs of infection. b. X-ray showing the inserted Steinman pins. The missing plantar calcaneal bone and the deep soft tissue void underneath can be seen. c. Three weeks post-surgery, following the use of the COD, skin began crawling from the side surface into the depth of the wound. Further coverage of the wound granulation tissue with epidermal tissue is seen after 7 weeks (d), 8 weeks (e) and 3.5 months (f) of COD treatment, resulting in 95% complete closure of the wound at 4.5 months (g). h and i. lateral foot and Axial calcaneal X-rays of the foot 4.5 months after surgery. Although large soft tissue void is prominent, it is filled with practically normal looking skin that crawled in. During all this period the foot was treated solely with COD.

post-surgery). At surgery and thereafter the wound was dressed with COD, which was changed weekly. While relatively rapid granulation seemed to fill the depth and walls of the large cavity, normal looking skin began crawling from the side surface into the depth of the wound. **Figure 6c**, taken 3 weeks post-surgery demonstrated epithelization beginning at the superficial wall of the cavity (arrows). This phenomenon is further demonstrated in the photos taken at 7, 8 weeks (**Figure 6d** and **e**), 3.5- and 4.5-months post-surgery (**Figure 6f** and **g**). The corresponding x-rays at 4.5 months are shown in **Figure 6h** and **i**.

2.4.3 Reduction of post-operative swelling and inflammation

62-year-old man suffered from degenerative changes of the 1st metatarsophalangeal joint (Hallux Rigidus) and metatarsalgia. The forefoot deformities included hallux valgus Interphalangeus, subluxed lesser MTPJ's, hammer 2nd toe and Bunionette deformity (**Figure 7a**). Surgery included cheilectomy of the first metatarsal head, Akin-Moberg osteotomy of the base of the proximal phalanx of the big toe, Weil osteotomies of the 2nd and 3rd metatarsals, Chevron osteotomy of the 5th metatarsal and PIPJ arthrodesis to correct the 2nd hammer toe (**Figure 7b**). The later was fixed with Kirschner wires (KW) and so was the 5th metatarsal. The 2nd and 3rd metatarsals were fixed with a screw and the bog toe proximal phalanx osteotomy was secured with absorbable suture. The foot was dressed with COD immediately after surgery with first dressing change after 3 weeks. At that time, surgical wounds were without any sign of infection or inflammation (**Figure 7c**). Despite having 4 metatarsal osteotomies and one toe arthrodesis in any of these sites, there was no swelling to the degree that normal skin wrinkles could be observed (**Figures 7c-e**). This is in contrast to the usual significant swelling that is observed for several months after foot osteotomies.

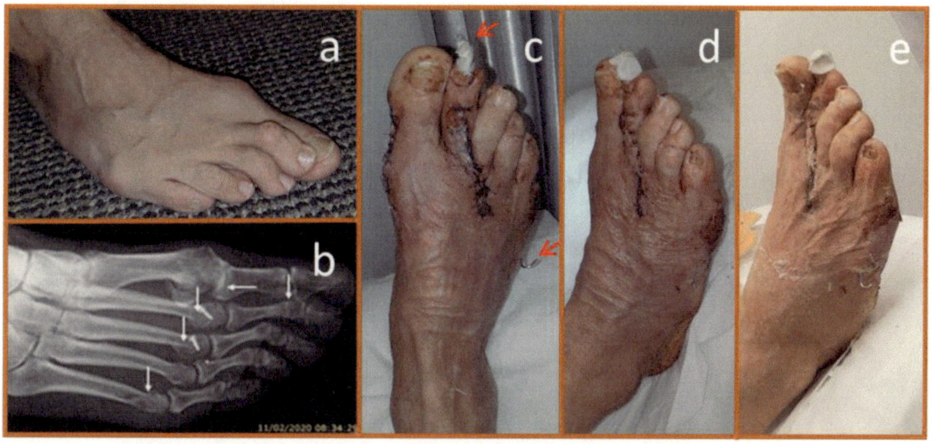

Figure 7.
Reduction of swelling after forefoot surgeries and osteotomies. a. Forefoot deformities in a 62-year-old man. Hallux valgus, hammer second toe, subluxed 2nd and 3rd metatarsophalangeal joints and Bunionette deformity are observed. b. X-ray image taken 2 months after surgery demonstrates osteotomy of the base of the proximal phalanx of the big toe, Weil osteotomies of the 2nd and 3rd metatarsals, Chevron osteotomy of the 5th metatarsal and PIPJ arthrodesis of the 2nd hammer toe (arrows). c. Clinical photo of the foot at first dressing change three weeks after surgery (COD dressings were applied during surgery). Surgical wounds are without any sign of inflammation and lack of swelling and skin wrinkles can be seen. The tip of the KW's fixing the 2nd toe and the 5th metatarsal are seen and marked with red arrows (the second toe KW is wrapped with plaster to prevent accidental pullout) d. Oblique view of the same foot at the same visit after stitches removal demonstrates clearly the reduction of swelling. e. Clinical photos taken at 5 weeks post-surgery. Skin wrinkles and no swelling is again evident.

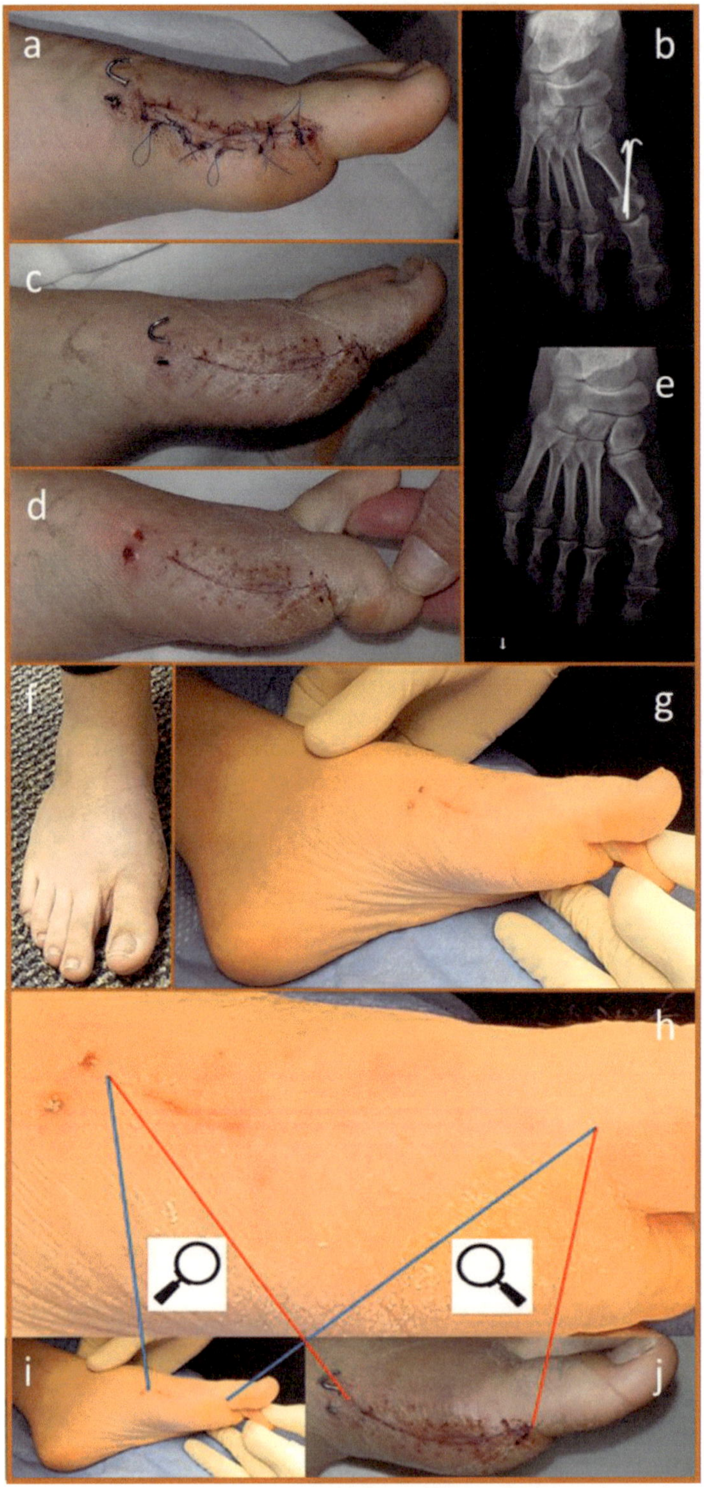

Figure 8.
Reduction of scar formation – Case Report 1. a. Bunion surgery that included Chevron type osteotomy of the 1st metatarsal and fixation with two KW's. b. X-Ray of the foot following surgery. c. Surgical incision appearance at two weeks post-surgery. d. Surgical incision appearance at four weeks post-surgery. e. X-Ray of the foot at 7 weeks post-surgery. f. Clinical appearance of the foot at seven weeks post-surgery. g. Surgical incision appearance at seven weeks post-surgery. h. Enlargement of the surgical site at seven weeks post-surgery. Comparison between the scar appearance after 7 weeks (i) and 2 weeks (j) post-surgery shows that most of the scar has disappeared and was not detectable even at high magnification (h).

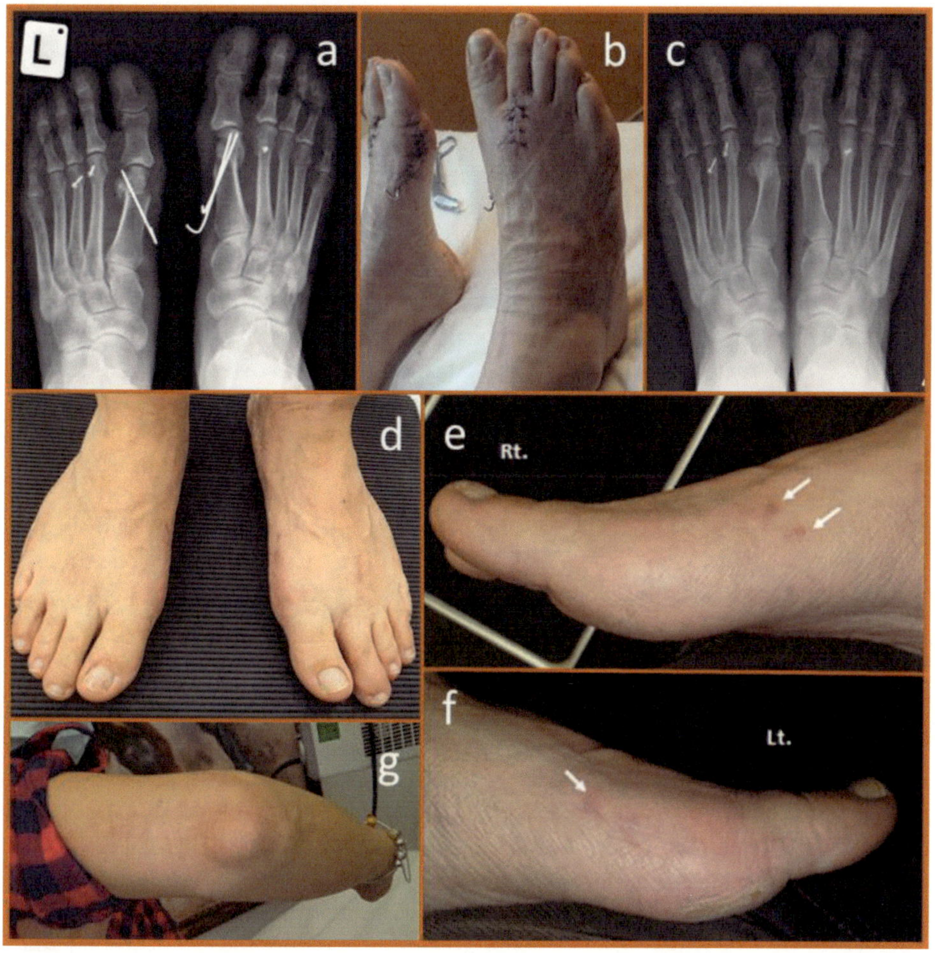

Figure 9.
Reduction of scar formation – Case Report 2. a. X-ray of both feet showing 1st and 2nd metatarsal osteotomy due to hallux valgus and metatarsalgia. b. Surgical incision appearance at 2 weeks post-surgery. c. X-ray and d. photographs of both feet one-year post-surgery showing successful foot positioning. e. Surgical incision appearance of right foot one-year post-surgery. f. Surgical incision appearance of right foot one-year post-surgery. g. Hypertrophic scar 25 years post-surgery due to elbow fracture.

2.4.4 Reduction of scar formation

Reduction of scar formation may be difficult to prove or demonstrate since the final surgical incision healing is a function of surgical technique as well as the patient own tendency to produce hypertrophic scar or even keloid. We have therefore elected to present the reduced scar formation in two cases of bunion surgery. **Figures 8** and **9** with unexpected rapid healing in one patients and very good healing despite basic tendency to hypertrophic scar in another patient.

2.4.4.1 Case report 1

The first one is a 20-year-old healthy woman who had bunion surgery which included Chevron type osteotomy of the 1st metatarsal and fixation with KW (**Figure 8a**). The surgical incision and the KW's are seen at two weeks post-surgery (clinical photos and x-rays, (**Figure 8a** and **b**). The KW's were removed at 4 weeks. By that time nice healing of the surgical incision seems to have taken place (**Figure 8c** and **d**). At 7-weeks post-surgery, the osteotomy has healed and clinical appearance is satisfactory (**Figure 8e** and **f**). The surgical scar is very delicate (**Figure 8g**). A comparison between the original incision and its appearance after 7-weeks shows that ~80% of the incision scar is not observed even in high resolution and magnification photography (**Figures 8h–j**). This implies that either direct epithelization has occurred or remodeling of the scar took place. The superb cosmetic results at 7-weeks seems to be beyond a "successful case" and we attribute it to the beneficial effect of copper oxide on wound healing.

2.4.4.2 Case report 2

The second case is of a 49-years-old healthy woman who underwent bilateral hallux valgus surgery, which included distal first metatarsal osteotomy, fixed with KW's and Weil ostetomies of the 2nd (+ 3rd) metatarsals (**Figure 9a**). The feet were dressed with COD. Two weeks post-surgery swelling was minimal and even skin wrinkles could be seen (**Figure 9b**). One year post surgery the foot position is very good (**Figure 9c** and **d**). The dorsal incision scarring is minimal (**Figure 9d**), the medial scar on both feet is hardly visible (**Figure 9e** and **f**). The patient said she has a tendency to create hypertrophic scars, for example a scar following open reduction and internal fixation of elbow fracture 25 year ago (**Figure 9g**).

3. Discussion

Copper is a natural mineral, which is an essential element of nutrition due to its role in many of the physiological processes in all body tissues [12, 13]. We have reviewed the beneficial effect of copper in wound healing based on abundant basic science research as well as our cumulative experience with the use of COD. Copper has been known for its antimicrobial properties including against all common wound pathogens and resistant bacteria. Similar properties are attributed to silver. Indeed, silver-containing wound dressings are widely used in wound treatment to reduce the risk of wound and wound-dressing contamination [43]. It is desirable, of course, to have a wound dressing that also promotes wound healing. Previous research has shown the beneficial effect of copper on skin and integumentary system [14] as well as on wound healing in diabetic mice [41]. The mechanism by which copper exerts its positive roll has been shown to be through up-regulating the level of Hif-1α, which is a key protein in tissue generation, especially in conditions of ischemia, like in hard to heal wounds. In this regard copper differs from silver, which exerts the opposite effect on wound healing, probably by downregulating Hif-1α [44]. Therefore, the usefulness of silver-based dressing in promoting wound healing is questionable, among others due to cellular toxicity [45, 46].

However, since copper has potent biocidal properties [37], but in contrast to silver, is an indispensable trace element extremely well metabolized by the human body [12], we hypothesized that it could substitute silver in wound dressings. This would be justified for the goal of reducing bio-contamination. But, even more importantly, are the key roles copper plays in skin generation and angiogenesis. We further hypothesized that the inability of wounds to heal in individuals with compromised peripheral blood supply (e.g., with vascular diseases or diabetics), is partially due to low levels of copper in the wound site [47]. We suggested that by using a copper oxide-containing wound dressing we would slowly release *in situ* copper ions needed for angiogenesis, skin regeneration and wound healing.

Based on the above, we prepared wound dressings containing copper oxide (COD, **Figure 1**). The COD, which possess potent biocidal properties (**Figures 2 and 3**), were found to be safe in animal studies, showing no skin irritation and no local damage to open wounds or systemic pathological alterations in a porcine full-thickness wound model (unpublished data). Indeed, the risk of adverse reactions due to dermal contact with copper is extremely low [48, 49]. Furthermore, wounds inflicted in diabetic (db/db) mice under sterile conditions and kept covered throughout the study with sterile wound dressings demonstrated a statistically significant enhancement of wound closure when the dressings contained copper oxide [41]. Enhanced wound healing was nearly that anticipated from wild-type mice, where similar full-thickness dorsal skin wounds reach complete closure 7–10 days earlier than in db/db mice [50]. In contrast, commercially-used silver-containing wound dressings did not accelerate wound healing in this model [41]. Following the clearance of the COD to be used clinically, we have found, as described in some representative cases in the article, the significantly better results obtained with the COD than SOC dressings, including silver-based wound dressings.

The demonstrated cases (**Figures 5–9**) show the several effects of COD on different stages and aspects of wounds healing. The effects were reduction of colonized bacteria and superficial infection, as well as increased granulation and epithelization, as demonstrated in **Figure 5**. **Figure 6** shows rapid epithelization of normal looking plantar skin into the cavity underneath the calcaneus. In addition to wound closure, we see in **Figures 7–9** improved healing process on primary closed clean surgical incisions, which expresses itself in improved scar formation and reduces swelling.

Due to the effect of COD on the various stages of wound healing, we now often use the COD continuously during the various phases of wound treatment. For example, we apply them on debrided wounds after partial foot amputation due to diabetic foot infection (instead of povidone-iodine or chlorine based dressings), and as healing progresses, we use them to assist in filling the wound with granulation tissue (for example, instead of using Negative Pressure Wound Therapy (NPWT)). Once the wound has filled with new tissue, we use the COD to help epithelization until full wound closure is achieved.

Another advantage of COD is the few dressing changes it needs, usually once or twice weekly. This makes it convenient to the patient and savvy for the health care system. In the hospital, COD may replace chlorine-based dressings (e.g. Eusol or Daikin solutions), which needs changes 2–3 times daily, and thus reduce the workload on the nursing staff as well as diminishing the risk of spreading resistant bacteria and cross contamination in the Ward.

Additional studies are needed to further elucidate the exact mechanisms by which copper stimulates wound healing. It is clear, however, that copper directly or indirectly stimulates many factors, some of which are impaired in diabetics and are important for keratinocytes and fibroblasts proliferation, epithelization, collagen synthesis, extracellular matrix remodeling and angiogenesis. Indeed, by utilizing COD dressings on chronic wounds, which had failed to heal or healed slowly with other well-recognized wound care protocols, we found improved wound healing kinetics and wound closure in most patients.

4. Conclusions

As demonstrated by the murine diabetic model [41], the positive effect of the copper oxide-containing dressings is not related solely to its potent biocidal properties, but to the direct stimulation of wound repair. No adverse events were recorded with the use of the copper dressings and all patients showed positive response to its application. Thus, copper dressings appear to hold significant promise in the clinician's ongoing struggle to heal both acute and chronic wounds. Additional randomized, controlled studies should be conducted to further validate the efficacy of topically applied copper oxide-impregnated dressings.

Author details

Gadi Borkow[1]* and Eyal Melamed[2]

1 MedCu Technologies Ltd., Herzliya, Israel

2 Foot and Ankle Service, Department of Orthopaedics, Rambam Health Care Campus, Haifa, Israel

*Address all correspondence to: gadib@medcu.com

References

[1] Richardson M. Acute wounds: an overview of the physiological healing process. Nurs Times. 2004;100(4): 50-53.

[2] Diegelmann RF, Evans MC. Wound healing: an overview of acute, fibrotic and delayed healing. Front Biosci. 2004;9:283-289.

[3] Philips N, Keller T, Gonzalez S. TGF beta-like regulation of matrix metalloproteinases by anti-transforming growth factor-beta, and anti-transforming growth factor-beta 1 antibodies in dermal fibroblasts: Implications for wound healing. Wound Repair Regen. 2004;12(1):53-59.

[4] Sorrell JM, Baber MA, Caplan AI. Clonal characterization of fibroblasts in the superficial layer of the adult human dermis. Cell Tissue Res. 2007;327(3):499-510.

[5] Gailit J, Clarke C, Newman D, Tonnesen MG, Mosesson MW, Clark RA. Human fibroblasts bind directly to fibrinogen at RGD sites through integrin alpha(v)beta3. Exp Cell Res. 1997;232(1):118-126.

[6] Kornblatt AP, Nicoletti VG, Travaglia A. The neglected role of copper ions in wound healing. J Inorg Biochem. 2016;161:1-8.

[7] Ferreira MC, Tuma P, Jr., Carvalho VF, Kamamoto F. Complex wounds. Clinics. 2006;61(6):571-578.

[8] Bowering CK. Diabetic foot ulcers. Pathophysiology, assessment, and therapy. Can Fam Physician. 2001;47:1007-1016.

[9] Abbade LP, Lastoria S. Venous ulcer: epidemiology, physiopathology, diagnosis and treatment. Int J Dermatol. 2005;44(6):449-456.

[10] Coelho S, Amarelo M, Ryan S, Reddy M, Sibbald RG. Rheumatoid arthritis-associated inflammatory leg ulcers: a new treatment for recalcitrant wounds. Int Wound J. 2004;1(1):81-84.

[11] Cullum N, Nelson EA, Nixon J. Pressure ulcers. Clin Evid. 2006;(15): 2592-2606.

[12] Uauy R, Olivares M, Gonzalez M. Essentiality of copper in humans. Am J Clin Nutr. 1998;67(5 Suppl):952S–959S.

[13] Vetchy MPJV. Biological role of copper as an essential trace element in the human organism. Ceska Slov Farm. 2018;67(4):143-153.

[14] Polefka TG, Bianchini RJ, Shapiro S. Interaction of mineral salts with the skin: a literature survey. Int J Cosmet Sci. 2012;34(5):416-423.

[15] Ozumi K, Sudhahar V, Kim HW, Chen GF, Kohno T, Finney L, Vogt S, McKinney RD, Ushio-Fukai M, Fukai T. Role of copper transport protein antioxidant 1 in angiotensin II-induced hypertension: a key regulator of extracellular superoxide dismutase. Hypertension. 2012;60(2):476-486.

[16] Tsai CY, Finley JC, Ali SS, Patel HH, Howell SB. Copper influx transporter 1 is required for FGF, PDGF and EGF-induced MAPK signaling. Biochem Pharmacol. 2012;84(8):1007-1013.

[17] Sen CK, Khanna S, Venojarvi M, Trikha P, Ellison EC, Hunt TK, Roy S. Copper-induced vascular endothelial growth factor expression and wound healing. Am J Physiol Heart Circ Physiol. 2002;282(5):H1821-H1827.

[18] Prudovsky I, Mandinova A, Soldi R, Bagala C, Graziani I, Landriscina M, Tarantini F, Duarte M, Bellum S, Doherty H, Maciag T. The non-classical export routes: FGF1 and IL-1alpha

point the way. J Cell Sci. 2003;116(Pt 24):4871-4881.

[19] Philips N, Samuel P, Parakandi H, Gopal S, Siomyk H, Ministro A, Thompson T, Borkow G. Beneficial regulation of fibrillar collagens, heat shock protein-47, elastin fiber components, transforming growth factor-beta1, vascular endothelial growth factor and oxidative stress effects by copper in dermal fibroblasts. Connect Tissue Res. 2012;53(5):373-378.

[20] Mandinov L, Mandinova A, Kyurkchiev S, Kyurkchiev D, Kehayov I, Kolev V, Soldi R, Bagala C, de Muinck ED, Lindner V, Post MJ, Simons M, Bellum S, Prudovsky I, Maciag T. Copper chelation represses the vascular response to injury. Proc Natl Acad Sci U S A. 2003; 00(11):6700-6705.

[21] Parke A, Bhattacherjee P, Palmer RM, Lazarus NR. Characterization and quantification of copper sulfate-induced vascularization of the rabbit cornea. Am J Pathol. 1988;130(1):173-178.

[22] Narayanan G, BS R, Vuyyuru H, Muthuvel B, Konerirajapuram NS. CTR1 silencing inhibits angiogenesis by limiting copper entry into endothelial cells. PLoS One. 2013;8(9):e71982.

[23] La MD, Arnesano F, Hansson O, Giacomelli C, Calo V, Mangini V, Magri A, Bellia F, Trincavelli ML, Martini C, Natile G, Rizzarelli E. Copper binding to naturally occurring, lactam form of angiogenin differs from that to recombinant protein, affecting their activity. Metallomics. 2016;8(1):118-124.

[24] Ogen-Shtern N, Chumin K, Cohen G, Borkow G. Increased pro-collagen 1, elastin, and TGF-beta1 expression by copper ions in an ex-vivo human skin model. J Cosmet Dermatol. 2020;19(6):1522-1527.

[25] Gerard C, Bordeleau LJ, Barralet J, Doillon CJ. The stimulation of angiogenesis and collagen deposition by copper. Biomaterials. 2010;31(5):824-831.

[26] Rucker RB, Kosonen T, Clegg MS, Mitchell AE, Rucker BR, Uriu-Hare JY, Keen CL. Copper, lysyl oxidase, and extracellular matrix protein cross-linking. Am J Clin Nutr. 1998;67(5 Suppl):996S–1002S.

[27] Sajithlal GB, Chithra P, Chandrakasan G. An in vitro study on the role of metal catalyzed oxidation in glycation and crosslinking of collagen. Mol Cell Biochem. 1999;194(1-2):257-263.

[28] Kothapalli CR, Ramamurthi A. Copper nanoparticle cues for biomimetic cellular assembly of crosslinked elastin fibers. Acta Biomater. 2009;5(2):541-553.

[29] Tenaud I, Sainte-Marie I, Jumbou O, Litoux P, Dreno B. In vitro modulation of keratinocyte wound healing integrins by zinc, copper and manganese. Br J Dermatol. 1999;140(1):26-34.

[30] Das A, Sudhahar V, Chen GF, Kim HW, Youn SW, Finney L, Vogt S, Yang J, Kweon J, Surenkhuu B, Ushio-Fukai M, Fukai T. Endothelial Antioxidant-1: a Key Mediator of Copper-dependent Wound Healing in vivo. Sci Rep. 2016;6:33783.

[31] Edwards R, Harding KG. Bacteria and wound healing. Curr Opin Infect Dis. 2004;17(2):91-96.

[32] Ovington L. Bacterial toxins and wound healing. Ostomy Wound Manage. 2003;49(7A Suppl):8-12.

[33] Robson MC, Stenberg BD, Heggers JP. Wound healing alterations caused by infection. Clin Plast Surg. 1990;17(3):485-492.

[34] Laato M, Niinikoski J, Lundberg C, Gerdin B. Inflammatory reaction and

blood flow in experimental wounds inoculated with Staphylococcus aureus. Eur Surg Res. 1988;20(1):33-38.

[35] Hodgkinson V, Petris MJ. Copper homeostasis at the host-pathogen interface. J Biol Chem. 2012;287(17):13549-13555.

[36] Porcheron G, Garenaux A, Proulx J, Sabri M, Dozois CM. Iron, copper, zinc, and manganese transport and regulation in pathogenic Enterobacteria: correlations between strains, site of infection and the relative importance of the different metal transport systems for virulence. Front Cell Infect Microbiol. 2013;3:90.

[37] Borkow G, Gabbay J. Copper as a biocidal tool. Curr Med Chem. 2005;12(18):2163-2175.

[38] Borkow G. Using copper to fight microorganisms. Curr Chem Biol. 2012;6(2):93-103.

[39] Kumar A, Pandit V, Nagaich U. Therapeutic evaluation of chemically synthesized copper nanoparticles to promote full-thickness excisional wound healing. Int J Applied Pharmaceutics. 2020;12(6):136-142.

[40] Ghosh D, Godeshala S, Nitiyanandan R, Islam MS, Yaron JR, DiCaudo D, Kilbourne J, Rege K. Copper-Eluting Fibers for Enhanced Tissue Sealing and Repair. ACS Appl Mater Interfaces. 2020;12(25):27951-27960.

[41] Borkow G, Gabbay J, Dardik R, Eidelman AI, Lavie Y, Grunfeld Y, Ikher S, Huszar M, Zatcoff RC, Marikovsky M. Molecular mechanisms of enhanced wound healing by copper oxide-impregnated dressings. Wound Repair Regen. 2010;18(2):266-275.

[42] Scherer SS, Pietramaggiori G, Mathews JC, Chan R, Fiorina P, Orgill DP. Wound healing kinetics of the genetically diabetic mice. Wounds. 2008;20(1):18-28.

[43] Leaper DJ. Silver dressings: their role in wound management. Int Wound J. 2006;3(4):282-294.

[44] Yang T, Yao Q, Cao F, Liu Q, Liu B, Wang XH. Silver nanoparticles inhibit the function of hypoxia-inducible factor-1 and target genes: insight into the cytotoxicity and antiangiogenesis. Int J Nanomedicine. 2016;11:6679-6692.

[45] Atiyeh BS, Costagliola M, Hayek SN, Dibo SA. Effect of silver on burn wound infection control and healing: review of the literature. Burns. 2007;33(2):139-148.

[46] Chambers H, Dumville JC, Cullum N. Silver treatments for leg ulcers: a systematic review. Wound Repair Regen. 2007;15(2):165-173.

[47] Borkow G, Gabbay J, Zatcoff RC. Could chronic wounds not heal due to too low local copper levels? Med Hypotheses. 2008;70(3):610-613.

[48] Hostynek JJ, Maibach HI. Copper hypersensitivity: dermatologic aspects--an overview. Rev Environ Health. 2003;18(3):153-183.

[49] Gorter RW, Butorac M, Cobian EP. Examination of the cutaneous absorption of copper after the use of copper-containing ointments. Am J Ther. 2004;11(6):453-458.

[50] Chan RK, Liu PH, Pietramaggiori G, Ibrahim SI, Hechtman HB, Orgill DP. Effect of recombinant platelet-derived growth factor (Regranex) on wound closure in genetically diabetic mice. J Burn Care Res. 2006;27(2):202-205.

Chapter 10

Contribution of Topical Agents to Wound Healing

Tadej Voljč and Danijela Semenič

Abstract

The process of wound healing is often accompanied by bacterial infection or critical colonization, which leads to an extension of the inflammatory response phase and delayed epithelization. In the review of scientific articles, we found the description and mode of action of topical antiseptic agents, including silver and sodium hypochlorite solution, to control the spread of microorganisms. The value of hyaluronic acid for wound healing is described. Furthermore, a novel treatment option with microspheres is mentioned. Attachment of cells to microspheres establishes a local cytokine response that acts anti-inflammatory, cell attachment results also in morphological and functional cell changes that reactivate healing.

Keywords: chronic wounds, wound infections, antisepsis, silver, microspheres, polystyrene microspheres, hyaluronic acid, sodium hypochlorite

1. Introduction

Chronic wounds represent a serious problem for both the patient and the physician.

As chronic wounds are considered venous ulcers, wounds due to peripheral arterial occlusive disease, diabetic neuropathic, diabetic ischemic, diabetic neuroischemic wounds, pressure sores and atypic chronic wounds.

Atypical chronic wounds comprise less than 5% of all chronic wounds [1, 2]. They may present with a clinical picture the clinician has not previously encountered, therefore raising a diagnostic dilemma and challenge. A full range of pathogenic categories, including vascular, autoimmune, inflammatory, infectious, neoplastic, genetic, and drug-related processes, can cause an atypical ulcer [1–3].

Also, every acute wound has a certain potential to become chronic, usually with co-infection or when associated diseases are present.

For the successful treatment of chronic wounds, it is necessary to know and treat the underlying cause and provide the wound appropriate method to optimize wound healing.

2. Silver active compounds

Metallic silver has been used in the treatment of infections from at least the 18th century [4]. More recently products containing silver have been developed for the topical treatment of chronic wounds due to its antiseptic and anti-inflammatory activity [5, 6].

While metallic silver is chemically largely inert, it readily releases an electron in contact with moisture, becoming more reactive and gaining significant biocidal properties. In its ionized form (Ag^+) silver can interfere with thiol (-SH) groups, promote the production of reactive oxygen species (ROS) and bind to bacterial DNA and RNA. Through these mechanisms it causes structural changes to the bacterial cell wall, intracellular and nuclear membranes, disrupts the production of ATP and inhibits replication, ultimately leading to the loss of function and cell death [4–8]. Silver ion-release products are effective against various bacteria, including methicillin-resistant *S. aureus* (MRSA) and vancomycin resistant enterococcus (VRE) [4], fungi and viral pathogens [9]. Silver containing wound dressings are able to reduce the number of viable bacteria in a matter of minutes [10]. Silver ions were shown to destabilize the biofilm produced by *S. epidermidis* [11]. As such it presents a good adjuvant treatment option to combine with surgical debridement for dealing with bacterial biofilm.

Bacterial resistance to silver has rarely been reported, likely due to its multiple mechanisms of bactericidal action [12]. However, most reported cases of bacterial resistance to silver stem from burn units, where large amounts of silver salts were used as wound antiseptics. Among the described silver resistant strains were *E. coli*, *Enterobacter cloacae*, *Klebsiella pneumoniae*, *Acinetobacter baumannii*, *Salmonella typhimurium* and *Pseudomonas stutzeri*. The outbreak of a silver resistant strain of Salmonella even caused the closure of a burn unit at the Massachusetts General Hospital after three patients have died of septicemia in 1973 [13, 14].

While ionic silver has the highest therapeutic capacity, it is also rapidly inactivated after being applied to a wound due to its high nonspecific reactivity [7]. Instead, nanoparticles of silver have been used in modern wound dressings, combining a large active surface area and a degree of control over the rate of Ag^+ release into the wound [7, 8]. Silver wound dressings have been developed in several ways, some binding nanocrystalline silver to carbon fibers, attaching it to polyurethane foam, attaching it to hydrocellular foam and coating it over polyethylene. Silver can either be presented at the surface of the product facing the wound, diffusing and acting on the wound itself, or be bound inside a foam or mesh acting on the pathogens absorbed into the material [15, 16]. In a favorable environment silver cations can be released into the wound for several days from a single dressing [17], avoiding frequent dressing changes and unnecessary wound manipulation. After an initial lag the rate of Ag^+ release can be constant [7].

The majority of review articles noted the poor quality of the published data on the use of silver in wound care. Many studies in this area are funded or performed by manufacturers of silver-containing wound dressings [12], adding to the risk of bias.

The therapeutic range of Ag^+ concentration is 30–60 ppm, above which a toxic effect on skin keratinocytes becomes increasingly likely. The goal is thus to have a silver wound dressing that can exert a concentration of silver cations in the wound within the therapeutic range (30–60 ppm) for a prolonged period of time (several days) [12, 13].

Traditional preparations of silver in wound care, silver nitrate and silver sulfadiazine, are as such of limited suitability, providing an initial Ag^+ concentration very much above the therapeutic range (3176 ppm and 3025 ppm respectively), with little residual activity [13].

Nanocrystalline silver incorporating wound dressings are able to provide a Ag^+ concentration of 50–100 ppm in a constant manner [12, 18]. As such they are more suited in the treatment of infected wounds compared to traditional silver preparations, albeit still providing a wound silver ion concentration above the target range. The effect of silver ions has been shown to have a synergistic effect with negative pressure wound therapy, with silver-coated polyurethane foam providing better results than the use of a polyurethane sponge alone [12]. In this way wound Ag^+ concentration of 20–40 ppm can be achieved, falling in the optimal range. A similar effect can be observed by adding a layer of silver-coated nylon between a polyurethane sponge and the wound [19].

Despite their broad spectrum of antimicrobial action and low incidence of bacterial resistance silver-containing products do not come without limitations. The use of silver sulfadiazine, a once very popular preparation of silver, especially in the treatment of burn wounds, is nowadays widely discouraged due to the comparatively high risk of negative effects on the viable wound tissue and little to no advantages when compared to nanocrystalline silver preparations [12, 13, 20]. Not only traditional preparations of silver but nanocrystalline silver, too, has been shown to have an inhibitory effect on epithelization, albeit to a lower extent [20, 21]. Considering this and other possible side effects of silver-releasing products they are thus not recommended for treating non-infected, clean wounds or closed surgical incisions [12].

Silver-releasing products have been shown to reduce the viability, induce oxidative stress and DNA damage in porcine ex vivo skin cells, as well as promote the production of pro-inflammatory IL-6 by monocytes and reducing the oxidative burst and viability of neutrophils in a dose-dependent manner [20]. It should thus come as no surprise that though an important tool in the fight against wound infections they should be used cautiously. The current state of research suggests they should be used on infected wounds for up to 2 weeks, after which the wound should be evaluated. If there is clear improvement with persistent signs of infection the use can be continued until a total of 4 weeks of silver-assisted therapy is reached. If there is no sign of improvement after two weeks the use should be discontinued immediately. Silver-releasing products should not be used for over 4 weeks without a good clinical rationale [22].

Topical application of silver in a nonadhesive wound dressing can be used not only for the treatment of typical chronic wounds, but also for un-usual wounds for example for the treatment of pyoderma gangrenosum ulcers [23]. Pyoderma gangrenosum (PG) is often associated with autoimmune disease and is a neutrophilic dermatosis, characterized by a wide range of clinical presentations, among which recurrent cutaneous ulcerations are the most characteristic [24]. Ulcers are very painful [23]. In addition to systemic immunosuppressant therapy, topical or intralesional drugs can be used [25].

3. Hyaluronic acid

Hyaluronic acid (HA) is a linear glycosaminoglycan (GAG) molecule composed of disaccharide units of GlcNAc and D-glucuronic acid linked together with β-1,4 and β-1,3 glycosidic bonds. The sequence can be repeated over 20,000 times [26]. Hyaluronic acid was first discovered in the vitreous humor in 1934 by Karl Meyer and John Palmer. They proposed the name "hyaluronic acid" lending from the Greek hyaloid (vitreous) and uronic acid, one of the two repeating monosaccharide units [26].

Most human cells have the ability to synthetize HA at some point in their cell cycle, leading to the presence of HA as a component of the extracellular matrix (ECM) in many tissues throughout the human body [27, 28]. The hygroscopic and viscoelastic properties of HA and its derivatives provide a lubricating environment for cells [29]. Its derivatives are an important role in HA's function. It is involved in various processes, from fertilization and development to cancer [26]. Hyaluronic acid and its signaling receptors play a role in initiating an inflammatory response, maintaining structural cell integrity, and promoting recovery from tissue injury [30]. Interestingly, high molecular weight HA displays an anti-inflammatory effect whereas low molecular weight HA acts immunostimulatory and pro-inflammatory [31–33]. High molecular weight HA has been shown to exhibit a cytoprotective effect [34].

HA stimulates the development of fibrin, phagocytic activity, neutrophil and macrophage mobility, assists in cellular infiltration and in the mobilization of proinflammatory cytokines [29, 35]. Hyaluronic acid plays a role in all stages of wound healing [35]. In the early granulation stage HA, abundant in the ECM, facilitates cell proliferation and migration into the temporary wound matrix, and helps with the organization of the granulation tissue matrix. At a later stage HA helps to stabilize the matrix by scavenging free radicals. In the proliferation stage HA plays a role in supporting and regulating basal keratinocytes [35]. A lower HA content has been observed in hypertrophic scars and in the keloid compared to ordinary scars [32].

Due to its many regulatory functions hyaluronic acid has seen significant use as a topical agent in wound treatment. Without yet a clear literature consensus on its efficacy there does seem to be an overall positive effect of HA on the healing of chronic wound ulcers of various etiologies, burns and epithelial surgical wounds no matter the form in which HA is applied (e.g., pad, cream or substrate) [36]. However, the low number of high-quality studies in this area limits any systematic review trying to determine HA's effects in clinical use. To illustrate, a marked increase in the healing rate of diabetic foot ulcers was described in a paper, even when compared to other forms of ulcers among chronic wounds [36, 37], while another systematic review found no advantage whatsoever in the HA group when compared to paraffin gauze [29]. Both systematic reviews were only able to include two papers studying the topic.

3.1 Combination of different active substances (Ag^+, chlorhexidine, hyaluronic acid)

Modern wound healing products combine different active substances in a single product, better adjusting the finished product to the clinical requirements of a certain wound type. An example is a combination of Ag^+ and chlorhexidine, both

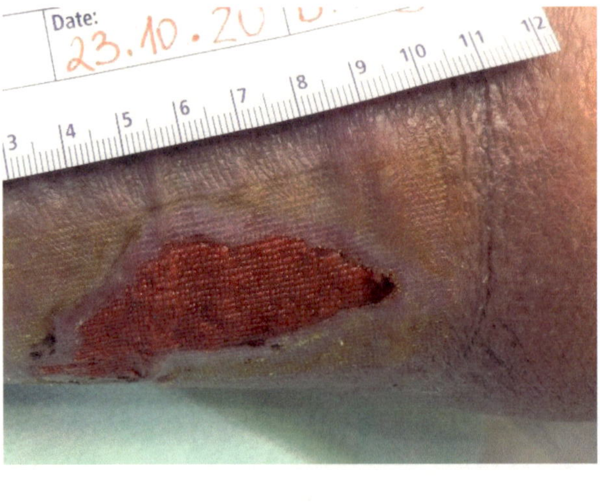

Figure 1.
Chronic wound before treatment with a combination of Ag+, chlorhexidine and hyaluronic acid in a spray.

DOI: http://dx.doi.org/10.5772/intechopen.97170

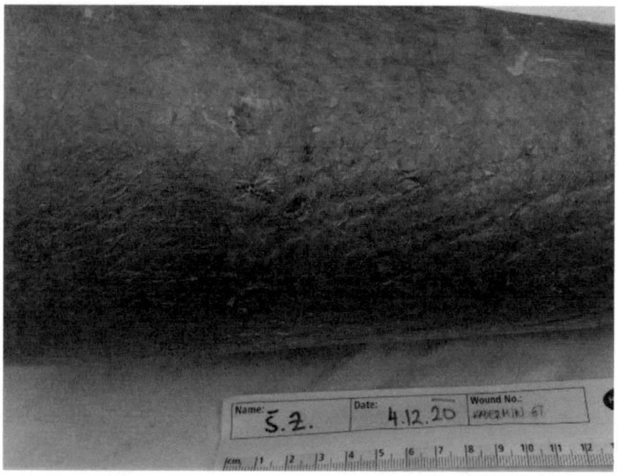

Figure 2.
The result of treatment with spray that contains Ag+, chlorhexidine and hyaluronic acid after 6 weeks.

antiseptic agents bound to silicon dioxide, with added hyaluronic acid to promote the healing process.

Figure 1 shows an example of a chronic wound treated in our institution. Written consent for publication by the patient was obtained.

Presented is a 73-year-old male patient, with diabetes, venous insufficiency, peripheral arterial disease, and heart failure, with consequent bilateral lower leg edema. The treatment was carried out with a combination of Ag^+, chlorhexidine and hyaluronic acid in a spray, every 2 days, covered by a non-adhesive modern dressing. The result of treatment is visible after 6 weeks (**Figure 2**).

Promising results for this combination have also been reported regarding the incontinence associated dermatitis related wound regression rate, moisture control and pain reduction in a study [38].

4. Sodium hypochlorite

Sodium hypochlorite is a strong oxidizing agent and was first discovered in 1787 in Paris by Berthollet. During World War I it was used by Alexis Carrel and Henry D. Dakin as an effective antiseptic agent for combat wounds, sparking its popularity as a wound antiseptic between the two world wars. The popularity of such use later declined with the rise of antibiotics, but it remained a popular household product – sodium hypochlorite is the active ingredient in bleach [39].

With an increasing awareness of the limitations of antibiotic drugs it is again being investigated as a viable option for the prevention and treatment of wound infections. Today a 0.5% sodium hypochlorite solution or more diluted preparations are used. Dakin's solution has been known to have a bactericidal effect against *S. aureus* (MRSA and non methicillin-resistant), *Pseudomonas aeruginosa*, *Escherichia coli*, *Proteus mirabilis*, *Serratia marcescens*, *Enterobacter cloacae*, group D enterococci, *Bacteroides fragilis*, *Streptococcus mitis*, *Staphylococcus epidermidis*, and a fungicidal effect on *Candida albicans* among others [39].

However, as a strong oxidizing agent it is certainly able to exert an important cytotoxic effect on healthy human cells, too. While lower concentrations of sodium hypochlorite have been shown to retain their bactericidal effect, it seems that the cytotoxic effect on human cells sees a stronger reduction with dilution [39]. This area is notably lacking in detailed research.

While sodium hypochlorite is currently not widely used as a wound antiseptic some institutions are reporting positive results with its use. It has been reported to be effective in the treatment of infected and open wounds [39]. In patients undergoing coronary artery bypass surgery it has been shown to be more effective as an irrigator for the prevention of post-sternotomy wound infections when compared to povidone-iodine [40]. It has also been investigated as an irrigator for drain tubes after breast and axillary operations, helping provide much lower rates of positive drain bulb cultures and a lower bacterial load when combined with a chlorhexidine disc at the drain exit site and compared to the standard of drain care (cleansing with alcohol swabs) [41].

5. Polystyrene microspheres

The microspheres are round in shape, located in a suspension of sterile water-soluble solution at a concentration of 0.025%, consist of polystyrene and have a diameter of 5 micrometers.

They are intended for topical application on the wound bed, applied in the form of drops (1–2 drops/cm2 of the wound bed). The mechanism of action is explained by both preclinical in vitro and in vivo studies [42], where the presence of microspheres shows increased cell proliferation, increased cell migration and also increased activity of membrane-bound enzyme proteolytic complexes on cells [43].

The property of the size and surface of the microspheres offers a supportive microenvironment on the surface of the chronic wound, as it serves as an additional surface to which epithelial, endothelial, and even inflammatory cells can attach and migrate [44, 45]. Microspheres have a negative charge on their surface, which accelerates the secretion of growth factors such as growth factor beta-1 [45], and an excess of proteolytic enzymes, which inhibit normal healing, metalloproteinases and human neutrophil elastase, also bind to their surface [42].

The purpose of treatment with microspheres is, in a way, to "de-chronicize" a chronic wound into an acute wound condition, by inducing changes in the microenvironment that would allow the best possible conditions for healing [46].

In a study where microspheres were administered to 54 patients with chronic wounds of various etiologies over a period of 4.5 weeks [42], an effective reduction in wound size and area was described. 39% of the wounds completely healed, and in the remaining cases, effective growth of granulation tissue of the wound bed was observed, which covered up to 75% of the surface of the wound bottom [42].

Accelerated growth of granulation tissue is an indicator that the wound is in the proliferative phase of healing. Granulation tissue is the basis for later re-epithelialization or surgical closure of the wound with suturing, skin graft or flap [47], and the healing indicator is a reduction in wound size, which means that epithelialization began from the edges of the wound [42]. Wounds where bone or tendon are exposed in depth are less responsive to healing [48, 49], but according to the results described in the literature, such wounds may also respond effectively to microsphere treatment [42].

From the possible side effects in the literature, pain and itching are the most common symptoms [42].

In a multicenter randomized double-blind study treating 66 patients with a chronic wound of various etiologies, complete wound healing was found in 20% of patients, in 80% of patients the wound bed was 3/4 covered with granulations after 12 weeks of treatment [46].

Treatment with the application of microspheres potentially accelerates the growth of granulation tissue and epithelialization. We also notice that after the

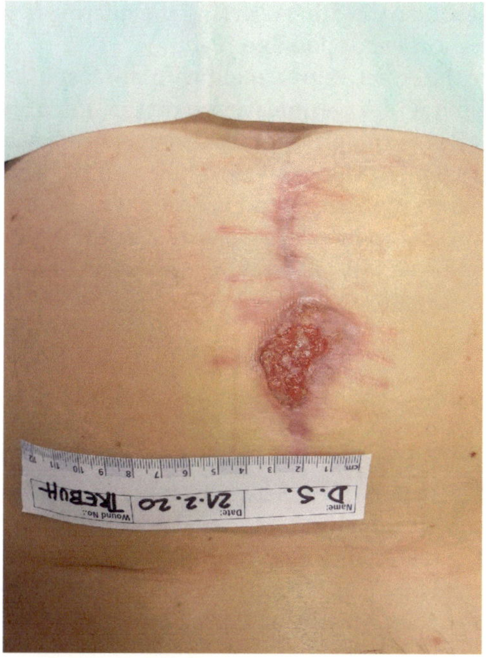

Figure 3.
Chronic wound before treatment with polystirene microspheres.

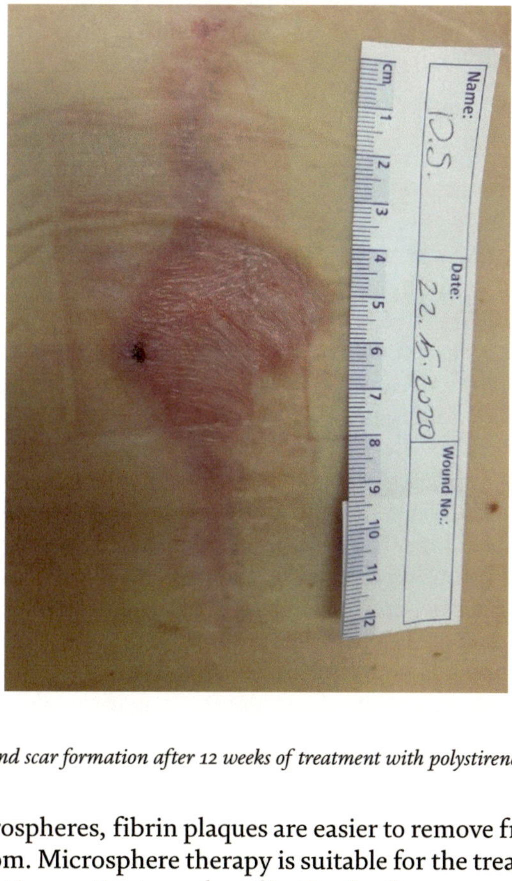

Figure 4.
Effective epithelization and scar formation after 12 weeks of treatment with polystirene microspheres.

application of microspheres, fibrin plaques are easier to remove from the surface of the wound bottom. Microsphere therapy is suitable for the treatment of both inpatient and outpatient patients, and application by the community health service is also possible. The secondary coating covering the microspheres must be non-adhesive and as non-absorbent as possible.

An example where the effective treatment with microspheres is presented is a 44-year-old male patient with a chronic wound on the skin of the abdominal wall after a hepatectomy, after hernioplasty and subsequent resection of the infected hernia mesh. Drops with microspheres were applied on the wound bed every 2 days, over which a non-adhesive modern wound dressing with a silicone contact layer and polyurethane foam was applied. The condition of the wound before treatment (**Figure 3**) and the condition after 12 weeks of treatment (**Figure 4**) with effective epithelization and scar formation [50].

6. Activated charcoal

With its biocompatibility and large surface area, activated charcoal acts as a useful adsorbent of fatty molecules. The most important raw materials for its production are rice, coconut shell and different types of wood. Activated charcoal is obtained by heating the material to around 1000°C in an oxygen-free environment and the subsequent breakdown of carbon-rich compounds. Through this process the material becomes porous, greatly increasing its surface area and its adsorbent capacity [51].

Commercial activated charcoal containing wound dressings contain between 85 and 98% active carbon, with the main difference being the material used to cover the charcoal cloth. Such materials include viscose rayon, alginate, polyethylene, polyamide and nylon [52]. *E.coli* was among the first cultures whose adherence to activated charcoal has been studied [53]. Gram-negative bacteria have been found to adhere stronger and wash out less easily from activated charcoal than Gram-positive bacteria [54].

7. Polyhexanide

Polyhexanide, also known as polyhexamethylene biguanide (PHMB), is a synthetic compound with a broad antimicrobial spectrum, including various types of Gram-positive and Gram-negative bacteria and some fungi (*Candida* spp., *Aspergillus* spp.). It acts as a strong base, binding to negatively charged phospholipid molecules in cell membranes of microorganisms, disturbing their integrity and leading to loss of viability. Its effect on neutral phospholipids of human cells is supposed to be negligible [55].

Betaine, with its amphoteric properties, acts as a surfactant and can be used in the cleaning of wounds. Often polyhexanide and betaine are used together in order to reduce the microbial burden and promote wound healing. As a combination they are available in a number of commercial products and were shown to be effective in reducing the number of viable bacteria in a formed biofilm produced by MRSA [55, 56]. Products containing both polyhexanide and betaine are currently often used in the management of pressure ulcers, venous ulcers and other chronic wounds, while further indications are under investigation [55].

8. Povidone iodine

Povidone iodine's broad spectrum of activity, ability to penetrate biofilms, lack of associated resistance, anti-inflammatory properties, low cytotoxicity and good tolerability have been cited as important factors, and no negative effect on wound healing has been observed in clinical practice [57].

The efficacy of povidone iodine on wound healing in the presence of biofilms has been reviewev [57, 58]. Studies have confirmed the *in vitro* efficacy of povidone iodine against *S. epidermidis* and *S. aureus* growth, as well as the inhibition of staphylococcal biofilm formation at sub-inhibitory concentrations [57–59].

9. Other topical agents

Different clinical practices are used according to different medical institutions in the world. However, several other compounds are also part a wound-care specialist's daily routine. According to the conclusion of infectious disease specialists and surgical infection specialist at the University Medical Center Ljubljana, antibiotic ointments for chronic wounds are not recommended, with purpose, to prevent possible acquired microbial resistance. Topical antibiotic ointment is occasionally used only for impetiginous skin lesions and dermatological indications, not for the treatment of chronic wounds.

The use of topical antibiotics should be discouraged if appropriate antiseptics are available [57, 60].

While the general principles of action remain similar across different substances, a chapter on topical wound healing agents would not be complete without a brief overview of other important agents.

9.1 Mafenide acetate

Mafenidine acetate has been developed as a topical Sulphonamide in 1966. It is effective in reducing the wound bacterial load through the inhibition of nucleoside synthesis and became especially popular in the treatment of burn wounds. First marketed as a 10% cream formulation it did not come without important side effects – both local (neoeschar formation, pain) and systemic (metabolic acidosis) [61, 62]. Its concentration has later been reduced to 5%, with a reduction in the incidence of side effects, but even with preparations used today inhibitory effects on skin DNA and protein synthesis remain a concern [61–63]. This and the high cost of mafenide therapy led to recent research interests on whether the mafenide concentration could further be reduced. While the 5% mafenide acetate cream remains an important agent in burn treatment, novel research indicates that a 2,5% mafenide cream could be equally efficacious as its 5% counterpart [61, 62].

9.2 Bacitracin

Bacitran is derived from *Bacillus Subtilis* and the *licheniformis* group of bacteria and is one of the most widely used topical antibiotics. Its bactericidal activity spans against several Gram-positive and Gram-negative organisms [64]. Bacitracin can provide a 90% reduction of bacterial viability in 1 hour after application and an important reduction of bacterial adherence, without important systemic effects being associated with topical use [65]. There is some evidence to support its use in the prevention of surgical wound infections, however, the use of bacitracin for superficial clean wounds is discouraged [66–69]. While having important antibiotic properties it has also been reported to cause allergic contact dermatitis in a range from 7.7 to 9.2% in a patch-test. As with many antibiotic agents topical products have been associated with an increase in microbial antibiotic resistance. The recommended alternative to bacitracin and other topical antibiotics for the treatment of superficial clean wounds is white petrolatum, with comparable wound infection and wound healing rates [68, 69].

9.3 Neomycin

With a largely similar profile of side effects to bacitracin, is another highly popular topical antibiotic agent [68]. It is classified as an aminoglycoside and inhibits bacterial protein synthesis by binding to ribosomal RNA. It is effective against Gram-negative bacteria, with the exception of *Pseudomonas aeruginosa*, against some Gram-positive bacteria, including staphylococci, but not against streptococci and anaerobes. Its use extends across the spectrum of the prevention and treatment of chronic and non-chronic wound infections, superinfections and burns [64]. The incidence of allergic contact dermatitis is higher compared to bacitracin (7–13% in a patch-test) [69]. Plasmid-mediated resistance to neomycin has been reported in several bacterial strains, including staphylococci, *E. coli, Klebsiella spp.* and *Proteus spp.* [64].

10. Conclusions

Hyaluronic acid, activated charcoal, chlorhexidine, sodium hypochlorite, polyhexanide and polystyrene microspheres serve as good examples of different already well established and potential up-and-coming topical treatment solutions. The advantage of these active ingredients is that no acquired microbial resistance, has been known so far.

By ensuring the optimal microenvironment of the wound, the transition from the inflammatory phase to the proliferative phase of healing is enabled.

The choice of treatment method must be both clinically and cost-effectively.

A short review chapter discusses the possibilities for managing the bacterial load in the wound bed, the advantages and disadvantages of different topical agents and their mode of action.

As with many already established formulations, new topical agents should be put through testing in the form of blinded randomized controlled trials, in order to provide valid support for the formulation's efficacy and safety. Only through this process can we achieve important and much needed evidence-based advances in regard to the treatment of wounds with novel and ever developing topical agents.

Conflict of interest

The authors declare no conflict of interest.

Author details

Tadej Voljč[1] and Danijela Semenič[1,2]*

1 University Medical Center Ljubljana, Ljubljana, Slovenia

2 Medical Faculty, University of Ljubljana, Slovenia

*Address all correspondence to: danijela.semenic@kclj.si

References

[1] Situm M, Kolić M. Definicija i podjela atipicnih rana [Atypical wounds: definition and classification]. Acta Med Croatica. 2012 Oct;66 Suppl 1:5-11.

[2] Semenič D, Aleksovska N. An Atypical Chronic Ulcer Caused by Acute Myeloid Leukemia. Wounds. 2019 Apr;31(4):E25-E28

[3] Hoffman MD. Atypical ulcers. Dermatol Ther. 2013 May-Jun;26(3):222-235. DOI: 10.1111/dth.12048

[4] Lansdown AB. Silver. I: Its antibacterial properties and mechanism of action. J Wound Care. 2002 Apr;11(4):125-130. DOI: 10.12968/jowc.2002.11.4.26389

[5] Wilkinson LJ, White RJ, Chipman JK. Silver and nanoparticles of silver in wound dressings: a review of efficacy and safety. J Wound Care. 2011 Nov;20(11):543-549. DOI: 10.12968/jowc.2011.20.11.543

[6] Lansdown AB. Silver in health care: antimicrobial effects and safety in use. Curr Probl Dermatol. 2006;33:17-34. DOI: 10.1159/000093928

[7] deBoer TR, Chakraborty I, Mascharak PK. Design and construction of a silver(I)-loaded cellulose-based wound dressing: trackable and sustained release of silver for controlled therapeutic delivery to wound sites. J Mater Sci Mater Med. 2015 Oct;26(10):243. DOI: 10.1007/s10856-015-5577-1

[8] Cho KH, Park JE, Osaka T, Park SG. The study of antimicrobial activity and preservative effects of nanosilver ingredient. Electrochimica Acta. 2005 51(5):956-960. DOI: 10.1016/j.electacta.2005.04.071

[9] Percival SL, Bowler PG, Russell D. Bacterial resistance to silver in wound care. J Hosp Infect. 2005 May;60(1):1-7. DOI: 10.1016/j.jhin.2004.11.014

[10] Wright JB, Lam K, Burrell RE. Wound management in an era of increasing bacterial antibiotic resistance: a role for topical silver treatment. Am J Infect Control. 1998 Dec;26(6):572-577. DOI: 10.1053/ic.1998.v26.a93527

[11] Chaw KC, Manimaran M, Tay FE. Role of silver ions in destabilization of intermolecular adhesion forces measured by atomic force microscopy in Staphylococcus epidermidis biofilms. Antimicrob Agents Chemother. 2005 Dec;49(12):4853-4859. DOI: 10.1128/AAC.49.12.4853-4859.2005

[12] Khansa I, Schoenbrunner AR, Kraft CT, Janis JE. Silver in Wound Care-Friend or Foe?: A Comprehensive Review. Plast Reconstr Surg Glob Open. 2019 Aug 12;7(8):e2390. DOI: 10.1097/GOX.0000000000002390

[13] Murphy PS, Evans GR. Advances in wound healing: a review of current wound healing products. Plast Surg Int. 2012;2012:190436. DOI: 10.1155/2012/190436

[14] McHugh GL, Moellering RC, Hopkins CC, Swartz MN. Salmonella typhimurium resistant to silver nitrate, chloramphenicol, and ampicillin. Lancet. 1975 Feb 1;1(7901):235-240. DOI: 10.1016/s0140-6736(75)91138-1

[15] Akhmetova A, Saliev T, Allan IU, Illsley MJ, Nurgozhin T, Mikhalovsky S. A Comprehensive Review of Topical Odor-Controlling Treatment Options for Chronic Wounds. J Wound Ostomy Continence Nurs. 2016 Nov/Dec;43(6):598-609. DOI: 10.1097/WON.0000000000000273

[16] Dalac S, Sigal L, Addala A, Chahim M, Faivre-Carrere C,

Lemdjadi Z, et al. Clinical evaluation of a dressing with poly absorbent fibres and a silver matrix for managing chronic wounds at risk of infection: a non comparative trial. J Wound Care. 2016 Sep;25(9):531-538. DOI: 10.12968/jowc.2016.25.9.531

[17] Fong J, Wood F. Nanocrystalline silver dressings in wound management: a review. Int J Nanomedicine. 2006;1(4):441-449. DOI: 10.2147/nano.2006.1.4.441

[18] Tredget EE, Shankowsky HA, Groeneveld A, Burrell R. A matched-pair, randomized study evaluating the efficacy and safety of Acticoat silver-coated dressing for the treatment of burn wounds. J Burn Care Rehabil. 1998 Nov-Dec;19(6):531-537. DOI: 10.1097/00004630-199811000-00013

[19] Karr JC, de Mola FL, Pham T, Tooke L. Wound healing and cost-saving benefits of combining negative-pressure wound therapy with silver. Adv Skin Wound Care. 2013 Dec;26(12):562-565. DOI: 10.1097/01.ASW.0000434518.86905.8a

[20] Nešporová K, Pavlík V, Šafránková B, Vágnerová H, Odráška P, Žídek O, et al. Effects of wound dressings containing silver on skin and immune cells. Sci Rep. 2020 Sep 16;10(1):15216. DOI: 10.1038/s41598-020-72249-3

[21] Innes ME, Umraw N, Fish JS, Gomez M, Cartotto RC. The use of silver coated dressings on donor site wounds: a prospective, controlled matched pair study. Burns. 2001 Sep;27(6):621-627. DOI: 10.1016/s0305-4179(01)00015-8

[22] Wounds UK. Best Practice Statement: The use of topical antimicrobial agents in wound management. 3rd ed. London: Wounds UK; 2013. 16 p.

[23] Semenič D, Bukovec P. Advanced Treatment Options of Pyoderma Gangrenosum Ulcers. Wounds. 2020 Feb;32(2):E1-E5

[24] Hafner J, Nobbe S, Partsch H, Läuchli S, Mayer D, Amann-Vesti B, et al. Martorell hypertensive ischemic leg ulcer: a model of ischemic subcutaneous arteriolosclerosis. Arch Dermatol. 2010 Sep;146(9):961-968. DOI: 10.1001/archdermatol.2010.224

[25] Miller J, Yentzer BA, Clark A, Jorizzo JL, Feldman SR. Pyoderma gangrenosum: a review and update on new therapies. J Am Acad Dermatol. 2010 Apr;62(4):646-654. DOI: 10.1016/j.jaad.2009.05.030

[26] Hascall VC. The journey of hyaluronan research in the Journal of Biological Chemistry. J Biol Chem. 2019 Feb 1;294(5):1690-1696. DOI: 10.1074/jbc.TM118.005836

[27] Chen WY, Abatangelo G. Functions of hyaluronan in wound repair. Wound Repair Regen. 1999 Mar-Apr;7(2):79-89. DOI: 10.1046/j.1524-475x.1999.00079.x

[28] Noble PW. Hyaluronan and its catabolic products in tissue injury and repair. Matrix Biol. 2002 Jan;21(1):25-29. DOI: 10.1016/s0945-053x(01)00184-6

[29] Shaharudin A, Aziz Z. Effectiveness of hyaluronic acid and its derivatives on chronic wounds: a systematic review. J Wound Care. 2016 Oct 2;25(10):585-592. DOI: 10.12968/jowc.2016.25.10.585

[30] Jiang D, Liang J, Noble PW. Hyaluronan in tissue injury and repair. Annu Rev Cell Dev Biol. 2007;23:435-461. DOI: 10.1146/annurev.cellbio.23.090506.123337

[31] Litwiniuk M, Krejner A, Speyrer MS, Gauto AR, Grzela T. Hyaluronic Acid in Inflammation and Tissue Regeneration. Wounds. 2016 Mar;28(3):78-88

[32] Aya KL, Stern R. Hyaluronan in wound healing: rediscovering a major player. Wound Repair Regen. 2014 Sep-Oct;22(5):579-593. DOI: 10.1111/wrr.12214

[33] Maytin EV. Hyaluronan: More than just a wrinkle filler. Glycobiology. 2016 Jun;26(6):553-559. DOI: 10.1093/glycob/cww033

[34] Wu CL, Chou HC, Li JM, Chen YW, Chen JH, Chen YH, et al. Hyaluronic acid-dependent protection against alkali-burned human corneal cells. Electrophoresis. 2013 Feb;34(3):388-396. DOI: 10.1002/elps.201200342

[35] Schneider HP, Landsman A. Preclinical and Clinical Studies of Hyaluronic Acid in Wound Care: A Case Series and Literature Review. Wounds. 2019 Feb;31(2):41-48

[36] Voigt J, Driver VR. Hyaluronic acid derivatives and their healing effect on burns, epithelial surgical wounds, and chronic wounds: a systematic review and meta-analysis of randomized controlled trials. Wound Repair Regen. 2012 May-Jun;20(3):317-331. DOI: 10.1111/j.1524-475X.2012.00777.x

[37] Chen CP, Hung W, Lin SH. Effectiveness of hyaluronic acid for treating diabetic foot: a systematic review and meta-analysis. Dermatol Ther. 2014 Nov-Dec;27(6):331-336. DOI: 10.1111/dth.12153

[38] Cassino R, Ippolito A, Cuffaro P, Corsi A. Argento tecnomolecolare nella cura della IAD. Acta Biomed. 2014 Jun;85(4):3-8.

[39] Ueno CM, Mullens CL, Luh JH, Wooden WA. Historical review of Dakin's solution applications. J Plast Reconstr Aesthet Surg. 2018 Sep;71(9):e49-e55. DOI: 10.1016/j.bjps.2018.05.023

[40] Mohd AR, Ghani MK, Awang RR, Su Min JO, Dimon MZ. Dermacyn irrigation in reducing infection of a median sternotomy wound. Heart Surg Forum. 2010 Aug;13(4):E228–E232. DOI: 10.1532/HSF98.20091162

[41] Degnim AC, Scow JS, Hoskin TL, Miller JP, Loprinzi M, Boughey JC, et al. Randomized controlled trial to reduce bacterial colonization of surgical drains after breast and axillary operations. Ann Surg. 2013 Aug;258(2):240-247. DOI: 10.1097/SLA.0b013e31828c0b85

[42] Govrin J, Leonid K, Luger E, Tamir J, Zeilig G, Shafir R. New method for treating hard-to-heal wounds: clinical experience with charged polystyrene microspheres. Wounds UK. 2010:6(4);52-61.

[43] Ritter VM, Rosenblat G, Maretski SH, et al. The role of PolyHeal microspheres in wound healing in patients with chronic ulcers. 2004.

[44] Wu L, Mockros NE, Casperson ME, Gruskin EA, Ladin DA, Roth SI, et al. Effects of electrically charged particles in enhancement of rat wound healing. J Surg Res. 1999 Jul;85(1):43-50. DOI: 10.1006/jsre.1999.5354

[45] Sasaki A, Mueller RV, Xi G, Sipe R, Buck D, Hollinger J. Mast cells: an unexpected finding in the modulation of cutaneous wound repair by charged beads. Plast Reconstr Surg. 2003 Apr 1;111(4):1446-1453. DOI: 10.1097/01.PRS.0000049451.38505.45

[46] Shoham Y, Kogan L, Weiss J, Tamir E, Krieger Y, Barnea Y, et al. Wound 'dechronification' with negatively-charged polystyrene microspheres: a double-blind RCT. J Wound Care. 2013 Mar;22(3):144-6, 148, 150-2 passim. DOI: 10.12968/jowc.2013.22.3.144

[47] World Wide Wounds, Should alternative endpoints be considered to evaluate outcomes on chronic recalcitrant wounds? [Internet]. 2004

Oct. Available from: http://www.worldwidewounds.com/2004/october/Enoch-Part2/Alternative-Enpoints-To-Healing.html [Accessed 2021-01-28]

[48] Brandi C, Grimaldi L, Nisi G, Silvestri A, Brafa A, Calabrò M, et al. Treatment with vacuum-assisted closure and cryo-preserved homologous de-epidermalised dermis of complex traumas to the lower limbs with loss of substance, and bones and tendons exposure. J Plast Reconstr Aesthet Surg. 2008 Dec;61(12):1507-1511. DOI: 10.1016/j.bjps.2007.09.036

[49] Chen X, Chen H, Zhang G. Management of wounds with exposed bone structures using an artificial dermis and skin grafting technique. J Plast Reconstr Aesthet Surg. 2010 Jun;63(6):e512–e518. DOI: 10.1016/j.bjps.2009.11.004

[50] Semenič, D. Stimulacija celjenja z vezavo celic na mikrosfere [Healing processes stimulatied with cell adhesion on microspheres]. In: Zbornik predavanj 50. podiplomskega tečaja kirurgije za zdravnike [Conference proceedings of the 50. postgraduate surgery course for medical doctors]; 20-21 November 2020; Ljubljana. Ljubljana: Slovensko zdravniško društvo; 2020. p. 453-456

[51] Kerihuel JC. Effect of activated charcoal dressings on healing outcomes of chronic wounds. J Wound Care. 2010 May;19(5):208, 210-2, 214-5. DOI: 10.12968/jowc.2010.19.5.48047

[52] Akhmetova A, Saliev T, Allan IU, Illsley MJ, Nurgozhin T, Mikhalovsky S. A Comprehensive Review of Topical Odor-Controlling Treatment Options for Chronic Wounds. J Wound Ostomy Continence Nurs. 2016 Nov/Dec;43(6):598-609. DOI: 10.1097/WON.0000000000000273

[53] George N, Davies JT. Adsorption of Microorganisms on Activated Charcoal Cloth: A Material with Potential Applications in Biotechnology. J. Chem. Tech. Biotechnol. 1988;43:117-129.

[54] Frost MR, Jackson SW, Stenes PJ. Adsorption of bacteria onto activated charcoal cloth: an effect of potential importance in the treatment of infected wounds. Microbios Letter. 1980;13:135-140.

[55] Wattanaploy S, Chinaroonchai K, Namviriyachote N, Muangman P. Randomized Controlled Trial of Polyhexanide/Betaine Gel Versus Silver Sulfadiazine for Partial-Thickness Burn Treatment. Int J Low Extrem Wounds. 2017 Mar;16(1):45-50. DOI: 10.1177/1534734617690949

[56] Davis SC, Harding A, Gil J, Parajon F, Valdes J, Solis M, Higa A. Effectiveness of a polyhexanide irrigation solution on methicillin-resistant Staphylococcus aureus biofilms in a porcine wound model. Int Wound J. 2017 Dec;14(6):937-944. DOI: 10.1111/iwj.12734

[57] Bigliardi PL, Alsagoff SAL, El-Kafrawi HY, Pyon JK, Wa CTC, Villa MA. Povidone iodine in wound healing: Int J Surg. 2017:Aug;44:260-268. DOI: 10.1016/j.ijsu.2017.06.073

[58] Percival SL, Finnegan S, Donelli G, Vuotto C, Rimmer S, Lipsky BA. Antiseptics for treating infected wounds: efficacy on biofilms and effect of pH. Crit. Rev. Microbiol. (2014), pp. 1-17. DOI: 10.3109/1040841X.2014.940495

[59] Oduwole KO, Glynn AA, Molony DC, Murray D, Rowe S, Holland LM, McCormack DJ, O'Gara JP.Anti-biofilm activity of sub-inhibitory povidone-iodine concentrations against Staphylococcus epidermidis and Staphylococcus aureus. J. Orthop. Res., 28 (2010), pp. 1252-1256. DOI: 10.1002/jor.21110

[60] European Wound Management Association (EWMA).Position

Document: Management of Wound Infection London (2006)

[61] Afshari A, Nguyen L, Kahn SA, Summitt B. 2.5% Mafenide Acetate: A Cost-Effective Alternative to the 5% Solution for Burn Wounds. J Burn Care Res. 2017 Jan/Feb;38(1):e42-e47. DOI: 10.1097/BCR.0000000000000425

[62] Ibrahim A, Fagan S, Keaney T, Sarhane KA, Hursey DA, Chang P, Sheridan R, Ryan C, Tompkins R, Goverman J. A simple cost-saving measure: 2.5% mafenide acetate solution. J Burn Care Res. 2014 Jul-Aug;35(4):349-353. DOI: 10.1097/BCR.0b013e3182a22715

[63] Zhang XJ, Heggers JP, Chinkes DL, Wolf SE, Hawkins HK, Wolfe RR. Topical Sulfamylon cream inhibits DNA and protein synthesis in the skin donor site wound. Surgery. 2006 May;139(5):633-639. DOI: 10.1016/j.surg.2005.10.013

[64] Spann CT, Taylor SC, Weinberg JM. Topical antimicrobial agents in dermatology. Dis Mon. 2004 Jul;50(7):407-421. DOI: 10.1016/j.disamonth.2004.05.011

[65] Beckman JM, Amankwah EK, Tetreault LL, Perlman SA, Tuite GF. Complications associated with bacitracin powder in surgical wounds. J Neurosurg Pediatr. 2015 Dec;16(6):719-725. DOI: 10.3171/2015.4.PEDS14699

[66] Chan JL, Diaconescu AC, Horvath KA. Routine Use of Topical Bacitracin to Prevent Sternal Wound Infections After Cardiac Surgery. Ann Thorac Surg. 2017 Nov;104(5):1496-1500. DOI: 10.1016/j.athoracsur.2017.04.017

[67] MacIver RH, Stewart R, Frederiksen JW, Fullerton DA, Horvath KA. Topical application of bacitracin ointment is associated with decreased risk of mediastinitis after median sternotomy. Heart Surg Forum. 2006;9(5):E750–E753. DOI: 10.1532/HSF98.20051187

[68] Jacob SE, James WD. Bacitracin after clean surgical procedures may be risky. J Am Acad Dermatol. 2004 Dec;51(6):1036. DOI: 10.1016/j.jaad.2004.05.022

[69] Draelos ZD, Rizer RL, Trookman NS. A comparison of postprocedural wound care treatments: do antibiotic-based ointments improve outcomes? J Am Acad Dermatol. 2011 Mar;64(3 Suppl):S23–S29. DOI: 10.1016/j.jaad.2010.11.010